Praise for *Prescriptions from Paradise...*

"*Prescriptions from Paradise* is chock full of practical information that everyone needs to know in order to become or stay healthy."

—Christiane Northrup, MD
Ob/gyn physician and author of *Women's Bodies, Women's Wisdom*

"With great mastery Dr. Viana has created this user-friendly work for the health-conscious individual to learn of the root causes of illnesses and remedies to enhance their health. Bravo!"

—Joseph Christiano
Author of *Bloodtypes, Bodytypes and YOU*

"The work of Dr. Viana is highly admirable and encouraging, contributing to the arduous task of reeducating the public. His example is like a flame that kindles other lights, guiding the way out of ignorance and suffering."

—Adriana Balthazar, MD, PhD
Internist and metaphysician

"In *Prescriptions from Paradise*, Dr. Carlos Viana lays out his comprehensive holistic approach to medicine in a clear style accessible to all readers. Highly critical of Western medicine's growing alliance with global pharmaceutical companies, Dr. Viana advocates a greater focus on individual well-being through common sense promotion of the body's natural healing processes."

—Armando Lampe, PhD
Priest and university lecturer

"Dr. Viana's *Prescriptions from Paradise* is a comprehensive yet easy-to-read treatment protocol for over sixty ailments. Thoroughly based on scientific research, these analyses combine the best of Chinese and Western medicine. It is high time for a book like this. If you are interested in a wonderful new holistic approach to healing, this is the book for you!"

—Dr. Kathleen E. Assar
Pima Community College

Hummingbird, according to Native American wisdom,
brings a special "medicine" to help solve the riddle of duality.
Health care today is fraught with the contradictions of duality:
conventional vs. alternative medicine, drug vs. herbal remedies,
physical vs. dental therapies.
Hummingbird inspires an integrative approach,
combining the many modalities into one "good medicine"—
the way of biocompatible medicine.

To Lori BRENNAN
May you Enjoy this book and
get great ideas

Carlos Viana

ARUBA

24 MAY 2012

PRESCRIPTIONS *from* PARADISE

INTRODUCTION TO BIOCOMPATIBLE MEDICINE
An A-to-Z Compendium

CARLOS M. VIANA, OMD (CHINA), CCN
Aruba's "Barefoot Doctor"

Healing Spirit Press
Merritt Island, Florida

Published by: Healing Spirit Press, Inc.
125 East Merritt Island Causeway
Suite 209-307
Merritt Island, FL 32952
www.healingspiritpress.com

Editor: Ellen Kleiner
Book design and typography: Janice St. Marie
Cover image: Steve Keith of Digital Fly

Printed in the United States of America

Publisher's Cataloging-in-Publication Data

Viana, Carlos M.
    Prescriptions from paradise : introduction to biocompatible medicine: an A-to-Z compendium / Carlos M. Viana. — 1st ed. — Merritt Island, FL 32952: Healing Spirit Press, 2008.

        p. ; cm.

        ISBN-13: 978-0-9789920-4-0
        Includes bibliographical references and index.

        1. Holistic medicine. 2. Inflammation—Alternative treatment.
    3. Alternative medicine. 4. Self-help techniques. I. Title

R733 .V53 2007   2006935528
613—dc22   0706

10 9 8 7 6 5 4 3 2 1

Dedicated to my inner circle of friends, who, like a medicine wheel of individuals representing the four directions, are all adamantly convinced of the effectiveness of my medical protocol and supportive in many ways:

At the green east gate of the circle stands Milushka Nahr, who acts as my eyes, looking into the material needed for new projects, while providing me with the spiritual resource of willpower.

At the red south gate is my soul mate Phyllis, the source of my joy and happiness, who inspires and supports me, helping me find my voice.

At the black west gate are Elaine Frazier and Ginger Corte, who have shown me new paths to take while imbuing me with the ability to let go and move on.

At the white north gate are the wise men Robert Bruzzi, Esq., and Dr. Bernard Epstein, who guide my ambition with their judicious counsel.

At the yellow center are all the people who have allowed me to teach them, especially my sons, Julio and Fernando, and Bethany Bruzzi, DO, whose questions prompt the reflection I need to stay current.

IN GRATITUDE...

Thanks to the owner, John Chemaly, Sr., the directors, and the staff members of the newspapers that print my weekly health column—*Aruba Today* and, the Papiamento version, *Bon Dia Aruba*. Their willingness to help me educate Arubans in alternative medical ideas is courageous and admirable. The articles from this column form the backbone of *Prescriptions from Paradise*.

I am also grateful to those involved in the birthing of this book, which, like all births, needs mother power. This book was conceived by my soul mate and mother of my children, Phyllis, who insisted I write it. Parvati Markus incubated hundreds of newspaper articles I had written into a cohesive manuscript. Under the tutelage of my editor Ellen Kleiner, the book, my medical protocol, and I myself have matured. *Prescriptions from Paradise* would not have existed without these mothers.

I am grateful as well to Dr. Kathleen Assar, for her guidance and help and, while sharing a lovely bottle of Cabernet Sauvignon, for composing the title *Prescriptions from Paradise*.

Here in Aruba, we are indebted to our suppliers, who take fiscal risks by bringing sophisticated blood tests and supplements to the island, despite the stiff evaluation charge levied on vitamin, mineral, and amino acid dietary supplements because they are considered medicines just like pharmaceutical drugs.

In addition, I wish to thank the holistic and conventional practitioners, dentists, and oral hygienists who work with us to provide biocompatible dental care in our community. In particular, biocompatible dental physician Hendrick "Henk" Marsman and I have collaborated in pushing the edge of biocompatible dentistry, to the benefit of our patients.

Thanks to our patients, especially, for their willingness to open their minds to complementary medicine. Phyllis and I realize that the success of our grass-roots clinic is a reflection of our patients' belief in our ability to provide simple and effective medical treatments. Our patients are open-minded individuals with the self-confidence to take responsibility for their health and the strength of mind to see beyond the limited views of conventional medicine to embrace a broader protocol of natural healing.

I am deeply thankful for the sacrosanct relationships in my life, especially with my family and dear friends.

Finally, I am ever grateful to my grandfathers. In American Indian spirituality, we learn in spirit from the council of grandfathers, who are not just biological relatives but guides illuminating the path of our calling. The following are my grandfathers, highly spiritual people as well as specialists in their fields, to whom I owe much:

MARK A. BREINER ~ Although very busy in his private mercury-free dental practice, Mark has guided me and provided an instrumental key to my detox protocol by showing me a safe method for the removal of toxic material from patients' mouths.

BERNARD EPSTEIN ~ Bernie, who has a successful practice in BioSET—a form of energy medicine that integrates acupuncture, chiropractic, homeopathy, and enzyme nutrition—has helped me coordinate many aspects of energy medicine and kept me "in the loop" regarding new medical data.

JAY HOLDER ~ Awarded the Albert Schweitzer Prize in Medicine, Jay lectures worldwide and is in his twenty-fourth year of addiction treatment practice, operating several clinics. Although I am not a chiropractor and thus don't meet the program requirements, Jay welcomed me into the American College of Addictionology and Compulsive Disorders, which trains and certifies professionals in addiction recovery worldwide, allowing me to study the latest treatment modalities.

H. L. "SAM" QUEEN ~ Founder and director of research for the Institute for Health Realities, "Sam" has unselfishly provided supporting information to assist me in better serving our patients. His explanation of how to extract medical information from individual blood tests was a major contribution to our clinic.

C. TOM SMITH ~ An internationally recognized authority on all aspects of clinical nutrition and cell regeneration, Dr. Smith was a homeopathic medical doctor and a consummate teacher whom I considered my mentor before he passed away.

CONTENTS

Foreword by Dr. Ernesto Rodriguez Robelto   13
Preface   15
Introduction   19

Acupuncture   25
ADD, ADHD, and Autism   28
Addiction   30
Adrenals   35
Aging   38
Anemia   39
Antibiotics   41
Anxiety or Panic Attacks   44
Arteriosclerosis   46
Arthritis   49
Asthma   53
Back Pain   57
Biocompatible Dentistry   59
Blood Type Diet   65
Cancer   69
Childbirth   71
Cholesterol   79
Chronic Inflammation   83
Climate Control   84
Colon Hydrotherapy   85
Constipation   88
Coral Calcium   90
Dehydration   93
Dementia   95
Diabetes Type II   97
Dieting   99
Diverticulitis   100
EDTA Chelation   103
Energy Refinery   106
Environmental Toxins   115
Eyesight   118
Fasting   121
Gallbladder and Liver Problems   123
Gout   125

Hair Loss   129
Headaches   131
Heart Attacks   133
Heartburn   137
Hormones   140
Hygiene   144
Hypertension   146
Liver Detoxification   149
Longevity   150
Nerve Problems   153
Obesity   157
Osteoporosis   159
Oxidative Stress   160
pH Balance   163
Rejuvenating Cell Replacement Therapy   169
Ringing in the Ears (Tinnitus)   172
SAMe   175
Seasonal Affective Disorder (SAD)   177
Sexual Relationships   178
Skin   184
Sleep   187
Stress   189
Sugar   191
Thyroid   195
Ulcers   199
Urinary Tract Infection   201
Yeast Overgrowth   205

Appendix A: The Biocompatible Treatment Protocol   209
Appendix B: Getting Back on Track: A Patient's Viewpoint   215

Notes   217

Index   229

FOREWORD

As a Cuban physician specializing in both family medicine and clinical laboratory immunology, I was fortunate to be trained by Dr. Viana in his biocompatible medicine protocol in 2005. While working with Dr. Viana in his Aruba clinic, I witnessed the amazing results of his protocol, which aims not only to improve the quality of life but also to prevent and even reverse the development of chronic diseases. Having been exposed to acupuncture and herbal medicine as part of my medical studies in Cuba, I immediately developed an intense interest in Dr. Viana's approach and scope of treatment.

Dr. Viana's protocol begins with a focus on a comprehensive diagnosis that includes an in-depth patient consultation. He first conducts a traditional Chinese medicine examination, checking both pulses on each wrist, examining the surfaces of the tongue, and inspecting the eyes and skin, as well as morphological signs of weight and height. Next he conducts a battery of laboratory tests to support the diagnosis. Saliva tests are used to determine blood type secretor status and hormone precursors. Extensive blood tests are utilized, for which Dr. Viana has developed a diagnostic procedure that goes far beyond any conventional medical one. Hair analysis is used to establish loss of bone minerals and the body burden of toxic heavy metals, to determine if patients have hemochromatosis, also known as liver loading disease. In addition, thermograms, used to detect subtle heat changes, reveal inflammatory areas in the bodies of patients suffering from chronic inflammation.

Of all Dr. Viana's clinical therapeutic treatments to which I was exposed, perhaps the one that impacted me most profoundly was colon hydrotherapy, which provides patients with immediate relief from a number of chronic symptoms. In this treatment, water slowly infused into the colon over a forty-minute period removes compacted fecal material from the colon walls, as well as gas and pathological bacteria, after which beneficial lactobacillus bacteria are reintroduced into the body. Other effective procedures include a food and chemical sensitivity/intolerance test that assists Dr. Viana in helping patients successfully overcome a wide variety of conditions resulting from food and chemical sensitivities, such as digestive disorders, migraines, obesity, chronic fatigue, skin disorders, and arthritis.

I invite readers to reap the rewards of this fascinating and informative book focused on improving health and well-being. It gives us a better understanding of how each day, through daily lifestyle and nutrition choices, we and our environment promote the components that create destructive inflammatory processes and disease. It provides a simple, clear, comprehensive guide to the steps and tools that can prevent, arrest, reverse, and cure chronic systemic problems, including the slowing down and reversing of the natural aging process.

Dr. Viana's biocompatible medicine protocol can put us and keep us on a path to healthy life and living.

—Dr. Ernesto Rodriguez Robelto

PREFACE

Some of my earliest experiences in life helped shaped my career in holistic medicine. At age seven, in 1955, I had the opportunity to attend school in the United States, which gave me greater exposure to a variety of subjects and career options. Landing at Miami International Airport, after a twelve-hour bumpy flight from Curaçao with stops in Port of Spain, Trinidad, Tobago, and Havana, I remember being flabbergasted at the opulence of runways separated by beds of grass, in stark contrast to the desert island landscape of Aruba.

The school I attended serendipitously set me on a course of learning that I otherwise might never have experienced. I had been labeled "mentally retarded" by a young Dutch school psychiatrist on Aruba who could not understand the mixed bag of five languages I had grown up speaking, and consequently, was sent to Miami Country Day and Residence School for Boys, with apologies that I was "unteachable." But as fate would have it, halfway to the school, "Doc" Abele, a founder who had picked me up, stopped at a convenience store and left me alone in the car alone staring at its fancy radio with enticing knobs. Being curious, I began playing with them, and after Doc returned he came to the conclusion that only a "normal" boy would fiddle with radio knobs, and turned me over to the school's other founder, Mr. Sommers, with reassurances that there was nothing wrong with me. This was my first experience in the limitations of a medical prognosis that fails to take into account the whole human being, social conditions, and cultural factors—and its potentially devastating consequences.

I learned another valuable lesson when my English teacher, Mr. Sommers's beautiful daughter, introduced me to a folktale from oral tradition entitled "The Blind Men and the Elephant," a story her father frequently referred to while teaching us to be tolerant of people with viewpoints different from our own. The story describes what happens as each of six men, all physically blind but very intelligent and wise, touch an elephant. The first touches its side and immediately announces the elephant is like a wall. The second feels the tusk and concludes the elephant is like a spear. The third grabs the trunk and boldly proclaims the elephant is like a snake. The fourth gropes around the knee and asserts the elephant is like a tree. The fifth touches the ear and states the elephant is like a fan. The sixth grabs hold of the tail and declares the elephant is like a rope.

The point is that each man draws an unshakable conclusion on the basis of a very narrow perspective instead of welcoming new information to broaden his impression of the whole animal. The story awakened me to the importance of looking at the whole picture and considering interrelationships of parts, precepts that came to guide my entire career in holistic medicine, from my training in traditional Chinese medicine and internship as an Oriental medical doctor in Shanghai's Longhua Hospital to my current focus on what I call biocompatible medicine, developed and practiced over fifteen years at our grassroots clinic in Aruba, the Viana Healing Center.

Other childhood experiences that influenced my later views on medicine pertained to vehicles. My father owned a car dealership and repair service. It was in the repair garage—with its heady mix of cars, smells, and people all mingled in a swirl of frantic activity—that I first became excited about fixing things. I watched, enthralled, as worried customers turned over their troubles to our head mechanic, Francisco the "Wizard," who understood the importance of all the interrelated parts and how they worked together to make the car run smoothly, a notion that ultimately informed my perception of holistic medicine.

Across the street from my father's business complex was a bus garage, where Hodge, a soft-spoken bus driver, escorted me into the alien world of diesel buses, with their smells and sounds so different from those of cars. Mechanics were always on hand inspecting the long yellow vehicles and taking care of the necessary repairs.

Later, during my teenage years, a fine-looking, big, red convertible was brought into my father's garage. Its owner, Toni, was open and fascinating, and another kind of "fixer"—a medical surgeon. It was his humanity toward his patients that instilled in me a passion for medicine.

A further experience also influenced my future work in medicine. In my mid-twenties I was invited to dinner by a dashing Englishman who enjoyed gardening. While leaving his house, I noticed a pot of dying orchids someone had thrown on the rubbish heap. On a whim, I asked for the dying orchids. Returning home with them, knowing nothing about orchids, I removed the wet rotten part of the plant and placed the remaining part in a dry pot. The plant thrived and was soon covered with flowers. As a result of this experience I had a revelation: you do not fix plants, you cultivate them. It was a concept I later found pertained to people as well.

Once back in the United States, I joined the staff of New York's Governor Hugh Carey, where, while serving on the executive staff of the New York Division of Alcohol Abuse and Alcoholism, I found I preferred doing medical research to working directly with people. I became involved in passing legislation that recognized alcoholism as a disease, mandating payment for alcoholism treatment by insurance providers, funding research on fetal alcohol syndrome, and increasing the legal drinking age, all the while working in community programs for the mentally ill. Eventually my attention was drawn to the social problems plaguing New York City's ethnic communities.

I later returned to Aruba to explore hyperbaric medicine, which utilizes high-pressure compression chambers to treat a variety of conditions. There I developed efficacious medical procedures while working with scuba divers, which enabled me to overcome my reluctance to work one-on-one with people.

Then in 1996 I was invited to Shanghai to enroll in an internship at Longhua Hospital, the largest traditional Chinese medicine (TCM) hospital in the People's Republic of China. There I was trained by Dr. Sun, considered one of the top TCM physicians. I assumed the program would strictly extend my theoretical knowledge of medicine, but I was forced to treat people in pain; finding I could help them feel better was enormously gratifying. Returning to Aruba, I began to treat family members and friends. People came in pain and left feeling better—then brought more people. Soon we were overwhelmed with so many people in pain we had inadvertently established a grassroots clinic, which became known as the Viana Healing Center.

Shortly afterward, a woman arrived in excruciating lower back pain. After I treated her, she thanked me and said she could now return to church to sing "Hallelujah." In that moment I realized that my calling was to help show people the road back to healing so they could once again praise the Healing Spirit that unites us all.

Prescriptions from Paradise: An Introduction to Biocompatible Medicine originated from a weekly health column I eventually published in the local newspaper *Aruba Today* and in the Papiamento, or native Spanish-based creole, version, *Bon Dia Aruba,* as well as from a weekly radio program called "Health Talk" that I broadcast on the Internet to Papiamento speakers scattered around the world. The column and radio show provided valuable vehicles for refining my views about the biocompatible protocol and for getting feedback from the public concerning health problems and treatments. More recently, surveyors have told us that "Health Talk," known for encouraging callers to ask questions and voice their opinions, is popular among listeners of all ages, from teenagers to elders. Since 2006, on the last Saturday of every month the show has been presented in English over the Internet, prompting listeners to call us from the Netherlands, the United States, and even Jakarta, Indonesia.

Also contributing to the contents of this book are conclusions drawn from my fifteen years of experience operating the Viana Healing Center, where we treat everyone from newborns to octogenarians. Our clinic enjoys a high success rate, most likely because from the beginning we have documented, through blood tests and hair analysis, both the medical conditions affecting our patients and the paths back to recovery made possible by the biocompatible treatment protocol. And while Aruba is a recuperative paradise of fresh air, sunshine, and ocean water, its population, like that of other developed nations, suffers from the abundant presence of toxic heavy metals and the disastrous health consequences of rejecting traditional foods for the convenience of fast, processed ones. Seduced by inexpensive simple carbohydrates, which, using the same pathways as cocaine, critically impact the brains of those with blood type O—the blood type of the majority of Native Arubans on the island—most indigenous Americans in Aruba are disadvantaged before they begin school. Currently about 90 percent of Aruban children in grades one through six are obese, 40 percent of whom are clinically obese. Considering these unfortunate realities, combined with the fact that hypertension and type II diabetes are being diagnosed at younger and younger ages, the future of our island's national health looks bleak.

Interwoven with information culled from my health column and radio interviews, as well as from one-on-one patient care, is a wealth of understanding extracted from an array of scientific sources including books, journals, lectures, and consultations with medical experts. These resources further substantiate the main premise of biocompatible medicine, which is that the ravages of environmental toxins, our unmanaged stress, and the food we ingest can result in oxidative stress, which leads to chronic inflammation, the foundation of all degenerative medical conditions. The carnage would continue were it not for the biocompatible treatment protocol, a proven method for identifying and removing the body's burden of toxic material then providing elements the body needs to regain its health.

The aim of *Prescriptions from Paradise* is to raise awareness of biocompatibility in general, assist readers seeking treatment modalities for specific conditions, and provide an easy-to-use resource tool for preventive care in stressful times. The book's alphabetical format is intended to help implement the treatment and prevention protocols. The A-to-Z listings of medical conditions and associated terms include descriptions, commentary, treatment options, explanations of causal and developmental factors from a biocompatible perspective, and hands-on advice. Designed for readers interested in an integrated holistic approach to health, this volume is simple enough for a layperson to use yet extensive and detailed enough for practitioners. In fact, although I define my biocompatible protocol as being "holistic," all the citations herein reference peer-reviewed medical journal articles, the gold standard of conventional medicine.

INTRODUCTION

Two sisters and their mother once came to the grassroots, holistic clinic I run in my native Aruba, the Viana Healing Center. They were filling out consultation forms when I came over to greet them, barefoot and wearing only a cotton scrub shirt and loose cotton shorts, reflecting my view that loose-fitting cotton clothing is the healthiest way to dress in our Caribbean climate and my desire not to differentiate between "us" professionals and the rest of humanity through the social ritual of wearing a uniform. The three women eyed me and, not taking the time to ask questions, uttered apologies and left. Weeks later, I heard from another patient that the ladies had confided to her that they "could never consult with Dr. Carlos because he wears no shoes!"

Although most people believe that going barefoot is undignified, a sign of poverty, or unhealthy, in the People's Republic of China a barefoot doctor is a positive role model since the Chinese know that only healthy people can walk barefoot, as I learned during my internship at Longhua Hospital in Shanghai. There, a barefoot doctor is a healthy doctor who can show you how to regain your health.

Oriental medical doctors are aware that the soles of the feet each have 7,200 nerve endings extensively interconnected through the spinal cord and brain to all areas of the body and that experiencing pain while walking barefoot can indicate health problems in the corresponding body parts. Such knowledge is widely used to advantage in medical disciplines such as acupuncture and reflexology. In acupuncture, the soles of the feet and palms of the hands are studied to verify diagnoses, and then needles are utilized to stimulate the function of the affected gland, organ, body fluid, or other body part. Certified practitioners of reflexology, which number about 25,000 worldwide, apply pressure to points on the foot to release blockages that inhibit energy flow and cause pain and disease, affecting internal organs and glands and breaking up lactic acid and calcium crystals that have accumulated around corresponding nerves. In Denmark, where reflexology is the number-one alternative health modality, producers of reflexology sandals maintain that the bumps in the soles of the sandals stimulate reflexology points.

Here in Aruba we have a constant reflexology provider: the ground. Because the soil is neither cold, wet, nor infested with parasites, there is no reason to continually protect the feet. In fact, to wear shoes is to miss one of our island's health benefits, since tight shoes can cause numerous difficulties, including corns, bunions, athlete's foot, plantar warts, heel spurs, foot odor, leg pains, and varicose veins. Interestingly, after twenty-five years the American Podiatry Association has reversed its position on wearing shoes and now recommends that people walk barefoot as much as possible, a view I have long held. Because of such perspectives, in tandem with my general orientation toward holistic medicine, I am referred to as the "barefoot doctor."

Over the years, my medical training and practice have convinced me of the value of a holistic approach to medicine, in contrast to relying solely on conventional Western medicine, which was my initial focus. While studying as an emergency medical technician in the United States, I learned how Westerners view the human body as a machine, a notion I could identify with after years of watching car repairs at my father's dealership. This mechanistic view originated with the French mathematician René Descartes, who theorized in *Principles of Philosophy*, written in 1644, that humans were isolated from nature and, like machines, could be separated into parts and governed by mechanical laws. Later, in the 1930s, the word *allopathic* came into usage. *Allopathic* means "to lighten your disease feelings"; the root "allo" comes from the Latin word *alleviat*, which means "to lighten," while "pathic," from the Greek, means "feeling disease." The so-called scientific model it subsequently spawned has since been adopted by health departments worldwide that now regard health as the absence of disease and risk factors for disease, including immunity to a full range of infectious diseases through inoculation.

Many doctors trained in conventional medicine have learned not only to view people as machines but also to act like mechanics fixing broken parts. This approach can work, as the miracles of Western emergency medicine illustrate, but it is not oriented toward teaching people how to regain their health or prevent disease, and it turns doctors into experts invested with authority over patients. Patients are encouraged to give away responsibility for their health care, turning their bodies over to the doctor in the same way they might deliver a car to a garage for repairs, an attitude ultimately seeding the mistaken notion that the power to cure comes from outside.

Further, current conventional medical research promotes the idea of resolving medical conditions through the development of "magical" drugs, surgical procedures, or equipment that can be sold worldwide. Although 80 percent of conventional drugs originate from herbal sources, when research indicates the potential for a natural cure it is often ignored in favor of developing products that can be patented and made more profitable. As a result of this emphasis on products, conventional doctors tend to treat all their patients alike, recommending a "standard" diet, "routine" medical care, and "common" over-the-counter pharmaceutical drugs.

An unfortunate outcome of this perspective is that every year in the United States approximately 107,000 people are hospitalized for aspirin, ibuprofen, or other nonsteroidal anti-inflammatory drug-related complications, thousands of whom soon die.[1] So prevalent are these casualties that death certificates state the cause of death as "natural." Actually, most pharmaceutical drugs are toxic to the body. For instance, antibiotics (a word that means "against life"), contrary to popular belief, do not eliminate pathogens but instead slow their growth, transforming acute infections into chronic ones.

Medical mistakes are another huge problem, according to a report issued by the Institute of Medicine, citing studies estimating that at least 44,000 hospitalized

Americans, and perhaps as many as 98,000 die every year from errors made by their doctors. Referred to as adverse drug events (ADEs), these errors are considered preventable. One study arrives at a yearly total of 380,000 ADEs—which exceeds the number of deaths each year either on the nation's highways, from breast cancer, or from AIDS[2]—while another states 450,000, both of which are believed by the Institute of Medicine to be understimates.[3]

So widespread are medical problems resulting from the use of common drugs and procedures that a new word has been coined to refer to them—*iatrogenesis*, meaning "brought forth by a healer." (*Iatros* means "healer" in Greek.) Iatrogenesis most often refers to the harmful consequences caused by physicians prescribing drugs, surgery, radiation, or chemotherapy. It can also result from recommendations made by other medical professionals, such as psychologists, therapists, pharmacists, nurses, or dentists. Ivan Illich, in his book *Medical Nemesis*, points out that "approximately one out of every five people admitted to a research hospital acquires an iatrogenic illness," ranging from depression to infection, disability, or dysfunction.[4]

As a result of these problems in conventional Western medicine, over the last ten years individuals have been flocking to medical providers who offer a variety of nontoxic treatments and procedures for healing, including acupuncture, chiropractics, homeopathy, shiatsu, nutritional therapy, environmental medicine, Ayurveda, massage, and meditation. Another advantage of these alternative approaches is that they, unlike conventional medicine, awaken an appreciation of the fact that we are beings of energy, or light, as is intimated in biblical references to the Creation ("In His image… according to our likeness" [Gen 1:26]) and that it is energy which keeps us healthy. Practitioners of holistic medicine view health as more than the absence of disease and its risk factors; to them, health means having the energy to live a full, high-quality life.

Many medical associations in the West are alarmed at the growing popularity of alternative medicine in developed countries. In the United States alone, between 30 and 70 percent of people say they have tried an alternative therapy such as acupuncture, vitamin supplements, or herbal treatments; and about 70 percent of older adults say they routinely use "alternative medicine."[5] In fact, the use of alternative medical therapies has become so prevalent that the National Institutes of Health (NIH) established the Center for Complementary and Alternative Medicine and began awarding grants of nearly $3 million for the study of these methods worldwide.[6] Of course professionally, the different medical methods are only diverse expressions of a larger medical picture. As Richard Dawkins, author of *A Devil's Chaplain*, puts it, "There is no alternative medicine. There is only medicine that works and medicine that doesn't work."[7]

Many alternative, or holistic, medical procedures are based on the view of Eastern philosophy that all life is part of nature, including the human being, who is seen as a miniature universe, reflecting the cosmos, or a garden with defined cycles and conditions. In keeping with this holistic paradigm, the role of a Chinese doctor, like that of a gardener who both nourishes plants and helps them resist disease, is to cultivate life energy by perceiving signs and symptoms of a patient and making diagnoses that sound like a gardener's assessments of plants, in terms of heat and cold, moisture and dryness, and the excess or deficiency of specific conditions. But it is also true that the very term "alternative medicine" implies the presence of a culturally biased point of view, because the practices considered alternative in the West are regarded in the greater part of the world as aspects of traditional medicine, such as Chinese medicine, Ayurveda, shamanic healing, or herbal therapy.

In the end, depending on personal perspective it is possible to view conventional and alternative, or holistic, medicine as complementary. For example, osteopathic medicine, which offers all the benefits of conventional medicine, including prescription drugs and the use of technology to diagnose disease and evaluate injury, provides the additional benefit of hands-on diagnosis and treatment through a manipulative therapy that releases blocked energy. In other words, osteopathic medicine bridges conventional and natural holistic medicine, integrating scientific research with the healing powers of nature.

In my view, the most comprehensive modality for overcoming the apparent contradiction between conventional and holistic medicine is biocompatible medicine, the protocol I use at the Viana Healing Center. Biocompatible physicians employ therapies that support and promote the body's natural healing process, leading to the highest state of wellness. Professionally, I oppose the use of pharmaceutical drugs, artificial vitamins, food-based supplements, and chiropractic adjustment to ameliorate symptoms, and advocate instead counteracting the foundational causes of disease. A major difference between biocompatible medicine and all other medical modalities is that biocompatible medicine identifies and corrects the factors negatively impacting the metabolic process of the body. In effect, biocompatible means *compatible with one's own biology* rather than with some standardized list of foods, supplements, activities, or procedures regarded as beneficial.

Biocompatible medicine also incorporates dental procedures involving nontoxic materials and aims to identify the source of and correct chronic inflammation in the body, a condition thought to be the foundation of all degenerative medical conditions, including cancer and premature aging. Although many other medical models claim to be holistic, taking into account a person's physical, mental, and social conditions, rather than just physical symptoms, no other approach integrates dental health. And yet, the condition of a person's mouth and teeth has a great impact on their well-being, and a dental examination, by a trained biocompatible dentist, presents a rapid, noninvasive way to evaluate their overall health.

Biocompatible medicine views the foundation of all degenerative medical conditions, including cancer and premature aging, as chronic inflammation from persistent acidity. The acidity develops from one or more of the following:

• Dehydration and eating the wrong foods for metabolic type, which includes your blood and secretor type, and which results in colon toxicities
• A body burden of toxic heavy metals that affect the biochemical metabolism
• Chronic infections

• Exposure to insecticides, pesticides, and fungicides
• Exposure to petroleum chemicals in the environment

In other words, your body can become persistently irritated, or inflamed, for a variety of reasons. First, dehydration and eating the wrong foods for your metabolic type (see "Blood Type Diet," p. 65) results in digestive problems and the production of poisons in the colon. Second, chronic infections treated by antibiotics—such as a *Helicobacter pylori* bacteria stomach infection, gum disease, or infections in the jawbones—lead to acid stress. Third, toxic heavy metals ingested from breathing polluted air, eating nonorganic fruits, vegetables, eggs, and meats, vaccines, or having mercury amalgams in teeth act as irritants. Fourth, insecticides and pesticides absorbed from food and the environment cause toxicity. And fifth, the 300,000 petrochemicals used in modern society add to body toxicity.

Chronic inflammation due to acidity decreases the body's ability to utilize oxygen efficiently. In an oxygen-poor, anaerobic environment, cancer and degenerative conditions establish a foothold and impair the body's natural ability to maintain health. Quickly a vicious cycle spirals us into accelerated aging, causing a gradual deterioration in various body parts, with a consequent incapacity to function adequately. The biocompatible protocol is therefore concerned primarily with identifying and detoxifying the body from the stressors that set the degenerative disease in motion. Once the body burden of toxicities has been removed and a healthy biochemical metabolism has been restored, the body's instinctive healing mechanisms can regain their functioning with amazing success. In a healthy body, free of infections and acidity, all the cells are well oxygenated and cancer resistive.

Following this approach in our clinic, we use high-tech hair analyses, blood tests, thermograms (regional temperature maps of the surface of the body, highlighting areas that are inflamed), and saliva tests to investigate beyond the biochemical parameters of conventional diagnostics, while integrating nontoxic dentistry and disciplines of traditional Chinese medicine, iridology, colon hydrotherapy, and psychiatric counseling. In biocompatible medicine, the boundaries between conventional Western medicine and holistic medicine have been eliminated; we offer just *good medicine*.

Over the last fifteen years at the Viana Healing Center, where our aim is to identify and eliminate the sources of chronic inflammation in the body, our patients have reported feeling better; having more energy and enthusiasm for work, family relationships, and hobbies; and enjoying a higher libido. Blood tests indicate they have healthier metabolic ranges and lower cholesterol, uric acid, and free blood calcium levels. Hair tests show that the body burden of toxic metals has been reduced. And thermograms reveal fewer inflamed areas in the body. These outcomes indicate that once we have identified and removed the toxicities producing acid stress, supported the body in recovering from various forms of poisoning, provided the right food, encouraged exercise and lifestyle improvements, and injected rejuvenating cellular material to restore and revitalize the affected tissues and organs, we have achieved true healing.

Unfortunately, in today's world the biocompatible protocol is often undermined by lack of education, as well as toxins in foods and the environment. For example, most people in our community still do not comprehend the primary health concept of basic nutrition, especially the distinction between simple and complex carbohydrates—an understanding that may mean the difference between living a healthy life and risking adult-onset type II diabetes. Over the last fifty years, the general shift away from the consumption of healthy fresh fruits and vegetables and complex carbohydrates (good starches and fiber foods) and toward a diet of simple carbohydrates (processed wheat products, sugar, white rice, corn, and convenient fast foods) has been largely responsible for today's epidemic of obesity, diabetes, cardiovascular problems, and rotten teeth. Likewise, the poisons in our environment have taken a huge toll, with aluminum increasing the incidence of Alzheimer's disease; lead reducing the scholastic grades of children by triggering learning disabilities; mercury causing decreased thyroid function, endometriosis, brain damage, cataracts, cerebral palsy, poor coordination, joint pain, kidney damage, and loss of self-control; cadmium inducing alcoholism; and copper contributing to allergies, anorexia, anxiety, arthritis, autism, migraines, mood swings, and multiple sclerosis.

Despite these hurdles, in our clinic we are making progress. In the early days, before Aruba established mandatory socialized medicine, patients would come in with minor health problems and, after uncovering more major ones beneath the surface, would return to their government-subsidized primary care practitioners, or "house doctors." Now people are taking advantage of the socialized medical benefits for their minor medical complaints and coming to us for more serious conditions, paying for the care themselves because word has gotten out about our cure rates.

True healing, we realize, can only be an endeavor reflecting physical, mental, social, and environmental priorities. With this in mind, we have made considerable progress in diagnosing and treating medical problems that originate in the mouth and have seen serious medical conditions disappear after an offending tooth was pulled. Presently we are making advances in diagnosing and treating sexual and addiction disorders and codependency issues. With respect to the environment, we encourage Aruban hotels to urge suppliers to import nontoxic cleaning products that are 100 percent biodegradable.

In this book, we will look at symptoms and diseases in terms of how energy may have become blocked, how the body may have absorbed toxins, and how the organism may be coping with stress and inappropriate diet—all with the aim of understanding natural ways to regain health. Aaron Sachs, professor of history and American studies at Cornell University and an award-winning environmental journalist, says, "Death is more universal than life; everyone dies but not everyone lives." We start truly living when we take inventory of ourselves and make a commitment to live a healthy life.

A

ACUPUNCTURE

Although pharmaceuticals have a valued place during a life-threatening emergency, they change the body's chemistry and are therefore not the treatment of choice for all medical conditions. Instead, alternative treatments are used by holistic physicians, who view humans as beings of light and evaluate disease from a broad perspective that takes into account many aspects of bodily processes, including energy patterns. As an Oriental medical doctor, one of my preferred treatment modalities is acupuncture, a Chinese medical procedure developed over four thousand years ago that is highly effective in addressing a wide variety of ailments. Based on the theory that conditions causing disease interrupt energy flow in the body, acupuncture aims to reestablish healthy energy flow through the insertion of thin sterile needles at specific points, along with the application of heat and pressure. The needles, which are used only once, are a finer gauge than even the finest hypodermic needles.

In the past, Western medical experts have been skeptical of acupuncture's therapeutic value, unable to believe that the simple act of inserting fine needles into tissue could elicit any positive, long-lasting response. The ancient practice, however, is now gaining increased acceptance in the Western world. In recent years, more people in the United States have consulted energy physicians than conventional doctors, prompting the American Medical Association to recommend that their member doctors either buy an existing complementary practice or attend an acupuncture certification course to maintain their business's cash flow.[1] In 2003, the number of acupuncturists in the United States without traditional medical degrees was estimated at eleven thousand, while those with medical degrees was three thousand—a number expected to quadruple by 2015.[2] Most likely it will, considering that a consensus panel convened by the National Institutes of Health in 1997 concluded that acupuncture treatment is effective for many medical and painful conditions.[3]

The key to acupuncture's therapeutic effect is not only the insertion of ultrafine needles at specific points on the body but also the manipulation of the needles to bring out a *deqi* response, as I learned at Longhua Hospital in Shanghai. A component of *deqi* is a phenomenon called "needle grasp," often described by acupuncturists as feeling like a fish tugging on a line and experienced by the patient as an aching sensation, heaviness, or an electric feeling flowing through the arm or leg. Generally during a treatment, which usually lasts twenty minutes, patients feel deep relaxation, in part caused by brain endorphins released during the procedure. Relaxation is further enhanced in our clinic in Aruba by the aroma of moxa herb burning on the handles of inserted acupuncture needles, mingling with the scents of orchids and other tropical plants.

Acupuncture works to stabilize energy among the organs, relieve pain, and reduce swelling. For example, at the organ level it can beneficially treat all symptoms of liver chi stagnation, which include fibromyalgia; migraine headaches; arthritic joints; symptoms of irregular periods; PMS; dark-colored menstrual blood with small clots; breast pain with distension; yeast infections; spleen dampness and liver heat; as well as irritability, depression, and frustration. In terms of pain management, the number of needles and specific treatment depends on whether the pain is acute or chronic.

Acupuncture is safe if practiced by trained acupuncturists. To evaluate a practitioner's potential, use the following points as a guide.

Ask medical doctors who are also acupuncturists how long they have trained in acupuncture, as well as where and how long they have practiced traditional Chinese medicine.

Among the many questionable acupuncturists, those to avoid outright are doctors who have been "certified" as acupuncturists after taking a weekend course. It is wise to be skeptical even about those who took a six-week course that did not include at least two hundred hours of clinical experience in acupuncture. Ultimately, a medical degree, anatomy courses, and clinical experience, all rooted in the West, are insufficient for acquiring an understanding of the concepts involved in traditional Chinese medicine, which is over four thousand years old and incorporates cultural attitudes foreign to the Western mind, though similar to basic views of shamanism, which I share as a Native American and a medical anthropologist.

Unfortunately, many acupuncturists have studied traditional Chinese medicine only in the West, at schools still teaching the medical knowledge brought to the West more than a hundred years ago. Oriental medical doctors trained in the People's Republic of China are the most up-to-date in modern acupuncture techniques—a point made clear to me during my internship at the largest traditional Chinese medicine hospital in the People's Republic of China. There, when asked by my new professors to show my needling technique of *xie* and *bu* manipulation, I could hear my colleagues laughing at my outdated information, making the first of my professors' tasks to rid me of the antiquated techniques I had picked up in the West that had not been used for years in the People's Republic of China.

Despite the fact that Oriental training can provide the most current knowledge of acupuncture techniques, however, it has one drawback: acupuncture is about releasing energy trapped in the body, which is enmeshed with suppressed emotions. Although Chinese physicians know all about how emotions correlate with specific organs, they do not integrate this information into treatments. It is as though the discussion of emotions in clinic is taboo. While interning in Shanghai, I never saw Chinese patients cry during acupuncture treatments, no matter how much pain they suffered. I was the only one who cried while being treated, exhibiting emotional releases that surprised my colleagues.

In the end, I believe that as Western practitioners of traditional Chinese acupuncture integrate emotional counseling with treatments, we are taking acupuncture to a higher level. The path to health is facilitated when there is recognition that the body, mind, emotions, and spirit are intertwined and affect one another.

Ask acupuncture practitioners how they develop their diagnoses.

Having been trained in Shanghai, I make my diagnoses in the traditional manner from the two wrist pulses, tongue, mouth, face, and nails. In our clinic, we do not use a lengthy questionnaire or ask about a client's symptoms. If a physician trained in acupuncture examines you, asks a couple of questions, and then tells you what you have been feeling, you have found a good one.

Inquire about the nature of the treatment environment.

The hospital where I interned in Shanghai had ten beds in each large treatment room, staffed by a professor, two medical interns, and two nurses—a very public place where patients could learn from one another, with no mind-numbing TV. The Chinese are very modest and, in such a public space, do not disrobe; rather, the acupuncture needles are stuck right through clothes, a method considered unsanitary in the West. Unlike the isolating treatment rooms often seen in the United States, treatment rooms in our clinic in Aruba place several people of the same sex in one treatment room so they can learn from one another, support one another, and not worry about sexual impropriety.

Overall, your best bet for finding a good acupuncturist is to ask people you know if they have consulted with a practitioner they would recommend. Then, when you call for an appointment, ask the questions listed above.

THE BIOCOMPATIBLE VIEW

Medical researchers dubious about things they cannot see or measure are often skeptical regarding acupuncture's ability to help reestablish healthy energy flow. Yet the difference between a living individual and a cadaver is in fact energy that cannot be measured via current medical technology but can be read from the pulse by traditional Chinese medicine physicians.

Biocompatible medicine recognizes this reality and also emphasizes the use of nontoxic materials in medical treatments. Toward that end, it supports the World Health Organization's position on acupuncture, stated as follows: "Generally speaking, acupuncture treatment is safe if it is performed properly by a well-trained practitioner.... Unlike many drugs, it is nontoxic, and adverse reactions are minimal." For example, while comparable to morphine preparations in its effectiveness against chronic pain, acupuncture lacks the narcotic's adverse consequences, including dependency, and is therefore a far safer option.[4]

- Arrive at your acupuncture session as lightly clad as possible while still feeling comfortable, so the needles will not have to be inserted through clothing. Also refrain from wearing perfume or heavy cologne, since body scent assists in the diagnosis.
- For purposes of hygiene, make sure your practitioner opens a new package of acupuncture needles when preparing for a treatment.
- Although acupuncture can trigger emotional release, it tends not to be physically painful. If you have needle phobia, mention your anxiety to the acupuncturist and, during your session, use your mind to achieve relaxation.

ADD, ADHD, AND AUTISM

The number of children said to be suffering from neurodevelopmental disorders, such as attention deficit disorder (ADD), attention deficit hyperactive disorder (ADHD), or autism, has reached epidemic proportions, and the increasing incidence of autism, in particular, is gaining widespread concern.[5] Such disorders, which have similar causes but whose consequences vary, affect 1 out of every 166 children. The reported incidence of autism alone, more prevalent among boys, has increased from 1 in 10,000 in the 1970s to 1 in 150 today, an increase of over 6,000 percent.[6] Additionally, many more children are diagnosed with other neurodevelopmental disorders considered to be on the same spectrum, including Asperger's syndrome and speech delay.

Signal traits and recommended treatments for ADD, ADHD, and autism are as follows. ADD, generally diagnosed in childhood, is characterized by a persistent pattern of impulsiveness, a short attention span, and often hyperactivity, all interfering with academic, occupational, and social performance.[7] ADD treatment options in regular medicine are routinely limited to psychostimulant medication combined with such behavior and cognitive therapies as self-recording, self-monitoring, modeling, and role playing.[8] ADHD is identified by distractibility, hyperactivity, impulsive behaviors, and the inability to remain focused on tasks or activities.[9] Treatment options, according to *The Merck Manual*, the world's best-selling medical textbook, are the same as those for ADD.[10] Autism, a pervasive developmental brain function disorder, is marked by problems with social contact, intelligence, and language, together with ritualistic or compulsive behavior and bizarre responses to the environment.[11] Treatment options include behavior therapy, butyrophenone (a neuroleptic drug), and speech therapy. Electric shock, used in the past, is no longer recommended.[12]

Neurodevelopmental disorders are associated with three distinctive behaviors, ranging from mild to disabling: difficulties with social interaction, problems with verbal and nonverbal communication, and repetitive behaviors or narrow, obsessive interests. The hallmark feature of autism is impaired social interaction. As early as infancy, a baby with autism may be unresponsive to people or focus intently on one item in the immediate environment to the exclusion of others for long periods of time. Some autistic children appear to develop normally then withdraw from social engagement at about the time they are immunized, underlining a link that many medical researchers suspect exists between autism and exposure to the mercury found in vaccines.[13]

Indeed, childhood vaccinations, including flu shots and B-complex injections, use as a preservative a mercury-containing compound called thimerosal (sodium ethylmercurithiosalicylate). Boyd Haley, PhD, a biochemist at the University of Kentucky and among the world's top experts on mercury toxicity, says, "I think that the biological case against thimerosal is so dramatically overwhelming anymore that only a very foolish or a very dishonest person with the credentials to understand this research would say that thimerosal wasn't most likely the cause of autism."[14] It is now thought that not only mercury but other metals and chemicals such as lead, arsenic, cadmium, insecticides, and pesticides contribute to the development of both autism and ADD.

Hair analysis tests, interpreted by a clinical nutritionist or toxicologist, can identify toxic heavy metals, and blood tests can reveal damage brought about by pesticides and insecticides. The best means for getting rid of these poisons seems to be glutathione, an antioxidant responsible for the excretion of mercury.[15]

To address the epidemic rise of neurodevelopmental disorders over the past decade, treatments have been advanced that greatly increase our ability to help such children. The latest news is that autistic children are improving with aggressive hyperbaric oxygen therapy, a medical treatment based on research identifying autism not as a diagnosis but rather symptomatic of an injury in the cortical and midbrain areas of the brain.[16]

Also, researchers have found strong evidence that in children with autism certain immune system components promoting inflammation in the brain are consistently activated.[17] Following a biocompatible protocol, our treatment of such children begins with recommendations for a healthy diet high in quality protein foods, such as eggs and lean meat, as well as vegetables and balanced essential fatty acids, and compatible with the child's metabolic type, which can be easily digested without causing constipation and can restore the bacterial environment necessary to temper inflammatory conditions. One reason we emphasize diet is because we have witnessed children with neurodevelopmental disorder symptoms caused by malabsorption and intolerances to certain foods, especially dairy products and gluten contained in wheat and grain products.[18] Since pasteurization turns milk casein into a dangerous molecule that can inflame and injure the brain, we sometimes recommend the elimination of milk from the diets of such children, after which parents have noticed positive changes.

Further, because ADD and autistic spectrum disorders have characteristics similar to those of chronic metal toxicity,[19] in our clinic children who suffer from neurodevelopmental disorders are screened for toxic heavy metals using hair analysis. In addition, knowing that toxic metals disable a growing body and brain by producing chronic irritation, we look for chronic inflammation (see "Chronic Inflammation," p. 83). We have consistently found symptoms of chronic inflammation in children exhibiting neurodevelopmental problems.

THE BIOCOMPATIBLE VIEW

Chronic inflammation in the brains of children exhibiting ADD, ADHD, autism, and other neurodevelopmental problems has been found to come from eating the wrong foods for metabolic type, particularly wheat and other grains; having a significant body burden of heavy metals, especially mercury, which is found as thimerosal in vaccinations; and toxicity from pesticides and insecticides.

WORDS OF ADVICE

- Do not be swayed by teachers or healthcare professionals who recommend that an active child be placed on psychotropic medication.
- Make sure the child eats the right foods for his or her metabolic type, focusing on a healthy diet of high-quality protein foods, such as eggs and lean meat, as well as vegetables and balanced essential fatty acids.
- Have a hair analysis performed by a clinical nutritionist or toxicologist to identify toxic heavy metals. Have blood tests to reveal any damage caused by pesticides or insecticides.

ADDICTION

An addiction is an activity or substance we repeatedly crave to experience, and for which we are willing to bear the negative consequences. In physical terms, addiction is a disease of the hypothalamus in the middle section of the brain, which is activated when we perform natural functions that help us stay alive, such as eating, and provides pleasurable feelings that lead us to repeat the activity.[20] Many drugs also stimulate this system and can induce even greater feelings of pleasure, in which case their influence on the reward circuit can lead the brain to bypass survival activities and repeat drug use. Addicted brains exhibit the disease in a variety of ways: through substance dependency (alcohol, cocaine, other recreational hard drugs, prescription medicines, nicotine); food disorders like bulimia, bingeing, or anorexia; or compulsive activities, including promiscuity, flamboyant eccentric behavior, zealous religious convictions, workaholism, and obsessive gambling.

In effect, addicts of all kinds have learned how to give themselves a quick "fix," or achieve an emotional high, to change how they feel or to escape their life problems. The disparity between an addict and an abuser is that an abuser uses an activity or substance to get high or feel different, while an addict uses an activity or substance to self-medicate or feel normal. Some abusers are considered "day after" people, because they do not have an addicted brain but simply feel sick or foolish after indulging in a potentially addictive behavior and don't often repeat it. Addicts, on the other hand, feel compelled to repeat addictive behavior even though they know that doing so will get them into trouble. Regardless of the type of addiction, the common denominator is that the chosen activity or substance has negative consequences on the person's work, family life, or health.

People whose brains become addicted are born with low levels of serotonin,[21] a neurotransmitting brain chemical that is metabolized from the amino acid tryptophan and widely distributed in tissues, especially in the middle section of the brain, functioning to constrict blood vessels at injury sites and profoundly

affect emotional states by making people sleep soundly. Serotonin converts into
dopamine, which causes pleasurable feelings and participates in the formation of
epinephrine, also known as the hormone adrenaline. Addictive substances such
as tobacco, alcohol, marijuana, and other drugs force the hypothalamus to release
more serotonin, making the individual feel better instantly. Drug abusers have
a limited "safe time" before they become addicted to the serotonin-stimulating
aspect of drugs and the brain loses its natural ability to produce serotonin.

Professionals know that denial lies at the heart of addiction and that once
addicts, or even abusers, face their dark secret they are ready to change and on
the road to recovery. A young man once stated on the questionnaire that is filled
out when someone first comes to our clinic that he was looking for help with his
anxiety and nervousness. When I read his pulse during the traditional Chinese
medicine exam, the hard pulse in the liver position and wiry pulse in the kidney
position said it all. "So, besides alcohol," I asked, "what other drugs are you
abusing?" After tensing up, then realizing that my tone had been factual rather
than judgmental, he answered, "Booze, marijuana, and cocaine for a couple
of years." He appeared surprised when I said, "Thank God you were able to
self-medicate." "What?" he asked. "Are you condoning what I did?" "Well," I
answered, "if the drugs allowed you to leave your house and lead a semblance
of a normal life, they helped you function." His nod affirmed that I had hit the
mark. And indeed, biocompatible medicine views the perpetual use of alcohol
and other drugs as an individual's desperate attempt to try to live a normal life.

Many researchers are looking for palliative measures to address nutritional
deficiencies among alcoholics, reduce the effects of alcohol toxicity, and even
diminish the craving for alcohol.[22] Some explore metabolic imbalances because
they know that metabolism and toxicity of heavy metals may be enhanced by
alcohol abuse.[23] Biocompatible medicine goes further, however, and looks at
metabolic imbalances resulting from a host of factors thought to lower serotonin
levels and drive people to alcohol and drug abuse, including dehydration; eating
the wrong foods for one's metabolic type, which can lead to colon toxicities;
the body burden of toxic heavy metals that affect the biochemical metabolism;
chronic infections; insecticides, pesticides, and fungicides; and the more than
30,000 petroleum chemicals that pervade our environment.

It has been shown, for example, that counties in the United States with industrial lead pollution in the form of manganese release, have higher than average
rates of alcoholism[24] and that alcohol use increases the deleterious effects of toxic
metals by interfering with the serotonin, dopamine, and other neurotransmitter
systems necessary for exercising self-control.[25] Researchers in biocompatible
medicine are finding that when such metabolic imbalances are corrected and the
body is receiving proper nutrients, the compensatory effects of alcohol, cigarettes,
or other addictive substances are no longer necessary.

Teenagers and Drugs
Many teens either abuse or are addicted to drugs. According to United States
statistics, one out of every four teenagers uses drugs, but, as with adults, some are

abusers while others are addicts.[26] Teen drug addicts, who are likely to have been born with a propensity for the problem, use drugs to feel normal and in control in an environment where there is pressure to act cool among schoolmates and members of the opposite sex. Unfortunately, unless such teens get professional help quickly, they will have a major drug problem.

Thus far, with teens, the "war on drugs" has been a failure. Both drug abusers and drug addicts laugh at the slogan "Just Say No!" or heed the advice only from Monday to Friday, when they attend school. In fact, teenage drug problems go undiagnosed far longer than those of adults, because parents and other responsible adults tend not to look closely at what teenagers are doing, mistake drug-related behavior for typical teenage behavior, or put off confrontations, hoping the teens will outgrow the problems. As a result, relevant treatment is usually not provided until teens get into trouble with the law or demonstrate problematic social behavior.

Once parents, other responsible adults, or teenagers themselves admit there is a problem, the next step is finding professional help. The most difficult part of getting help usually involves constructing a bridge for communication among parents, teens, and doctors. It is generally best for a teenager to confer with a physician privately, presenting, for example, with a complaint about sleeping problems, which is indeed a frequent complication of regular marijuana or other drug use. To encourage teenagers to eventually reveal what is really going on, without fear of disapproval or repercussions from any authority figure, they should be told that an addicted brain is a medical condition, no different from diabetes or a broken bone. Ideally, parents and professionals will explain that their purpose is not to get the teens into trouble but to identify possible drug problems before they become big medical and social problems.

Today, addicted teens are at risk of medical problems associated not only with the drugs themselves but with the poisons some have been sprayed with. For example, teens smoking marijuana run increased risk because, in Colombia, drug fields are sprayed with paraquat, a quaternary ammonium herbicide that is dangerous to humans if swallowed, and more so when inhaled.[27] This weed killer destroys green marijuana and cocaine plant tissue on contact, although marijuana that comes from such fields is still harvested and sold. In addition to the medical and social problems faced by drug abusers and addicts, in most parts of the world the use of drugs is against the law and can result in jail sentences.

Codependency
Addicts are usually part of an addictive family, since what keeps addictive behavior going is the interaction between addicts and their codependents. The term "codependency" was first used to describe the dysfunctional pattern of thought and behavior displayed by spouses and children of chemically addicted people, but we now know that others close to addicts, such as friends and coworkers, can also function as codependents. In fact, it is almost impossible to be an addict without the help of a spouse, boss, coworkers, employees, parents, children, or others who provide support for what professionals call "the addictive drama." From this vantage point, an addict's wife is invariably awarded best supporting

actress for her role in enabling him to continue the addiction. Even though she may claim that she is trying to help him stop, which may very well be the case, she is rarely effective enough to succeed or even walk offstage before the final curtain.

Living with a family member who has an addiction can be so traumatic as to rob a person of a stable and loving environment. Many codependents, especially children, quickly learn to lie to protect their family image and often remain in denial, not allowing anyone, including themselves, to become consciously aware that there is a problem. In such homes, children experience constant chaos, fear, abandonment, denial, and real or potential violence, making survival a full-time job. Common problems of children from homes with an alcoholic or drug addict include:

- Difficulty assessing what is normal or even having fun
- Tendency to judge themselves mercilessly
- Trouble with emotional relationships
- Feeling different from other people
- Propensity for impulsive behavior
- Inclination to be either superresponsible or superirresponsible
- Tendency to seek approval and affirmation
- Chronic anxiety
- Lack of self-discipline
- Compulsive lying
- Lack of self-respect
- Fear and mistrust of authority figures

The worst legacy of addicted adults is their children who, when they become adults, have difficulty feeling their emotions unless they are in crisis mode and thus often become addicts themselves. Since reality is painful in such dysfunctional families, a child has to hide from it to survive daily shame, anger, bitter disappointment, and feelings of abandonment, and rapidly learns to withdraw. To exercise some control over the situation, the child may stop trusting others, blame others for causing problems that exist, or follow strict rules and patterns that inhibit spontaneous behavior.

The following are common feelings and perspectives of codependents:

- My good feelings about who I am stem from being liked by you.
- My good feelings about who I am stem from receiving approval from you.
- Your struggle affects my serenity. My mental attention focuses on solving your problems or relieving your pain.
- My mental attention is focused on you.
- My mental attention is focused on protecting you.
- My mental attention is focused on manipulating you to do things my way.
- My self-esteem is bolstered by solving your problems or relieving your pain.
- My own hobbies and interests are secondary; my time is spent sharing your hobbies and interests.

- Your clothing and personal appearance are dictated by my desires, and I feel you are a reflection of me.
- Your behavior is dictated by my desires, and I feel you are a reflection of me.
- I am not aware of how I feel; I am aware of how you feel.
- I am not aware of what I want; I ask what you want.
- The dreams I have for my future are linked to you.
- My fear of your rejection determines what I say or do.
- My fear of your anger determines what I say or do.
- I use giving as a way of feeling safe in our relationship.
- My social circle diminishes as I involve myself with you.
- I put my values aside to connect with you.
- I value your opinions and way of doing things more than my own.
- The quality of my life is dependent on the quality of yours.

Recovery for both the addict and codependent involves facing the truth, implementing changes in behavior, seeking counseling to deal with issues left over from childhood, and for the codependent, making a concerted effort to raise self-esteem. A codependent on the way to recovery will stimulate change in the addicted partner, so that both learn how to dance to a different tune.

Addiction and Intimacy Problems

For a variety of reasons, addiction often goes hand in hand with intimacy problems. Intimacy involves two individuals revealing their thoughts and feelings to each other because they feel comfort and support, and may also entail physical closeness.

One of the symptoms of alcohol or other drug addiction is a breakdown in emotional maturation at the time the abuse began. Consequently, addicted individuals are characterized by a defect in their ability to form personal relationships or respond to others in an emotionally meaningful way, and thus often have intimacy problems. In relationship with their codependent partner, lust is often interpreted as love and once lust is satisfied there may be minimal interaction. Many addicts, on the other hand, show little desire for sexual experience. They may marry but then be sexually apathetic with their spouse, since sex can mean closeness and intimacy can require facing the truth of addiction. As a substitute for the intimacy they do not allow themselves, addicts often seek highs from chemical substances. And even though they may be surrounded by supportive friends and family, addicts will frequently turn to their isolating behaviors, many of which involve persistent patterns of dishonesty, distrust, suspicion, deception, misrepresentation, alienation, manipulation, coercion, violence, and attempts to control their partner.

Such circumstances are complicated by the fact that true intimacy is not often demonstrated in Western society. Rather, we are taught that getting the relationship is the goal, and that once people come together they live happily ever after—a relationship model depicted in everything from children's fairy tales of princes and princesses, to movies, TV programs, and books in which boy meets girl and the happy couple rides off into the sunset. Song lyrics such as

"I can't live without you" or "You are my everything" describe addictive love, in which the partner serves as the drug of choice, but in believing that someone else has the power to make us happy, we set ourselves up as victims.

By contrast, the ability to sustain real romantic love requires emotional maturity. With the development of emotional maturity comes a tendency to stop looking to another person for fulfillment and to begin satisfying one's own emotional needs, making sharing in relationship a bonus and not a necessity.

As a certified addiction professional educated in the self-perpetuating aspects of this disease, I will not treat an addict who is currently on chemicals. Nor will I counsel a couple in an addict-codependent relationship without both partners first entering into treatment for addiction.

THE BIOCOMPATIBLE VIEW

A biocompatible physician acts as a toxicity detective intent on identifying the metabolic stress that is driving a person's addictive behavior. For example, job pressures combined with financial problems, working single-handedly, and being isolated are typically presented as the triggers for today's high rate of alcohol addiction among dentists. Biocompatible medicine's approach is to look at mercury intoxication among dentists as the primary metabolic stressor and to treat alcoholism as a result of this toxicity, since low-level exposure has been found responsible for alcoholism, as well as a host of other problematic behaviors.[28] Recommending that an alcohol-impaired dentist enter a detoxification clinic would be shortsighted unless he simultaneously undergoes metal detoxification treatments.

We live in a toxic world. The toxins that act on our bodies by mimicking hormones have been implicated in a multitude of addictive behaviors.[29] Without detoxification, the destructive behaviors are likely to continue. Only by ridding the body of these substances is there a chance for recovery from addiction.

WORDS OF ADVICE

• Understand that a codependent's "excusing" activities prevent addicts from experiencing the consequences of their behavior and thus help sustain the addiction.
• Recognize that denial needs to be faced for recovery to occur.
• Expand your definition of addiction. It does not reflect a moral deficiency. It is a cerebral disease of low serotonin production caused by an underlying metabolic dysfunction associated with particular toxins.
• Encourage drug testing in adolescence to identify and treat individuals with a serotonin deficiency as soon as possible, before toxicity levels become extreme.

ADRENALS

Shaped like the Emperor Napoleon's three-cornered hat, an adrenal gland is perched on each of the two kidneys. Despite weighing only a fraction of an ounce, the adrenals secrete more than a dozen hormones into the bloodstream, influencing physical characteristics, growth, and development, and therefore profoundly impacting health.

Each gland can be divided into two distinct organs: the adrenal cortex and the adrenal medulla. The adrenal cortex, or outer layer, takes its instructions from the pituitary hormone ACTH and produces three main types of chemicals, called steroids: those that control the balance of sodium and potassium in the body, those that raise the level of sugar in the blood, and sex hormones. Thus, the adrenal cortex affects the way energy is stored and food is used, the chemicals in the blood, and characteristics such as hair and body shape. The adrenal medulla, or inner layer, takes its instructions from the nervous system and produces two types of chemicals in reaction to fear and anger, called "fight or flight" hormones. Thus, the adrenal medulla is part of the sympathetic nervous system and responds to physical and emotional stress. The basic task of the adrenal glands is to rush the body's resources into a "fight or flight" reaction to stress. When healthy, the adrenals produce cortisol, which can instantly increase heart rate and blood pressure, release energy stores for immediate use, slow digestion and other secondary functions, and sharpen the senses. When unhealthy, the adrenals overproduce cortisol, leading to numerous problems.

Medical problems of the adrenals include destruction by infection, autoimmune system attack, Addison's disease, and Cushing's Syndrome, an inherited condition preventing adequate secretion of hormones, which can be life threatening. Cushing's Syndrome, which causes the sufferer's face to become round, generates excess belly fat, and makes arms, legs, and fingers skinny, commonly occurs due to excessive levels of adrenal hormones as the result of a tumor, pharmaceutical therapy for rheumatoid arthritis, or drugs used to prevent the rejection of an organ transplant.

Unfortunately, the current focus on drugs tends to suppress early-stage symptoms rather than treat their underlying causes. As a result, conventional medicine detects only the extremes of these conditions, when damage to the adrenals has already occurred and Cushing's Syndrome or Addison's disease has developed. Within those extremes, you can feel miserable and still be told that your adrenals are normal.

The effects of adrenal dysfunction can be profound, including fatigue and weakness, suppression of the immune system and normal cell replacement, muscle and bone loss, moodiness or depression, hormonal imbalance, skin and digestion problems, impaired metabolic and mental functions, and autoimmune disorders, as well as being a factor in fibromyalgia, hypothyroidism, chronic fatigue syndrome, arthritis, and premature menopause. Fatigue affects many people in today's fast-paced world. Whereas traditionally the problem of adrenal fatigue was prevalent mostly among medical professionals, police officers, executives, and teachers, currently even stay-at-home moms suffer from adrenal fatigue. Largely this is because while the "fight or flight" reaction to stress caused by the adrenals was appropriate in the past to escape attack from saber-toothed tigers, the body's response is the same to something as minor as the frustration produced by a broken TV remote control. The most common triggers include psychological stress from emotional problems due to unresolved relationships and past hurts; sleep deprivation; physical trauma from surgery, accidents, or disease; self-destructive habits; and chemical exposure from heavy metals, pesticides, insecticides, latex, street drugs, or prescribed pharmaceutical drugs. Unfortunately, many people suffer adrenal fatigue without showing glandular problems, making diagnosis challenging.

Not all stress is bad; some is needed to keep the mind sharp and the body alert. Problems start when we experience constant stress and lose the ability to cope, since the stress response takes priority over all other metabolic functions.

In biocompatible medicine, the first step in treating adrenal fatigue is taking control of the negative stressors in your life and ruling out other diseases by checking your hormone levels via a cortisol/DHEA saliva test. If saliva test results are normal in the morning but drop to low levels in the afternoon and evening, low adrenal reserve and adrenal fatigue are indicated. This is usually caused by stressors, a cortisol precursor deficiency (pregnenolone and progesterone), or nutritional deficiencies (low vitamin C and B_5, low-protein diet).

Another type of treatment that helps many people cope with stress is acupuncture. Additional forms of stress management include proper nutrition for metabolic type, adequate sleep, exercise that is not too intense, naps, meditation, increased protein in the diet, natural hormones, adrenal extracts, natural food-based supplements, zinc and selenium, and herbs such as deglycyrrhized licorice. In our clinic we have seen patients with mild to moderate cases of adrenal fatigue improve significantly through dietary changes that enrich nutrition while reducing carbohydrates and stimulants. We also recommend high-quality nutritional supplements, including essential fatty acids from fish oil and dried organs with vitamin B_6, pantothenic acid, and L-tyrosine. These treatments can help all but the most extreme cases of adrenal fatigue improve dramatically within about four months, and mild to moderate cases much faster.

THE BIOCOMPATIBLE VIEW
Adrenal fatigue lowers the immune response, increasing one's susceptibility to illnesses. It also makes it difficult for the body to get rid of toxic heavy metals, so adrenal fatigue must generally be corrected before detoxifying. Conversely, toxic metals can be implicated in adrenal fatigue.

Adrenal fatigue affects an estimated 80 percent of people living in industrialized countries at one time or another in their lives, yet it has been ignored and largely untreated by the medical community.[30] Biocompatible medicine, however, has been able to achieve positive outcomes through early identification and treatment of the responsible toxicities.

WORDS OF ADVICE
• Take control of the negative stressors in your life by getting more exercise, relaxation, and sleep to lower the risk of adrenal fatigue and dysfunction.
• Get acupuncture treatments to cope with physical and emotional stress.
• Check with a clinical nutritionist to make dietary changes that enrich nutrition, reduce carbohydrates and stimulants, and promote adrenal health.

- Take high-quality dietary supplements, including essential fatty acids from fish oil, dried organs with vitamin B_6, pantothenic acid, L-tyrosine, and deglycyrrhized licorice to nourish fatigued adrenals.
- To restore healthy adrenal function, eliminate bacterial imbalances, low-grade intestinal infections, and debris build-up in the intestines through colonic hydrotherapy treatments.

AGING

Mark Twain once said, "Life would be infinitely happier if we could only be born at the age of eighty and gradually approach eighteen." My father, Manuel, often repeated the old adage "Youth is wasted on the young!" Once at our clinic, a husband and wife in their late forties who had gained too many pounds, stopped exercising, began taking lots of medications for countless health problems, and acknowledged that their sex life had deteriorated, remarked, "When age catches up with you, this is what you get!" They reminded me of people standing at the bus stop waiting for an inevitable journey with unfortunate resignation.

At the other extreme, in today's youth-oriented society many people do try to do something about aging, which usually means hiding its detrimental effects on the outside of the body—coloring the hair, using expensive lotions and potions, and having plastic surgery. In fact, the demand for anti-aging products reached $30 billion in 2009.[31] Many such products, however, are associated with unsubstantiated claims about their ability to delay or reverse the aging process. Unfortunately, susceptibility to false promises of this nature can lead to further frustration and disappointment.

The second half of life need not be a steady decline in physical or mental capabilities. While we cannot avoid aging, we can learn to slow the process, age gracefully, and maintain optimal health for as long as possible. What we can realistically strive for is to be disease resistant, mentally sharp, physically fit, and functioning with high self-esteem so that we can interact positively with our environment, delay the onset of age-related disabilities, and focus instead on quality of life issues.

Accelerated aging starts not with the outer effects but on the inside of the body, at the cellular level. Interestingly, hygienists since biblical times have maintained that aging starts in the colon, and colon toxicity is indeed one of the main contributors to acid stress—the hallmark of chronic inflammation and the foundation of degenerative conditions. Researchers now propose that uncontrolled oxidation is a cause of aging at the cellular level (see "Oxidative Stress," p. 160).[32] And one thing that speeds up the oxidation leading to aging, especially in the later part of life, is toxins, making identification and reduction of heavy metals a necessity to ward off degenerative conditions.

In our clinic, age management is focused on regaining and maintaining optimal physical, mental, and emotional health through identifying and removing from the body heavy metals and bio-toxic materials and then replacing essential healing constituents; finding a suitable exercise routine; engaging in counseling for emotional changes; and maintaining a healthy lifestyle. Although following all the aspects of this protocol will boost vitality and can extend one's life span, I am not as concerned about increasing longevity as I am about building disease resistance, preventing premature disability and death, and enhancing the quality of life.

The following measures can slow down the aging process by bolstering health for the long term:

- Identify and remove toxins from the body.
- Drink sufficient water.
- Avoid artificial sweeteners.
- Eat according to metabolic type.
- Replace trans fats with fish oil.
- Take natural antioxidant supplements.
- Learn to make insulin more efficiently (see "Diabetes," p. 97).
- Exercise and get one hour of sunshine each day, preferably in the early morning or late afternoon.
- Improve your sleep habits.

In addition, having an optimistic attitude and taking interest in new experiences also helps slow the aging process. For example, my wife, Phyllis, who works hard at maintaining a healthy lifestyle, celebrated her fiftieth birthday by skydiving. Endless new adventures are possible for people, depending on mobility, health, and positive attitude.

THE BIOCOMPATIBLE VIEW
While many people believe that aging is an inevitable part of life over which they have no control, biocompatible medicine asserts that positive outcomes can be gained through self-investigation and self-education. It is possible to learn that accelerated aging, for instance, is the result of chronic inflammation, whose root cause is usually multifaceted and can include any of the following factors: eating the wrong foods for metabolic type, infections in the body, a body burden of heavy metals, the presence of insecticides and pesticides in the body, or the detrimental effects of petroleum products.

WORDS OF ADVICE
- Exercise five times a week, no matter how old you are.
- Check with a certified nutritionist to be sure you are getting the right antioxidant foods and supplements for your body.
- Utilize the results of hair tests, thermograms, advanced blood tests, bone density tests, and hormone tests to make the most of your physiological age.

ANEMIA
Anemia, one of the more common blood disorders, occurs when the number of healthy red blood cells in the body decreases. Typical signs of anemia are paleness of the skin, the lips, the lining of the eyelids, and the nail beds; irritability;

fatigue; dizziness; and rapid heartbeat. Depending on the condition causing the anemia, other symptoms may also occur, such as jaundice (yellow-tinged skin), dark tea-colored urine, easy bruising or bleeding, and enlargement of the spleen or liver. The causes of anemia range from nutritional deficiencies, some of which are hereditary, to environmental poisons. The only way to be sure of a proper diagnosis and type analysis is to evaluate your complete red blood cell count. When your red blood cell size is smaller than normal (microcytic), it indicates a deficiency of B-complex vitamins and folic acid, which is a B vitamin. A larger than normal red blood cell size (macrocytic) signifies exposure to environmental poisons, which can be treated with selenium, vitamin E, and glutathione supplements.

Another potential nutritional contributor to anemia is milk. Dr. Benjamin Spock, a world-renowned leading authority on childcare, advocated against giving cow's milk to children, saying it could cause anemia, allergies, and diabetes, leading ultimately to obesity and heart disease—the number one cause of death in the United States.[33]

Unfortunately, some doctors who diagnose anemia prescribe the wrong treatment. When blood tests determine anemia is due to low hemoglobin, many physicians prescribe iron supplementation, failing to appreciate that blood has a narrow range of iron it can use to help produce red blood cells and that too much iron causes symptoms resembling those of anemia. Also, the staff at blood banks tend to believe that hemoglobin and iron are the same, giving lists of foods high in iron to donors with low hemoglobin, invariably saying, "Your iron is low." Hemoglobin, however, is not iron but rather the unique molecule in red blood cells that carries oxygen to the body's tissues. When patients are anemic, iron, instead of going into hemoglobin, can be stored, causing iron overload. Many people of African descent have a tendency toward iron overload and need iron removed, as well as treatment with B vitamins, especially B_{12}, B_6, and folic acid.[34] The B vitamins should be taken as part of a complete B complex, with specific B vitamins added on an individual basis by a trained clinical nutritionist.

Certain inherited tendencies can contribute to anemia. First, many individuals with type A blood have a deficiency in stomach acid that prevents them from absorbing the iron from their food, leading to anemia. Second, many descendants from Mediterranean countries, including numerous Arubans and Americans who can trace their family tree to Portuguese, Spanish, Italian, or Greek roots, have inherited glucose-6-phosphate dehydrogenase (G6PD) deficiency, a condition in which either the red blood cells do not make enough of the enzyme G6PD or the enzyme they produce is abnormal and inefficient, causing the body's red blood cells to undergo extra stress or premature destruction. Red blood cells suffer stress, for instance, when such people have an infection and take sulfa medicine, are exposed to camphor, or eat fava beans, a staple in several Mediterranean locations.

In effect, G6PD provides the "glue," or structural integrity, of the skin of red blood cells, and with G6PD deficiency—the most common human enzyme deficiency, affecting an estimated 400 million people worldwide—the skin of red blood cells becomes very fragile, allowing them to fall apart prematurely. And while the life cycle of a normal red blood cell is four months, people who suffer from G6PD deficiency must recycle their red blood cells more often. Interestingly, G6PD deficiency confers a resistance to malaria, but G6PD crises result in anemia, also known as G6PD anemia or hemolytic anemia.

Although G6PD deficiency was discovered in 1956, it still often goes either undetected or improperly treated. And individuals with reduced G6PD activity who receive improper treatment are at risk for several potentially life-threatening pathologies. Sulfa drugs can contribute to an immediate anemia crisis. Other drugs also cause problems. Similarly, iron supplementation, far from helpful, stresses the red blood cells even more. Fortunately a simple blood test can let a person know if they have this deficiency.

A Venezuelan proverb states, "Blood is inherited, and virtue is acquired." Viewed in this context, although individuals with type A blood and people who have inherited iron overload or G6PD deficiency cannot alter their blood, they can acquire the virtue of health.

THE BIOCOMPATIBLE VIEW

Contrary to the practices of many conventional doctors, biocompatible physicians recognize that blood has a narrow range of iron it uses to help produce red blood cells. A lack of iron can cause anemia, but too much iron is problematic as well, causing a condition that resembles anemia. Biocompatible physicians also point out that a low hemoglobin count does not indicate a need for more iron-rich foods, since hemoglobin is not iron but rather transports oxygen to the body's tissues.

WORDS OF ADVICE

- If you are of African descent and have symptoms of anemia, you may need to have iron removed rather than supplemented, and to be treated with B vitamins, especially B_{12}, B_6, and folic acid.
- If you are of Mediterranean descent and seem to be anemic, get screened for G6PD deficiency.
- If you have type A blood, be aware that you have a deficiency in stomach acid that prevents absorption of iron from food, and request advice from a biocompatible doctor about how to get sufficient iron.
- Children should avoid drinking cow's milk, which has been implicated in anemia as well as allergies and diabetes.
- If you have been diagnosed with anemia, do not settle for iron supplements. Have a biocompatible physician find and treat the root cause of your anemia.

ANTIBIOTICS

Doctors frequently prescribe antibiotics, which, while at times lifesaving, are more often unnecessary and harmful. It is important to understand that the term "antibiotic" means "against life" and that antibiotics kill not only the bad but also the good bacteria, without which people cannot live. The World Health Organization (WHO) has repeatedly warned against the misuse of antibiotics, saying that by 2010 it could lead to the creation of "superbugs" that render ineffective the antibiotics currently being used and take the world "back to the time when minor infections killed."[35]

It is also essential to remember that although antibiotics affect bacteria they do not influence viruses. Bacteria, relatively large organisms, tend to reproduce outside of cells and have metabolic functions that antibiotics can target, either killing microorganisms or stopping them from reproducing, allowing the body's natural defenses to eliminate them. Viruses, on the other hand, are tiny and replicate inside cells using the cells' own metabolic functions, where antibiotics cannot reach them.[36] Therefore, the use of antibiotics in a nonbacterial illness does not shorten its duration, as is sometimes hoped, but instead contributes to the destruction of susceptible bacteria and an explosion of resistant bacteria, furthering the spread of drug-resistant bacteria.

Antibiotics used erroneously are most commonly prescribed for fever, sore throat, or diarrhea caused by viruses. Indiscriminate use of antibiotics for fever adds to the cost of therapy, increases adverse effects, contributes to drug resistance, and may also mask the signs of bacterial infection, making a proper diagnosis difficult. Instead, the majority of fevers can be brought under control with colonics or enemas. A survey of physicians in seventeen European countries shows fever from tonsillitis resolving itself in two to three days with or without antibiotic treatment.[37]

The antibiotics often prescribed for a sore throat of unknown origin are generally "broad spectrum" meaning that they affect many different bacteria. By contrast, in our clinic we send patients with persistent sore throats to a lab that will culture the pathogen; indicate if it is serious, such as group A streptococci; and if so, name the antibiotic that will eliminate it. As it turns out, only about 10 to 20 percent of people who visit our clinic with a sore throat have group A streptococci. Research shows that strep throat is almost unknown in children before age two and uncommon before age four; such a sore throat is most common in children between the ages of five and fifteen, although it can occur in younger children and also adults; and while children younger than three can get strep infections, these usually don't affect the throat.[38]

Antibiotics overprescribed for diarrhea is equally unjustifiable, since reversing the condition usually requires only adequate rehydration and replacement of beneficial colon bacteria. In our clinic, we use colon hydrotherapy to wash away the infection then recommend that the patient take a simple over-the-counter beneficial bacteria supplement. The following are two examples of supplements that can be used. In the case of urinary bladder infections, a simple sugar (D-Manos) naturally found in unsweetened cranberry juice will coat the bacteria so it cannot "stick" to the bladder walls and cause problems. To eliminate a serious stomach bacterium, *Helicobacter pylori* (HP), that causes stomach ulcers and cancers, in our clinic we have successfully used kelp seaweed called bladderwrack, which contains a simple sugar (D-fucose) that HP bacteria love to eat. The bacteria will leave the walls of the stomach and embed in the bladderwrack herb to feed on the D-fucose, then when the bladderwrack leaves the stomach it carries the HP bacteria with it.

In addition, antibiotics are generally prescribed for all ear infections, regardless of appropriateness. Finally, antibiotics have absolutely no effect on colds, which are caused by viruses. During a cold, it is normal for mucus to thicken and change color, a symptom that does not indicate the presence of a bacterial infection. Nor do most children with thick or green mucus have a bacterial sinus infection; such mucus production may instead be caused by milk or cheese. In fact, at least three-quarters of the infections most pediatricians see in their offices are viral, requiring only that the child get adequate fluids and eat healthy foods.[39]

It is important to acquire the information and self-confidence necessary to decline inappropriate antibiotic treatment. Such therapy should be reserved only for medical emergencies when it has been determined that the cause of symptoms is bacterial. This can often be determined by tests, which you should request to verify the need for antibiotics. For example, a bacterial illness such as strep throat can be diagnosed by taking a throat culture to see if strep bacteria are present. Also, any pathological condition associated with bacterial infection, inflammation, or tissue destruction is accompanied by elevation of the C-reactive protein (CRP) level in the person's serum, which can be detected within six to twelve hours of the onset of the inflammatory process.

In cases where antibiotics are indicated, the entire course of medication must be taken, even if the individual begins to feel better sooner, because just as overuse of antibiotics leads to resistant bacteria, so does using only a partial dose. Any antibiotic treatment should be supplemented with beneficial bacteria (normally found in the colon), also known as probiotics, acidophilus, or bifadolphilus, which are available at health food stores.

THE BIOCOMPATIBLE VIEW

Contrary to popular belief, antibiotics do not eliminate a pathogen completely but instead reduce its numbers, often considerably. As a result, one of three outcomes may ensue. If the antibiotic has sufficiently reduced the numbers of bacteria, the person's immune system will finally cure the infection by killing off the remaining bacteria before they multiply. If not, the bacterial infection returns and another round of antibiotics is needed. The third scenario takes place when the remaining bacteria colonize and become held in equilibrium by the immune system. This equilibrium produces a subclinical chronic inflammation that exerts unremitting stress on the immune system. The blood chemistry protocols of biocompatible medicine clinically demonstrate the presence of such chronic inflammation, which is most often found in infections in the jaws.

WORDS OF ADVICE

- Never take antibiotics haphazardly or without a doctor's supervision.
- Develop self-confidence to question a prescription of antibiotics for fever, sore throat, or diarrhea, which are usually caused by viral not bacterial infections.
- Ask your doctor to verify the presence of a bacterial infection via a laboratory-run low-sensitivity C-reactive protein (CRP) test or other tests before prescribing antibiotics.

- If you are diagnosed with a urinary bladder infection, drink cranberry juice to coat the bacteria that caused it, preventing them from multiplying, or take D-mannose, the sugar found in cranberries that repels infecting bacteria.
- To eliminate the stomach bacterium *Helicobacter pylori* that causes stomach ulcers and cancers, take bladderwrack, a seaweed containing the simple sugar D-fucose that attracts and eradicates the HP.
- If you are on antibiotic treatment, avoid alcoholic beverages and supplement with probiotic lactobacillus to replace the friendly bacteria in the intestines.
- A susceptibility to suffering from repeated infections is a symptom of oxidative stress and should be regarded as a warning that there exists a major metabolic imbalance.

ANXIETY OR PANIC ATTACKS

Anxiety disorders, characterized by excessive, irrational dread of everyday situations, are the most common form of mental illness. Anxiety or panic attacks, on the other hand, are intense periods of fear and discomfort caused by the body's energy going too much in one direction. During such an attack, a person may experience a pounding heartbeat, pain or other discomfort in the chest, sweating, shaking, difficulty breathing, dizziness, tingling sensations, cold or hot flashes, a choking sensation that produces nausea, as well as fear of losing control, going crazy, or dying—all symptoms that can be produced by an underactive thyroid.

Many people experience an anxiety or panic attack at some time in their lives, and while it may be disconcerting it doesn't result in an anxiety disorder. To be classified as a medical problem, the attack has to be followed within a month by one or both of the following: major behavioral change related to the attack, or constant worry about having another attack, or a heart attack.

One cause of panic attacks in women is hormone imbalance due to the menstrual cycle, which explains why attacks are twice as common in women as in men. In our clinic, we see women who suffer from these symptoms during the week before and a few days into their menstrual cycle, or while transitioning into menopause.

Men more often suffer from anxiety attacks attributed to different causes. Many men have high uric acid that makes joints painful and reduces the blood's ability to carry oxygen, forcing them to hyperventilate and possibly have an anxiety attack.

Symptoms of an anxiety or panic attack can also be triggered by the person's immediate surroundings. For example, many schoolchildren in our community have symptoms of anxiety during school exams, including stomachache, nausea, sleep problems, and headaches. Chronic stomach problems in older children are usually associated with homes where a parent is abusing alcohol or drugs. Likewise, symptoms of an anxiety or panic attack can affect one's surroundings, such as a workplace, where colleagues and clients may be influenced by an individual's inability to focus on tasks or by their fear of failure, flying, entering an elevator, or public speaking.

To control the symptoms, frequency, and severity of anxiety or panic attacks, doctors usually prescribe pharmaceutical drugs, especially antidepressants or antianxiety medication. This protocol becomes counterproductive, however, since, especially at the beginning of treatment or when doses are changed, individuals on such drugs can develop an increase in anxiety, panic attacks, irritability, insomnia, impulsivity, hostility, and mania. As stressed by the Food and Drug Administration (FDA), it is especially important to watch for these behaviors in children, who may be less able to control their impulsivity than adults and therefore at greater risk for suicide.[40]

If you are suffering from anxiety or panic attacks, first visit your doctor for a checkup to rule out physical causes. Hopefully your doctor does not treat all anxiety and panic attacks with psychotropic drugs used for psychiatric disorders. In our clinic, for example, we do not start with the supposition that individuals having anxiety disorders are crazy. Having an acidic body produces sluggishness because of the markedly lowered ability to circulate oxygen throughout the body. The less than optimal oxygen circulation then produces the same symptoms as those experienced by people who travel to higher elevations, including hyperventilation, shortness of breath during exertion, increased urination, change of breathing pattern at night, frequent waking at night, and weird dreams. Biocompatible medicine doctors therefore treat anxiety or panic attacks by reducing acid stress, making more oxygen available throughout the body.

In our clinic, we use acupuncture treatments effectively to treat anxiety disorders and reintroduce balanced states. Whereas excessive caffeine, medication, a thyroid disorder, or low blood sugar is known to cause shakiness and sweating, eliminating stimulants, increasing your physical exercise, or using relaxation techniques such as listening to music, praying, or meditating can be immediately beneficial.

THE BIOCOMPATIBLE VIEW
Biocompatible medicine treats anxiety or panic attacks by reducing acid stress, making more oxygen available throughout the body.

WORDS OF ADVICE
- If you are suffering from anxiety or panic attacks, first visit your doctor for a checkup to rule out physical causes.
- Eliminate caffeine and other stimulants, and increase exercise to reduce symptoms of anxiety.
- Take time out from hectic schedules and daily concerns to participate in relaxing and rejuvenating activities, such as playing sports, swimming, listening to music, reading, praying, or meditating.
- Learn how to breathe from your abdomen. Many people do not breathe this deeply and thus do not exchange lung gasses efficiently, leading to a buildup of carbon dioxide that causes them to gasp for breath, a symptom associated with anxiety. An introductory yoga lesson can show you how to breathe properly.

• Avoid situations that have caused panic in the past or that you fear might cause panic, such as going to crowded places.
• If panic sets in, escape as soon as you can, even if this means rushing through the supermarket aisles to get out as quickly as possible.

ARTERIOSCLEROSIS

Arteriosclerosis is obstructed blood flow caused by the formation of plaques on the inner surfaces of arteries. This condition often begins with chronic inflammation of the body (see "Chronic Inflammation," p. 83), which increases the calcium floating in the bloodstream, damaging arterial walls. Then, like the building of calluses on a palm, the body deposits calcium, cholesterol, heavy metals, and bound insulin on the irritated arterial walls.

When such vascular transformations occur, the veins and arteries are not fully able to circulate blood to all parts of the body. Cells that normally get a proper supply of glucose, oxygen, and other nutrients have the raw material necessary to make adenosine triphosphate (ATP), the "gasoline" that keeps the human body functioning. Cells, like batteries that need to be recharged, give off heat and other forms of energy, then must receive ATP to provide more energy. However, when veins and arteries are blocked and unable to circulate a steady supply of blood, your cells, unable to receive adequate ATP, start dying and becoming stiff.

Blockage preventing adequate blood flow through the arms and legs is called peripheral arterial disease (PAD), which may at first present no obvious symptoms but, over time, produces a cramping pain, usually in the calves, that is induced by exercise and relieved by rest. Blood circulation problems of the arms are less common than of the legs but may be more incapacitating, resulting in pain, weakness, stiffness, nerve-related symptoms, and general difficulty using the hands. Blood circulation problems to the brain, common among older populations of developed countries, typically affect the carotid artery, which carries most of the brain's blood supply. Blocked arteries of the heart, coronary artery disease (CAD), and other blood circulation problems are present with PAD, increasing the risk of infection. People suffering from PAD are also at increased risk of dying from a heart attack or stroke.

Severe obstruction of the arteries, which decreases blood flow to the extremities (hands, feet, and legs) to the point of severe pain and even nonhealing skin ulcers, is called critical limb ischemia (CLI). The pain caused by CLI, known to wake the sufferer up at night, is called "rest pain." It can be relieved temporarily by getting up and walking around. CLI is a very serious condition that requires comprehensive treatment since it will not improve on its own.

For instance, darkening legs, which indicates blood circulation problems, is an ominous sign that heart bypass surgery may be required to replace plugged heart arteries. People who have had heart bypass surgery, however, must also realize that arteries do not selectively get plugged, and a heart starved for circulating blood reflects other body parts that are similarly in need of fresh oxygenated blood.

Unfortunately, the pharmaceutical drugs prescribed for arteriosclerosis, such as statins, antiplatelet drugs, and aspirin, have an alarming array of side effects, including fatigue, nausea, gastrointestinal problems, and muscle weakness and pain—surely one reason up to 75 percent of people who take statins eventually discontinue their use.[41] Also, antiplatelet drugs inhibit vitamin K-dependent blood coagulation, an outcome that may be counteracted by eating foods rich in vitamin K, such as green leafy vegetables, alfalfa, egg yolks, soybean oil, and fish livers.

By contrast, biocompatible physicians use natural substances to increase the blood flow to veins. They also recommend controlling risk factors such as cigarette smoking; treating cholesterol problems, high blood pressure, and diabetes; sticking to special diets; exercising; and employing natural remedies and therapies. Specifically, ginkgo biloba extract has the ability to reduce major symptoms of cerebral vascular insufficiency. The plant *Coleus forskohlii*, a member of the mint family, is the source of the compound forskolin, which has been shown to widen or dilate blood vessels to allow more blood flow. Also, horse chestnut, a longtime folk remedy for varicose veins and hemorrhoids, relieves common symptoms of chronic vascular insufficiency, such as pain and swelling of the legs and itching and cramping of calf muscles, while horsetail assists in the reduction of water swelling, the edema commonly associated with chronic vascular insufficiency. In addition, foot ulcers, commonly caused by diabetes or vascular insufficiency, can be cleansed at home or in the sea and healed by regained healthy blood flow.

Our clinic protocol for arteriosclerosis also focuses on adequate hydration and sodium elimination (see "Dehydration," p. 93). Most people are extremely dehydrated, especially older individuals who either have problems with bladder control (in women from urinary incontinence, in men from having to wait a long time or straining to begin urination) or get nauseous after drinking water. With little digestive fluid in the stomach, even a small amount of water will further dilute the stomach acid and produce heartburn and nausea, a problem that can be alleviated by adding the juice of half a lime (approximately 5 ml) to 1.5 liters, or quarts, of water. When older people drink water and have to urinate almost immediately, they believe they are ridding the body of the water they just drank, but this is not true. Rather, when a person who is dehydrated drinks ten ounces of water, the body signals the kidneys to expel ten ounces of salty, excess fluid from between tissue cells, which is transparent, like water. By contrast, people with a well-hydrated body can drink a liter of water and not have to urinate for over an hour.

Dehydration leads to edema from excess serous fluid, a body fluid resembling serum that is loaded with sodium waste from the cells. The salty fluid, lodged between tissue cells, swells the body, especially the lower legs, obstructing the flow of blood by literally squeezing the blood vessels closed. The problem with salty water is that the kidneys are programmed, especially in people of African descent, not to remove sodium from the blood. Unfortunately, patients suffering from edema often are given diuretics ("water pills") that stimulate the kidneys to expel water and potassium but not the sodium, which makes the problem worse, since the amount of sodium in the body increases and traps even more water in the body.

By contrast, in our clinic we take all patients suffering from edema off diuretics and send them to the ocean to perform a therapy I developed during the years I was teaching scuba diving, which we call head out immersion (HOI). The patient drinks at least one liter, or quart, of water and soaks in the ocean, immersing the body up to the neck for forty minutes to one hour. People not near the ocean can soak in a shallow pool or bathtub. The difference in the water pressure against the adrenal glands, located on top of the kidneys, and the subsequent lack of pressure on the sinuses, signals the kidneys to dump sodium. After HOI patients urinate in the water, they notice an immediate difference in their once-swollen limbs, which can be verified by measuring them with a tailor's cloth tape before and after immersion. Indeed, the amount of sodium excreted from immersion can amount to between 200 and 300 percent of preimmersion levels.[42] The reduction in blood serum sodium can make some patients become very tired afterward, so when performing HOI therapy we make sure to have an assistant present.

To further remove sodium from the body, we also recommend taking supplements such as vitamin B_2, vitamin A, and magnesium (see "Energy Refinery—Magnesium," p. 108), since magnesium deficiency can lead to increased sodium and fluid retention. With magnesium present, potassium is taken into the cells, where it is needed for the energy producing Krebs cycle, and sodium is pumped out.

In addition, we use hair analysis to test individuals with arteriosclerosis for heavy metals. Once we have identified the contributing metals and renovated the mouth to remove toxic mercury fillings, we recommend using EDTA (ethylenediaminetetraacetic acid) to detoxify the body (see "EDTA Chelation Therapy," p. 103). Finally, we recommend acupuncture as an important part of arteriosclerosis treatment since it stimulates movement in the meridians.

THE BIOCOMPATIBLE VIEW

Arteriosclerosis starts with an increase in the chronic inflammation of the body caused by eating the wrong foods for metabolic type (see "Blood Type Diet," p. 65); infections in the body; a body burden of heavy metals; the presence of insecticides and pesticides in the body; and the detrimental effects of petroleum products.

WORDS OF ADVICE

• Use the natural substances gingko biloba, *Coleus forskohlii*, horse chestnut, and horsetail to increase the flow of blood in veins and arteries.
• Drink sufficient water to avoid problems with blood flow associated with dehydration.
• Avoid using diuretics ("water pills") that stimulate the kidneys to expel water and potassium but not sodium, making arteriosclerosis worse.
• To eliminate sodium from the body, use head out immersion (HOI) treatment at the ocean or in a bathtub.
• Take the supplements vitamin B_2 and vitamin A—all the natural carotenoids, not just carotene—to help remove sodium from the body.
• Take supplements of magnesium to avoid deficiency, which can lead to increased sodium and fluid retention.
• See a biocompatible physician to have EDTA chelation therapy to detoxify heavy metals from your body and have mercury fillings removed from your mouth.

ARTHRITIS

Arthritis is a constellation of different forms of chronic joint inflammation resulting in pain and stiffness, whose origin, according to conventional medicine, is not officially known. It is the number-one cause of physical disability in the United States, affecting 21 percent of adults,[43] including people of both sexes and all races, socioeconomic levels, and geographic areas, although women are those most affected by rheumatoid arthritis, an autoimmune disease in which the body attacks itself, causing inflammation and damage. Typically arthritis is initially treated with salicylates and other nonsteroidal anti-inflammatory drugs (NSAIDS), causing many patients to end up either in wheelchairs or in surgery to remove the excess tissue that develops from progressive joint damage.

Traditional Chinese medicine does not combine under one name the dozens of different medical ailments that cause pain, stiffness, and swelling in the joints, but instead recognizes seven conditions that can produce "steaming joints"; divides them into three categories of increasingly severe joint damage; and identifies patterns of disharmony that produce joint problems. In traditional Chinese medicine, the condition most similar to arthritis, as it is known in the West, is called "Bi syndrome." This category of joint damage presents as pain, soreness, or numbness of the joints due to an "invasion" by wind, cold, dampness, or heat.

Wind Bi, resulting from unprotected exposure to wind over a prolonged period of time, is characterized by the movement of soreness and pain from one joint to another. Range of motion of the affected joints is limited, and there is often fever, as well as an aversion to wind. A thin white tongue coating and a floating pulse are signs that help Chinese medicine practitioners diagnose wind Bi.

Cold Bi is characterized by severe pain in a joint, which is relieved by applying warmth to the area and intensified with exposure to cold. Movement of joints is limited. Signs of cold Bi include a thin white tongue coating, combined with a wiry and tight pulse.

Damp Bi is characterized by pain, soreness, and swelling in a joint with a feeling of heaviness and numbness in the limb or all extremities. The pain, aggravated by damp weather, has a fixed location.

Heat Bi, which can develop from any of the other forms, is characterized by severe pain and hot red, swollen joints, often due to infection, especially in the mouth. The pain is generally relieved by applying cold to the joints. Other symptoms include fever, thirst, anxiety, and an aversion to wind. A yellow, dry tongue coating and slippery, rapid pulse are seen with heat Bi.

The next category of increasingly severe joint damage identified in traditional Chinese medicine comprises internal disorders contributing to mucus or phlegm in the joints. The most severe category is associated with blood stagnation due to a history of trauma.

To understand the causes of arthritis, it is necessary to first comprehend how joints work. Healthy joints have a rubbery material called cartilage that covers the bone and acts as a shock absorber to cushion the impact of movement and keep the ends from grinding against each other. The joint is then held together by ligaments and tendons. Tendons are strong, flexible cables that attach the muscles to the bones and allow movement in various directions. The bone ends, cartilage, ligaments, and tendons are enclosed by the synovial membrane, which lubricates the joint so it can move smoothly.

This membrane includes the synovial lining, or inner layer, and the subintimal area, or lower layer. In normal joints, the synovial lining serves as an important source of nutrients for cartilage, which has no blood vessels. The synovial lining is normally only one to three cells thick, but in rheumatoid arthritis it increases to eight to ten cells thick, eroding the bone and cartilage. As such, it can be thought of as a tumor-like tissue, although metastasis does not occur. Chronic dehydration and consequent nutritional deficiencies rob the synovial lining of the nutrition needed by a healthy joint. And, with the reduced function of the synovial lining, waste products from the metabolism of the joint cannot be carried away, which is why an affected joint becomes bigger.

In addition, the subintimal area, where the synovial blood vessels are located, normally has very few cells, but in people with rheumatoid arthritis it is infiltrated with inflammatory cells, including T- and B-lymphocytes, macrophages, and mast cells, all of which, as "soldiers" of the immune system, respond to a "steaming joint" as if it were a foreign invader. When there is an infection, T- and B-lymphocytes, the two main types of white blood cells, are the first to arrive. Next, macrophages, large scavenger cells common in connective tissue and certain body organs, arrive to engulf and destroy what they perceive as bacteria and other foreign debris. Finally, mast cells, containing numerous basophilic granules, arrive and release substances such as heparin and histamine, their natural reaction to injury or inflammation of bodily tissues. Unfortunately, if this immune response goes on for an extended period of time, the activity starts destroying the connective structure of the joint.

Joint Pain and Dehydration

At our clinic, we have an arthritis protocol that has proven effective in the treatment of joint pain, guided by the Nei Jing, the Yellow Emperor's 4,700-year-old classic treatise of internal medicine, which states: "The meridians move the energy and blood, regulate yin and yang, moisten the tendons and bones, and benefit the joints." As medical theory, this description was well ahead of its time, considering that circulation of the blood was not discovered in the West until thousands of years later. We recognize that painful, stiff joint symptoms occur in connection with mild dehydration since joint cartilage is composed mainly of water (70 to 80 percent). In moderate chronic dehydration, we see most of the symptoms of arthritis, including high cholesterol, high blood pressure, heart problems, diabetes, and water retention, or edema. Yet chronic dehydration is a problem doctors and our Public Health Department normally do not address until it has become life threatening (see "Dehydration," p. 93).

When the body becomes dehydrated, chemicals called pain factors (P-factors) are produced that shift water from muscles and other cells to brain cells. Since the brain is the control center for the body, the body sends whatever water it has to the brain as its first priority. When water is lacking in the muscles, the chemical reactions that govern the muscle contraction-relaxation cycle become less efficient and are thrown out of balance, causing what we perceive as stiffness in the joints that are moved by these muscles, leading to a misalignment in bone structure, such as in the spine, which can be very painful. Chiropractic treatment can resolve the effects of misalignment of bone structure, especially in the spine. But since the primary source of the pain is body dehydration and a lack of water in the muscle cells, to hold bones in their proper place it is necessary to hydrate the body and reestablish balance in the muscle contraction-relaxation cycle.

Albumin and Arthritis

People with rheumatoid arthritis often have decreased levels of albumin, the most abundant protein found in blood plasma, accounting for 55 to 60 percent of serum protein. Sufficient albumin is necessary for healthy functioning in several ways. First, albumin has antioxidant potential, helping to rid the body of oxygen-free radicals, which have been implicated in inflammatory diseases and aging.[44]

Second, healthy amounts of albumin help regulate the acid base balance, preventing the body from becoming too acidic, which would rob calcium from bones and teeth and lead to excessive deposits of uric acid in the soft tissue of joints. Uric acid crystals, which are sharp as razors, demolish soft tissue, produce pain, and accelerate joint destruction.

In addition, albumin is capable of attracting heavy metals. As such, it plays a role in removing toxic heavy metals from the body.

Blood tests showing low values of albumin can signal the potential for serious illness years before any medical condition develops. When blood serum albumin is low, the synovial membrane will not have sufficient protein to transfer into the joint. So as part of our arthritis protocol, we try to determine what is reducing the blood albumin level.

Heavy Metals and Joint Pain

A low level of albumin indicates that heavy metals may be in the body. Certainly, individuals with severe joint problems tend to have a considerable body burden of toxic heavy metals.

Heavy metals enter our bodies through the food we eat, the air we breathe, and the water we drink. They enter the water supply because our water, devoid of minerals, leaches copper from water pipes and lead from solder. In Aruba, because our "soft" water leaches out the copper from our water pipes we have an abnormally high exposure to this metal. Metals such as lead, mercury, arsenic, chromium, cadmium, and nickel are toxic even at low concentrations and cannot be degraded or destroyed. In trace amounts, some heavy metals, such as copper and zinc, are essential to maintaining good health and metabolism, but in higher concentrations they prove to be poisonous. Symptoms associated with excessive exposure to copper are joint and muscle pain, depression, irritability, tremors, hemolytic anemia, learning disabilities, and behavioral disorders.

What makes heavy metals particularly dangerous is their tendency to accumulate, to occur in increased concentrations, over time. They do this naturally because heavy metals absorbed from the environment are stored faster than they are metabolized or excreted from the body, especially when the amount of albumin in the blood is low.

An excess, deficiency, or maldistribution of heavy metals in the body can be determined by hair analysis, since the amount of an element that is incorporated into growing hair is proportional to the level of the element in other body tissues. Although individuals vary greatly in sensitivity to toxic metals in the body, clinical research indicates that hair levels of potentially toxic elements such as mercury, lead, arsenic, and cadmium correlate highly with the presence of pathological disorders. Mercury, for example, contributes to immune problems by binding or sequestering selenium, which is critically important to a well-functioning immune system. Sources of mercury include contaminated seafood, hemorrhoid preparations, skin lightening agents, certain instruments (thermometers, electrodes, batteries), the combustion of fossil fuels, and dental amalgams. Because the baseline hair mercury level for individuals with dental amalgams is higher than those without amalgams, we recommend that physicians trained in biocompatible dentistry remove dental amalgams made of 50 percent mercury.

Regarding teeth, at our clinic we have found that the inflammatory effects from periodontal disease, a chronic bacterial infection of the gums and infections in the jaws, called cavitations, cause oral bacterial by-products to enter the bloodstream and trigger the liver to make proteins that inflame arteries and joints. To identify infection, we use the blood test C-reactive protein (CRP), a substance found in the liver when arteries are inflamed. We are seeing reduced joint pain after treating people's teeth and gums using the biocompatible protocol. In fact, more than three hundred patients went into total remission of their hot, painful joints after receiving our biocompatible protocol.

Joint Problems and Metabolic Type

In our clinic, we have been finding a relationship between people's joint problems and their metabolic type, identified by blood type and Lewis blood group antigens. Generally, we find that people with type A blood tend to get a puffy, inflamed arthritis, a more aggressive form of rheumatoid arthritis, while people with type O usually get a harder, more persistent type of arthritis.

In addition, certain aspects of nutrition specific to blood type can cause joint pain. For example, the sugar of wheat germ lectin is highly specific to blood types A and O in causing joint pain, and adopting a wheat-free diet appears to have a positive effect. The two sugars most commonly used in alternative medicine to treat arthritis, glucosamine and chondroitin, may in fact be effective due to their lectin-blocking action.[45] It is worth noting that glucosamine binds wheat germ lectin very effectively, while chondroitin is the blood type A antigen in very long linkages. In either case, it is likely that both interact with lectins and prevent them from reacting with inflamed tissue. In fact, glucosamine and chondroitin may chemically mimic the effect of a low-lectin diet. The aberrant antibody in rheumatoid arthritis, galactose-free immunoglobulin, has also been shown to have a high degree of reactivity with the lectin found in lentils.[46] A good experimental model of human rheumatoid arthritis can be produced in laboratory rabbits by injecting their joints with the lentil lectin. Considering the effects of nutrition on arthritis, we put all our patients at the clinic on the diet modified for individual blood type. Research has shown that individuals following the type O diet, for instance, experienced significant beneficial changes in their blood test results, including total cholesterol, HDL, and triglycerides.[47]

Some studies also point to a causal connection between emotional stress and rheumatoid arthritis since people who have the disease tend to be more high strung and prone to emotional stress.[48] Considering the effect of stress on the body, high-strung people with type A personalities who have rheumatoid arthritis should incorporate relaxation techniques into their daily routines to reduce the negative effects of stress.

THE BIOCOMPATIBLE VIEW

Arthritis patients present all the factors that make an individual susceptible to chronic inflammation: eating the wrong foods for metabolic type, infections in the body, a body burden of heavy metals, the presence of insecticides and pesticides in the body, and toxicity resulting from exposure to petroleum products.

WORDS OF ADVICE

The following preventive techniques for arthritis, are usually helpful:

- Keep your body hydrated.
- Have your doctor check your blood albumin level, and if it is low (<4mg/dl) consider the following possible causes then act accordingly to raise it: chronic inflammation from any or all of the factors listed above; a lack of dietary protein, which can be reversed by eating more protein; excessive use of simple carbohydrates, which can be reversed by greatly reducing your intake of simple carbohydrates; or a deficiency of protease enzyme activity, which can be reversed through a regular walking program and early morning breathing exercises.
- Check your body pH (see "pH," p. 163) and raise it if it is too acidic.
- Have dental amalgams that are 50 percent mercury removed.
- If you have type A blood, incorporate relaxation techniques into your daily routine.

ASTHMA

Asthma is a disease of the respiratory system, often caused by allergies. The number of adults suffering from asthma has more than doubled in the last several decades.[49] The risk of adult-onset asthma is almost three times higher in obese people.[50]

With regard to childhood asthma, nearly a third of all cases may go undiagnosed.[51] For example, in Aruba, where 90 percent of children in elementary school are obese,[52] many parents and doctors erroneously attribute children's postexercise wheezing or shortness of breath to a general lack of physical fitness, while parents who smoke rarely seek a doctor's advice regarding the negative effects of secondhand smoke on pulmonary inflammation. Childhood respiratory problems, including asthma, also may be linked to inhaling the mixture of chemicals emitted from disposable diapers.[53] Medical research shows as well that children under age three who receive a flu vaccine have a fourfold increase in the incidence of asthma within six weeks following the vaccine.[54] Also, babies delivered by cesarean section appear to be at greater risk for developing childhood asthma than those born via natural childbirth.[55]

According to other studies, the main reason for the increase in asthma is due to allergies to chemicals, foods, or dust and mold in the immediate environment.[56] One chemical cause of asthma is acetaminophen, the active ingredient in Tylenol and other pain medicines, which helps explain why asthma is more prevalent in Western countries than elsewhere.

Consumption of fish contaminated with mercury may also cause asthma. Japanese people who eat fish at least once or twice a week are more likely to have asthma than their peers who consume fish less often, and it is assumed that waterways contaminated with mercury from burning coal for electricity may be a contributing factor. A surprising Japanese study found that schoolchildren who ate the most fish had the highest rates of asthma.[57]

I believe the culprit in such instances is the heavy metal vanadium, which is high in water near offshore oil rigs and refineries. Inhalation of excess vanadium produces respiratory irritation and bronchitis, while ingestion of it can also result in decreased appetite, retarded growth, diarrhea and gastrointestinal disturbances, kidney toxins, and blood problems.

Treatment of asthma generally focuses on prescriptions for inhaled steroid medications or other drugs, the sales of which have increased more than sixfold over the last few decades.[58] Unfortunately, death from asthma has been associated with this increase in the use of inhaled corticosteroids, as has the intensified use of antibiotics, which have themselves been linked to asthma,[59] since they kill off beneficial bacteria in the colon and allow the yeast *Candida albicans* to grow out of control, resulting in a chronic cough. Asthma drugs also double the risk of heart attack, although some researchers now believe that it is not the drugs but the inflammation that increases cardiovascular damage.[60] The use of inhalers has been shown to cause erosion of tooth enamel as well, an effect that can be minimized by brushing the teeth and rinsing the mouth after treatment.

Biocompatible methods for treating asthma rely not on pharmaceuticals but on the elimination or drastic reduction of toxic chemicals used in homes and businesses; elimination or reduction of processed foods; increased intake of antioxidants; elimination of milk from the diet; elimination of tobacco smoke, poisons, and molds from the environment; treatment of yeast infections due to *Candida albicans*; and reduced stress. In particular, using nontoxic, biodegradable products for cleaning and gardening, as well as frequently scouring air-conditioning filters, reduces exposure to toxins. Avoiding processed foods and consuming flavonoid-rich foods such as apples, onions, tea, and red wine, as well as taking antioxidant vitamins and trace elements that act as antioxidants—such as selenium, zinc, and copper—also lowers asthma risk. Eliminating all milk and milk products from the diet further reduces the risk of asthma, especially in children, since when infants younger than four months old consume milk other than breast milk their risk of developing asthma increases dramatically.[61] Moreover, good ventilation and sunlight kill molds and bacteria, even the tough bacteria that cause tuberculosis. Because centralized heating ducts and air-conditioning filters can be breeding grounds for bacteria, mold, and viruses, they should be cleaned regularly. Also, in some situations an ultraviolet light source can be placed into a central air system that will reduce or neutralize pathogens.[62]

In addition, many people suffering from asthma, especially the obese, have *Candida albicans* (see "Yeast," p. 205), which can be treated in adults with at least 250 mg of magnesium a day, probiotics, or beta carotene if the person has never been a smoker.

Finally, we recommend the use of saltwater as a natural antihistamine. In Aruba, we advise patients to wash their sinuses in the ocean. People who are not near the ocean can use 1 tablespoon of sea salt in a quart of water. There are also over the counter (OTC) saline nasal solutions, but check the label for any ingredients that may be harmful.

THE BIOCOMPATIBLE VIEW

Asthma is a disease of the respiratory system often caused by allergic responses to eating the wrong foods for metabolic type; infections in the body; a body burden of heavy metals; the presence of insecticides and pesticides in the body; or the detrimental effects of petroleum products on health.

WORDS OF ADVICE

• Eliminate or drastically reduce the chemicals used in your home or business, and substitute nontoxic, biodegradable products for cleaning and gardening.
• Refrain from eating highly processed foods.
• Stop consuming milk and milk products and wheat products.

B

BACK PAIN

Back pain is the most widespread cause of disability in people under age forty-five.[1] And yet my mother, Nora, who suffered for years from lower back problems related to an automobile accident, at her eightieth birthday party walked effortlessly and honored me with the first of many dances, a testament that lower back pain need not be a life sentence.

Upon hearing a complaint about back pain, physicians usually order an X-ray, maybe via an advanced atomic machine that shows your insides in Technicolor, to supposedly reveal the offending vertebral disc or pinched nerve. In the many years our clinic has provided primary care, every patient who has come to us after seeing a previous doctor for lower back pain has had a diagnosis of a disc problem—either a herniated disc, meaning a rupture in the wall of a disc or between two vertebrae, or "pinched" nerves—and has been prescribed pain medication along with the general advice to "take some time off to relax." Unfortunately, such diagnoses and treatment have limited value since they are based only on an evaluation of structural problems, which does not even include how extensive the pain is or other sources of the pain, such as energy blocks. It is important to track down the source of any lower back problem in which the pain is spontaneous or regularly recurring.

Lower back pain can result from a combination of problems related to different parts of the back: injuries caused by either major trauma or many minor traumas occurring over time, or an energy imbalance, such as a rotated pelvis, a short leg, or an increased or decreased curve in the lower back, signifying areas of heightened tension that are more vulnerable to irritation. When an injury takes place, there is usually a muscle spasm and swelling, indicating inflammation of the discs or nerves. Muscles cause dull aches, while nerves cause sharp pain.

Nearly all lower back problems present with numbness, weakness, stiffness, tightness, or sciatica. *Numbness* can result when nerve impulses are not traveling properly from the skin to the brain, while weakness occurs when signals do not travel properly from the brain to the muscles or from problems in the muscles themselves. I see many patients suffering from type II diabetes with leg numbness or weakness.

Stiffness is seen in patients suffering from an inflammatory condition. Physical and emotional traumas alike seem to tighten and rigidify the muscles and facial tissues of the body, bringing on a loss of vitality, flexibility, and balance.[2] Ongoing stiffness of the body that is not attended to can limit the range not only of physical flexibility but of emotional flexibility as well.

Tightness in the back, neck, arms, or legs is most often due to changes in the muscles. Most neck and back problems are a result of tight, achy muscles brought on by years of bad posture. Additionally, joint stiffness and pain can be a risk factor for degenerative osteoarthritis, a condition occurring more frequently today due to sedentary lifestyles.

The term "sciatica" refers to pain that moves along the sciatic nerve from the lower back into the leg. While this condition can be treated successfully with acupuncture, we also check the health of the prostate in male patients and screen women of childbearing age for urinary tract or vaginal infections. In postmenopausal women, lower back pain, difficulty initiating stool or urination, urinary incontinence, and pelvic pain or pressure usually come from a weakening of the supporting structures of the vagina and uterus. During the childbearing years, the female hormones continuously stimulate the sex organs, but later in life without a replacement form of stimulation (Kegel exercises, continued sex, or masturbation), the muscles and ligaments weaken and are no longer able to hold the organs in place.

When there is no structural problem, a biocompatible physician looks for the cause of back pain in blocked energy or another physical condition not necessarily linked to the back. In our clinic we consider a map of the body to determine the origin of back pain and pinpoint where the energy is blocked, since every spinal vertebra and its discs are associated with different parts of the body. For back pain caused by energy blocks, acupuncture is an efficacious treatment. It facilitates the unblocking of energy responsible for the pain and many times helps in releasing corresponding emotional traumas and correcting underlying medical problems.

We also look for links between the back pain and causes that might not be immediately apparent. For example, if a patient comes in complaining of a stiff neck, we ask about the person's digestion and arrange for a blood test to check for *Helicobacter pylori*, a stomach bacterium, because stiff necks are often the result of stomach problems. If the patient's blood type is A and she frequently suffers from a stiff neck, deficient stomach acid is likely causing the problem, and to relieve the pain she needs more than a physical therapist; she needs a certified clinical nutritionist who uses blood tests to develop dietary recommendations. For example, protein is very effective in reducing joint inflammation. Consequently, at the clinic we recommend an increase in the type of protein that is beneficial for the patient's metabolic type (see "Blood Type Diet," p. 63).

And while surgeons often recommend back operations for L4/L5 back pain even though the outcome is less than satisfactory, biocompatible physicians focus more on the fact that the hypogastric plexus nerve exiting the spine at vertebrae L4/L5 commands the colon, bladder, rectum, and genital organs, and test them for possible problems. When back pain is found to be related to constipation, colon hydrotherapy proves to be highly effective in ameliorating the situation. In fact, I have never treated person with lower back pain, especially one with a supposedly herniated disc at L4/L5, who did not also suffer from constipation (see "Colon Hydrotherapy," p. 85).

In addition, biocompatible physicians take into account the mental and emotional bodies. Since according to traditional Chinese medicine, the organs controlled by the hypogastric plexus nerve are associated with elimination, if there are problems in vertebrae L4/L5 we look at the emotional aspects of elimination—namely, the letting go of past emotional traumas. Because in the energetic body emotional pain equals physical pain, holding on to emotional pain can produce an energetic block that causes pain at L4/L5. To find relief from lower back pain of an emotional nature, the patient does not need to completely resolve the issue, but the trauma does have to be acknowledged.

Drinking sufficient water (see "Dehydration," p. 93) is critical to treatment of back pain, since discs and other cartilaginous tissue in the back are composed of over 90 percent water. When dehydrated, the body first robs the lubricating fluid from joints and restricts the water available to cartilage. Along with adequate water intake, we recommend supplements such as glucosamine, MSM, magnesium, and zinc.

Finally, since weak stomach muscles contribute to lower back pain, our clinic protocol includes stress reduction and an appropriate exercise program that focuses on strengthening the abdominal muscles.

THE BIOCOMPATIBLE VIEW
Most physicians evaluate back pain by attempting to identify structural problems, while biocompatible physicians look for metabolic and emotional imbalances that are targeting areas of the back. For example, people with type A blood who eat the wrong foods for their metabolic type tend to have neck pain, as do people with emotional problems due to issues emerging from their subconscious. We also consider the connections between back pain and other medical problems. For instance, most individuals who have lower back pain also suffer from constipation. And because the lower back L5/S1 and below has holes where the nerve from the sex organs connects with the sciatic nerve, we check the prostate of men and order a PAP test for women to check for dysfunction in the sex organs.

WORDS OF ADVICE
• Get medical attention if you have any of the following symptoms: pain worsening when you cough or sneeze, pain or numbness traveling down one or both legs, pain awakening you from sleep, or difficulty maintaining control of urination or bowel movements.
• To ease back pain, drink plenty of water; dehydration robs lubricating fluid from the joints.
• Before electing surgery for back pain, look for alternative treatments like colon hydrotherapy and acupuncture that can effectively treat underlying conditions.

BIOCOMPATIBLE DENTISTRY
Imagine how strange it would be to consult with a medical physician who would examine, diagnose, and care for your whole body except for your right foot. Unfortunately, this is too often the scenario in modern medicine, except the body part being ignored is the mouth. Yet each tooth is connected to an organ, endocrine glands,

bones, muscles, and even energy production (see "Energy Refinery," p. 106). Moreover, gum disease has been overshadowed as a risk factor in heart disease and other health problems by more commonly acknowledged factors such as smoking, cholesterol, lack of exercise, and obesity. In Aruba, there is a folk saying, "Because of its mouth the fish dies!" meaning that if a fish would be a little more careful of what it puts in its mouth, it might live longer—and the same can be said of people.

The fact that the mouth is closely connected with other parts of the body and thus can affect general health is clear upon considering its structure. Much like a hammock hung between two trees, each tooth is suspended in the bone by periodontal ligaments, part of a periodontal complex of structures that support teeth, including cementum, alveolar bone, and the gingiva, or gums. Warm, dark, salty, wet mouths provide a rich environment for bacteria, which reside in the crevices between gums and teeth. The type and amount of bacteria in the mouth are the foundation of many health problems.

Connections between periodontal disease and other chronic diseases were addressed at a biocompatible dental seminar hosted on April 5 and 6, 2002, by the International Academy of Oral Medicine and Toxicology (IAOMT).[3] As an early member of IAOMT, my protocol includes the safe removal of amalgam fillings that this organization supports. In a lecture, "Sam" Queen, of the Institute for Health Realities, focused on how periodontal, or gum, disease is an early indication that health is deteriorating long before problems in standard medical tests show up, stating, "The mouth, then, is an excellent noninvasive window for viewing what is likely going on elsewhere in the body (even though the normally utilized disease indicators may not yet have manifested themselves)." In fact, having periodontal disease before age fifty is the biggest predictor that a person will die young.[4]

Queen also listed six common denominators of every chronic disease, remarking that all six are present in periodontal disease, as he has outlined in his training video for dentists entitled *A Mouthful of Evidence*.[5] In his experience, periodontal disease grows progressively worse as the body experiences the following six processes:

- Lack of physical exercise and eating the wrong foods for your metabolic type make the body more acidic as less oxygen is delivered to the cells.
- The body then develops anaerobic metabolism as an alternate way to produce energy, which requires less oxygen but produces many free radicals, speeding the aging process.
- Trying to balance the excess acid, the body pulls calcium out of the bones, causing too much free calcium to circulate in the blood.
- This calcium produces chronic inflammation, as a result of which the body constantly has to fight infection.
- The "glue," or connective tissue, that holds the body and teeth together starts to break down.
- The body loses the ability to neutralize free radicals, accelerating aging and allowing cancer a foothold.

The biocompatible protocol strives to offset these six processes, initially by controlling the body's acid-base balance (see "pH," p. 163), ensuring that the metabolism uses oxygen and recommending supplements to control the oxidant/antioxidant balance.

Periodontal disease, called gingivitis, develops when bacteria cause inflammation in the gums; untreated, it can lead to periodontitis, which occurs once the infection has begun "eating" the jawbone. Unfortunately, periodontal disease frequently is not detected in routine dental examinations and often is not associated with pain that would concern a person, especially in its early phases. Nevertheless, the following symptoms can be an indication of periodontal infection:

• Oral discomfort or abnormal coloring of the gums.
• Bleeding of ulcers or wounds in gum pockets from activities such as flossing, brushing, irrigating, rinsing, or chewing.
• Red, swollen, or tender gums.
• Abscesses, or swellings, on the gum surface that can either appear suddenly or grow gradually, and feel hot and painful. (If the area is irrigated with an antimicrobial solution and the discomfort goes away, the source of the pain is most likely periodontal infection. If the discomfort is a throbbing pain relieved by cold, however, the infection has probably moved into the nerve and the tooth needs immediate attention.)
• Gums that pull away from the teeth.
• Loose teeth or a change in the way teeth or partial dentures fit together when you bite.
• Persistent bad breath, usually caused by bacterial waste products known as hydrogen sulfide compounds, which can be identified by flossing and then smelling the floss to check for an odor like rotten eggs or spoiled food.

One of the best ways for a dentist to assess your periodontal health is to look at a sample of your tooth plaque under a microscope to determine the number of white blood cells or the type and number of bacteria.

Although gum disease has been overshadowed as a risk factor in heart disease, recent studies report a link between the severity of gum disease, measured by the amount of jawbone loss, and risk of heart disease and hardening of the arteries.[6] Apparently, bacteria from dental plaque enter the circulation and lodge in blood vessels, where they help produce arteriosclerotic plaque (fatty deposits). Other studies link periodontal disease to the inability to control blood sugar in diabetes,[7] low birth weight in premature babies,[8] pneumonia,[9] and especially arteriolosclerosis.[10]

Gum disease can also cause the loosening of dental implants, artificial tooth roots inserted in the jaw to hold replacement teeth. Because dental implants preserve teeth better than traditional bridgework, since they do not rely on neighboring teeth for support, they are still an ideal option for people in good general oral health who have lost a tooth to injury.

Fluoride

Recent data from the Environmental Protection Agency (EPA) indicate that fluoride is the sixth most emitted hazardous air pollutant in the United States, with total air emissions at about 155,000 tons and emissions into lakes, rivers, and oceans estimated to be as high as 500,000 tons a year.[11] In the United States, air is contaminated by fluoride from the production of iron, steel, aluminum, copper, lead, and zinc; phosphates, essential to the manufacture of agricultural fertilizers; plastics; gasoline; brick, cement, glass, ceramics, and the many other products made from clay; electrical power generation and all other coal combustion; and uranium processing. Water is filled with hazardous pollution from the fluoride trapped in the scrubbers of the producers and processors of glass, pesticides, fertilizers, chemicals, steel, aluminum, and other metals.

For the last fifty years in the United States, industries, the media, and the government have manipulated facts and opinions about fluoride to make the public believe that it is not only safe but beneficial, and that it reduces cavities, especially in children. As a result, manufacturers add fluoride to toothpaste and municipalities put it in the public's drinking water. But fluoridated toothpastes and dental products or ingestion of fluoridated water, either directly or by drinking juices reconstructed with fluoridated water or eating processed foods, dramatically increases the level of lead in children's blood since fluosilicic acid leaches lead from plumbing.[12] This outcome was graphically demonstrated when two cities temporarily stopped fluoridating their water systems—Tacoma, Washington, in 1992, where the lead level dropped from 32 ppb (parts per billion) to 17 ppb (compared to the EPA's maximum contaminant level of 15 ppb), and Thurmont, Maryland, in 1994, where the lead level dropped from 30 ppb to 7 ppb.[13] In both instances, fluoride was held responsible for the initial high lead level.

Ingestion of fluoride has other negative consequences as well. It causes a condition marked by mottling, yellow spots on the teeth. It also accumulates in the bones, making them brittle and more likely to fracture, and in the pineal gland, where it inhibits the production of melatonin, which helps regulate the onset of puberty, and confuses the immune system, causing it to attack the body's tissues. In addition, high levels of fluoride can cause learning disorders and brain damage, and can even kill a young child who consumes an entire tube of toothpaste all at once, which is why there is an FDA warning on fluoride toothpastes that reads: "Keep out of reach of children under six years of age. In case of accidental ingestion, seek professional assistance or contact a poison control center."

To avoid ingesting or using products containing fluoride, read labels of any food or tooth care products, such as toothpastes, mouthwashes, processed foods, vitamins, and beverages like fruit juice, soda, and tea. For tooth care, start using baking soda as toothpaste or nonfluoride toothpaste, which can be purchased at biocompatible dental offices and health food stores. Instead of products containing fluoride, we use natural care products that contain an extract of phytoplenolin, an essential oil derived from a bush known as "sneezeweed," or "old man's weed," native to Australia, where aborigines have used it for burns, wounds, skin infections, diarrhea, and rheumatism. As an Oriental medical doctor, I was taught in the

People's Republic of China to use this plant for treating colds, nasal allergies, asthma, malaria, and amoebic infections, but its anti-protozoan efficacy also makes phytoplenolin a valuable oral health aid in times of wellness.

Mercury

The American Dental Association (ADA) continues to maintain that dental amalgams, comprised of 50 percent mercury, the second most toxic element in the world after plutonium, pose no threat to human health.[14] But today's use of amalgams with mercury, first introduced in France in the early 1800s, is outdated. The formula itself was developed in 1819 in England by a man named Benjamin Bell and contained mercury that bound but did not seal the metals at room temperature. Even early practitioners expressed concerns about mercurial poisoning, because it was already recognized that mercury exposure resulted in many symptoms, including dementia and loss of motor coordination. In the 1920s, scientific concerns about amalgam safety were expressed in Germany but did not result in a resolution. Eventually, advocates for the formula prevailed, and the ADA, founded in 1859, argued that the mercury amalgams were safe and desirable for filling teeth.

There are also economic reasons for promoting amalgams as a replacement for safer materials such as gold, ceramic, and composites. Amalgams bring dental care within the financial means of a wider section of the population, and they are easy to install, so the dentist's technique does not have to be perfect, takes less time than with other materials, and does not require the use of special curing lamps. In many Western European countries amalgam tooth material is hardly used by dentists and no longer taught as a restorative material in dental schools.

Since the 1980s, new dental composites have been developed. The new materials can be used safely in the front or back teeth. Although they have become less expensive in recent years, making them more accessible, these composites require application by a skilled dentist.

Today, mercury is the filling material preferred by 92 percent of dentists in the United States, despite the controversy. The ADA has countered criticism surrounding the use of mercury fillings by pointing to their popularity and longtime use, claiming that mercury, when mixed, forms a biologically inactive substance and indicating that dentists have not reported adverse side effects in patients.[15] In addition, to make them sound less dangerous, mercury fillings sometimes have been referred to euphemistically as "silver fillings," an expression that connotes value ("sterling" silver). In reality, amalgams typically contain approximately 35 percent silver, 9 percent tin, 6 percent copper, a trace of zinc, and 50 percent mercury.[16]

Regardless of any economic and practical advantages of mercury fillings, they remain controversial and are considered toxic by biocompatible practitioners. Research has shown there is a sustained release of mercury and other metals from amalgams that can damage cells; cross the placenta into a developing fetus; induce autoimmune diseases; burden the kidneys; enhance the prevalence of antibiotic-resistant intestinal bacteria; increase the risk of lowered fertility; and cause bleeding gums, loosening of teeth, excessive salivation, abdominal cramps, constipation, diarrhea, *Candida albicans*, heart problems, chronic headaches, dizziness, ringing in the ears, persistent coughs, emphysema, allergies, asthma, thyroid problems, fatigue, and edema.[17] Mercury toxicity also produces psychological disturbances, including depression, anger, anxiety, and attention deficit, especially in children.[18]

In our clinic, countless test results have shown that what Hippocrates, the Greek physician who became known as the father of medicine, said in 500 BCE about disease in general also applies to dentistry: "Diseases are crises of purification, of toxic elimination." Consequently, for patients with problems in the mouth I look for ways to eliminate toxins and how such problems may be connected to other parts of the body. During a medical examination, I count the number of teeth the person has left and the number of amalgam fillings they contain, estimate how many different metals are there, and determine the number of root canals there are under the caps. In my clinical experience, I have found at least six out of ten whole tooth caps to have root canals. Evaluating a person with a skin rash, I may include on a list of recommendations a panoramic X-ray of the mouth because, among other pathways, toxic mercury from dental fillings finds its way out of the body through the skin. Mercury toxicity can also be confirmed by a hair test that measures the body's burden of toxic heavy metals.

Today, biocompatible physicians, who are trained not to use toxic materials in the mouth, are practicing dentistry of the future. Biocompatible dental, medical, and research professionals seek to promote mercury-free dentistry and raise the standards of dental treatment.

THE BIOCOMPATIBLE VIEW

Biocompatible medicine is the only medical diagnostic model that includes the mouth. Biocompatible physicians evaluate a patient's mouth as part of every consultation, believing the mouth to be an excellent noninvasive window for assessing what is likely going on elsewhere in the body. An indication of acid stress leading to chronic inflammation or periodontal disease can signal that a person's health is deteriorating before problems show up on standard medical tests. The biocompatible dental approach looks at:

- Focal, a tooth-specific infection from periodontal disease, a tooth abscess, or a tooth root abscess.
- Bone cavitation, area of dead bone in the jaw caused by a lack of blood flow to that part of the bone.
- Mercury tooth fillings and aluminum tooth caps.
- A corrected bite or occlusion, simply the contact between teeth. Trained dentists need to make sure the relationship between the upper and lower teeth when they approach each other, as occurs during chewing or at rest, are corrected.
- Other dental implications, such as impacted wisdom teeth or teeth that are being "eaten" or reabsorbed by the body. Both dental conditions can disrupt the tooth-body energy connection.

- If you experience oral discomfort, abnormal coloring of teeth, swollen gums, bleeding wounds in gum pockets, abscesses on the gum surfaces, or persistent bad breath, locate a biocompatible physician to check for periodontal infection.
- Find a mercury-free biocompatible dentist for regular teeth cleaning to reduce the risk of developing gum disease and to decrease exposure to mercury by safely replacing amalgams containing mercury.
- Since fluoride is a lethal poison that can accumulate in the body, check labels of food or tooth care products carefully to see if they contain it, including toothpastes, mouthwashes, processed foods, vitamins, and beverages like fruit juice, soda, and tea.
- Brush your teeth with nonfluoride toothpaste or baking soda.

BLOOD TYPE DIET

With their strong backgrounds in biochemistry, clinical nutritionists believe that the standard food pyramid does not work for everybody and that biochemical aspects must be considered. The main tool clinical nutritionists use to specify personal dietary recommendations is the individual's laboratory blood test results. In fact, research conducted over the course of many years shows that particular foods can be beneficial, neutral, or hazardous to a person's health, depending on their blood type.

For example, Dr. James D'Adamo, a naturopathic physician working in European spas, observed reactions to diets by people of different blood types. In 1980, he published his findings in the book *One Man's Food (Is Someone Else's Poison)*. In 1982, his son, Peter D'Adamo, for his dissertation in naturopathic studies at John Bastyr College in Seattle, focused on the theory in connection with medical research to see if there were correlations between blood type and certain diseases, finding that there was a scientific basis for his father's observations on the relationship between blood type, diet, and health.[19] By way of further confirmation, over the past fifteen years in our clinic, we have found eating according to blood type to greatly improve the blood test values of our patients, who report feeling much better.

The theoretical foundation of blood type diet, also known as metabolic diet, is based on the fact that food lectins can cause problems for people with specific blood types. All foods contain lectins, complex proteins that cause reactions in the blood. The nonprotein part of lectin is a carbohydrate usually produced by plants as a primitive immune system for protection against bacteria and fungi. Normally, cooking destroys many lectins, but some resist destruction and are taken into the body if foods are eaten raw.

Eating food containing a lectin that reacts negatively with your blood type is like receiving a blood transfusion of the wrong blood type during a medical emergency, which would produce thickening of blood in the blood vessels. This in turn could lead to circulation problems, such as the formation of blood clots that block blood flow to the heart or brain. With loss of blood flow, tissue can become gangrenous.

Lectins that react negatively to a specific blood type will cause blood cells to stick together, a condition called agglutination. In fact, plant lectins are hemagglutinins, substances that cause agglutination. Hemagglutinins other than lectins include antibodies, blood group antigens, autoimmune factors, bacterial, viral, or parasitic blood agglutinins. Tests for lectins can show whether or not the foods we eat are beneficial or harmful for our metabolic type—rendering information that can help us avoid doing what William Shakespeare described in *Anthony and Cleopatra*: "Now I feed myself the most delicious poison."

Wheat Intolerance
One food category that affects certain blood types negatively is wheat, a gluten-containing grain that people have been led to believe forms, together with other grain products, the foundation of a wholesome diet. Less refined grains, often in combination (such as granola and whole wheat breads fortified with bran, coarse flours, and other additives), are now eaten in large quantities because they have been presented as health foods. Unfortunately, wheat and its close relatives—barley, rye, and oats—have been proven to cause health problems for many people. Wheat intolerance or allergies rank second only to milk allergies when we analyze our patients' medical complaints in our clinic.

Grains are popular foods because of their ability to react with live yeast—a capacity attributed to proteins collectively called gluten. But many people, especially individuals with blood type O or A, are allergic to gluten. Grains can also cause many other problems, including negative reactions to the pesticides, preservatives, and molds that may be present in them.

The most-recognized form of gluten allergy is celiac disease, with symptoms ranging from diarrhea, weight loss, and malnutrition to isolated nutrient deficiencies with no gastrointestinal symptoms; other hidden symptoms include irritable bowel syndrome with iron deficiency anemia, involving little or no diarrhea. Celiac disease is thought to be most prevalent among people of northern European descent, but it also affects Hispanic, Black, and Asian populations. Richard J. Farrell, MD, and Ciaran Kelly, MD, director of the Celiac Disease Center at Beth Israel Deaconess Medical Center in Boston, in a clinical review of the pathology of celiac disease, state, "[T]here is increasing evidence that most people with gluten sensitivity have latent celiac disease with such mild manifestations (in the digestive tract) that the diagnosis is never made."[20]

Wheat intolerance also is associated with a variety of autoimmune disorders, carcinomas of the gastrointestinal tract, and lymphomas, suggesting the possible role of food antigens in causing this immune hypersensitivity.[21] In particular, celiac patients have an increased incidence of diabetes, autoimmune thyroid disease, sarcoidosis, vasculitis, pulmonary fibrosis, encephalopathy, and cerebellar atrophy.[22] Simply put, wheat can cause a host of serious health problems.

We have had patients with inflammatory arthritis who improved dramatically when we removed milk and grain products, especially wheat, from their diet. High cholesterol, skin disorders, and obesity can also result from wheat allergies.[23]

To ensure that their patients get sufficient fiber without eating gluten-containing grains, biocompatible physicians have them eating brown (whole grain) rice, which is not known to cause health problems in any blood type, is full of nutritious B vitamins, and if eaten daily, keeps the colon clean and healthy.

Unfortunately, public health departments are not disseminating the information that people are metabolically different and that tests for lectins can show whether or not the foods we eat are beneficial or harmful to us. In their book *Biochemistry: A Functional Approach*, Robert W. McGilvery, PhD, and Gerald W. Goldstein, MD, offer possible reasons for withholding this information, stating: "Recommendations made to influence the eating habits of a population must be distinguished from recommendations made to a particular individual. The first are, often to the chagrin of the authors, political decisions; the second are, if properly designed, a summation based on biochemical and personal considerations....Put another way, it would take an explosive expansion of row crop farming, one of the more demanding forms of agriculture, to make vegetables, fruits, and so forth major energy sources in the American diet. A shift in eating habits towards breads and other flour products would be easier to manage."[24]

Blood Type and Diet

The following medical facts about blood type and diet, based on the observations of Dr. James D'Adamo and others, contain information that we confirm daily in our clinic. As such, it is included here as a general guideline for blood type diet.

Type O Blood

In people with type O blood, wheat products can slow metabolism, leading to insulin-resistant obesity—the foundation of adult-onset type II diabetes. Worldwide 41 percent of people have type O blood, are obese, and have a high rate of adult-onset diabetes. To a lesser degree, corn, potatoes, and some beans also provoke a negative reaction. Milk and milk products can result in thick blood, leading to potentially dangerous circulation problems, indicated by darkening feet. Such individuals could lower their health risks for heart attacks or stroke by not eating foods that are thickening their blood and by eliminating drugs that are detrimental to their livers. A diet high in vegetables and protein from meat (except pork, which is harmful to people of all blood types), fish, and nuts speeds up metabolism and is extremely beneficial for individuals with type O blood.

To lose weight, type O individuals do well on very low carbohydrate diets, which minimize body fat, along with oregano and bladderwrack (a type of kelp) to burn more fat, and brisk, regular exercise three or four times a week, such as aerobics, weight training, or contact sports, to burn fat, build muscle, and release stress.

The worst thing anyone can do while dieting is to become less active. With decreased caloric intake and reduced exercise, the body cannibalizes muscles for energy instead of fat cells. Increasing physical activity forces the body to increase muscle and use fat stores.

Type A Blood

People with type A blood lack the stomach enzymes needed to digest complex proteins and are the only individuals who do well living a vegetarian lifestyle. When such people eat meat, it remains undigested, leading to intestinal imbalances that produce toxic substances in the intestines—namely, polyamine and indicant—which inhibit proper gastric function and block the absorption of nutrients. Fish, chicken, and turkey are nearly the only acceptable protein sources from meat. Milk and milk products are as detrimental to type A as to type O individuals. Some refined wheat products are neutral, so they may not be harmful, but whole wheat products are detrimental.

To lose weight, individuals with type A blood should omit meat and wheat products, eat well for breakfast and lunch then light in the evening; supplement the diet with magnesium, zinc, and CoQ10, which is critical for energy metabolism; and exercise in moderation. Effective forms of exercise include yoga, Tai Chi, and a limited amount of cardiovascular workouts two or three times a week.

Type B Blood

Many people with type B blood eat a lot of chicken, which unfortunately may thicken their blood, while other meats may not. In addition to chicken, the following foods, among others, contain lectins that will coagulate type B blood: peanuts, corn, lentils, tomatoes, sunflower seeds, and apples. Two percent cow's milk is beneficial and provides optimal amino acids for this blood group. People with type B blood can also tolerate some refined wheat, but should avoid whole wheat. The slow-moving metabolism they can develop is often seen in fatigue, dry skin, cold hands and feet, lower libido, constipation with water retention, and lightheadedness while standing.

To lose weight these individuals should avoid refined wheat but include low-fat milk and cheese in the diet and take supplements of magnesium, zinc, and CoQ10, along with participating in physical and mental activities that involve other people, such as tennis, martial arts, cycling, hiking, or golf.

Type AB Blood

People with type AB blood should avoid foods that are harmful to individuals with either type A or type B blood . Following dietary suggestions for both type A and B also helps AB blood types lose weight. For exercise, such people should alternate between calming activities, such as yoga, and more vigorous activities like aerobics.

THE BIOCOMPATIBLE VIEW

Eating the wrong foods for your blood type is the most common way to start a vicious cycle of metabolic problems leading to inflammation. Colon toxins produced from not properly digesting these foods can exacerbate the problems.

WORDS OF ADVICE

• Determine your blood type and follow the dietary recommendations for it.
• If you have type O or A blood, avoid all grains except brown rice.
• When you are stressed or not feeling well, learn to eat only the foods that are beneficial for your blood type.
• If you are feeling well and do not anticipate stressful events in the immediate future, allow one meal each week to consist of the foods you have eliminated yet still crave.

C

CANCER

Cancer, a medical condition in which a malignant tumor arises when cells multiply uncontrollably and destroy healthy tissue, has surpassed heart disease as the top killer of Americans under the age of eighty-five.[1] A third of all cancers are related to smoking, and another third are related to obesity, poor diet, and lack of exercise. It is likely that depression plays a causative role as well.[2] Cancer occurs when the respiration of oxygen in normal body cells is replaced by the fermentation of sugar, which is why control of insulin, exercise, and eating right for metabolic type all serve as preventives. Cancer is thus a message from the body to examine one's life and determine the factors that have contributed to the illness.

There are many options for treating cancer beyond conventional surgery, radiation, and chemotherapy, which can be used alone or in conjunction with conventional treatments. For monitoring purposes, we utilize cancer-specific blood tests, hair analysis, panoramic dental X-rays, hormone saliva tests, and thermography (use of an infrared camera to evaluate sites of abnormal tissue growth or inflammation), together with conventional diagnostic tools and traditional Chinese medicine techniques. Treatment may also require reevaluating lifestyle preferences, the work or home environment, and personality traits.

Protocols for prevention and treatment of cancer include the following:

Acupuncture (see "Acupuncture," p. 25).
Biocompatible dentistry (see "Biocompatible Dentistry," p. 59).
Blood type. Find out your ideal diet based on your blood type and eat accordingly, maintaining an appropriate weight. Eliminate foods that contain caffeine—such as green or white tea, coffee, and chocolate—as well as chicken and beef from nonorganic sources in the United States. (See "Blood Type Diet," p. 65.)
Colon hydrotherapy (see "Colon Hydrotherapy," p. 85).
Controlled insulin levels. One of the most powerful ways to reduce your cancer risk is to control insulin levels by eating enough vegetables. Ideally, you should be eating five portions of fresh, organic vegetables a day; however, fresh conventionally grown vegetables are healthier than no vegetables at all. The amount of vegetables needed also depends on blood type. People with type A blood may need up to 300 percent more vegetables than individuals with type O blood.[3] Because depression can contribute to cancer, counseling for emotional stress

may be helpful in preventing the illness or in dealing with emotional issues that accompany cancer diagnosis, including fear and anger.[4]

Herbs and supplements. Antioxidants, acidophilus, mushrooms that increase the quantity of natural killer cells, the glutathione precursors SAMe and 5 hydroxy tryptophan (5-HTP) can all be helpful in preventing and treating cancer. Crystalline powders, liquids, sublinguals, and suppositories provide easier absorption for those who cannot tolerate pills. Reduced glutathione therapy is best taken intravenously, in rectal suppositories, or sublingually.

Lifestyle changes. Research shows that nine and a half hours of sleep in total darkness is required to completely recharge the immune system.[5] By getting enough high-quality sleep, it possible to boost the pineal gland's production of melatonin, a protective hormone. When taken as a natural supplement to reset the sleep cycle, melatonin can slow breast cancer growth by 70 percent, findings that may explain why nurses who work the night shift have a high rate of breast and colon cancer.[6] Exercise, too, is important, for several reasons. First, it drives the insulin level down. Second, it raises the heart rate to levels that give the cardiovascular system a good workout. And third, exercising outdoors in the early morning and late afternoon has the added bonus of exposure to ultraviolet rays that safely optimize your vitamin D level, providing a natural antiviral remedy. People who do not have regular access to the sun can take fish oil as the primary source of omega-3 fats. It would be best to monitor your vitamin D level and normalize it with cod liver oil.

Poly MPV. This is a natural supplement that helps reduce cancerous tumors.

THE BIOCOMPATIBLE VIEW

Biocompatible medicine regards the proliferation of cancerous tumor cells as an adaptive strategy cells have taken on to survive in an oxygen-poor (hypoxic) environment. The level of acidity in the body determines the amount of oxygen that is circulated. A mere .15 pH point reduction in the body's acidity means the body is becoming slightly more acidic yet the blood, as a consequence of this shift, will circulate 64.9 percent less oxygen throughout the body.[7] Constant excessive acidity contributes to chronic inflammation, a precursor to cancer, arterial disease, and other degenerative conditions. Making the body less acidic and more alkaline improves the oxygen delivery system throughout the body.

WORDS OF ADVICE

- Eat the right foods for your metabolic type.
- Have a biocompatible physician help you eliminate infection from the gums and jaws.
- Get regular colon hydrotherapy treatments to remove toxic material from the colon.
- Have a hair test performed to identify your body burden of heavy metals, and detoxify for heavy metals using EDTA suppositories.
- As much as possible, avoid touching or eating foods containing insecticides and pesticides.

- Avoid contact with petroleum products.
- Begin an exercise program to oxygenate the body.

CHILDBIRTH

Views of childbirth differ depending on cultural norms. As a medical anthropologist who has witnessed children being born in traditional societies and in modern hospitals, I have seen how medical beliefs and practices are defined by cultural context, although no medical procedure is more shared around the world than assisting in the birth of a new community member.

A Historical Perspective

From our earliest history, childbirth has been viewed as a natural rather than a medical procedure. Women worldwide gave birth naturally for centuries until routine anesthesia was introduced one hundred and fifty years ago. In former times, most births took place at home, without even the assistance of a midwife, attended only by family members or close friends.

As most societies evolved, however, one of the first specialties to emerge was that of midwife.[8] The word *midwife* is a combination of Old English *wíf*, meaning "woman, wife," and *mid*, "with," combined to signify "with the woman." Historically, midwifery has been one of the few medical practices dominated and carried out by female practitioners.

In preliterate societies, the midwife had knowledge and skill in an area of life mysterious to most people, and it was widely assumed that her powers came from supernatural sources. Consequently, the fact that a midwife had both technical expertise and a mystical aspect resulted in the midwife being sometimes revered, sometimes feared, sometimes acknowledged as a society leader, and other times tortured and killed, especially if a birth entailed the death of the mother or child.

During the Middle Ages in northern European countries, witch burning, promoted by both religious and civic authorities, led to the deaths of up to several million women, many of them midwives and healers. By the eighteenth century, however, European women who could afford to birth their children at home had a great advantage over those having to go to a hospital, who, due to poverty, illegitimacy, or birth complications, suffered a mortality rate of 25 to 30 percent.[9] Even so, as much as a hundred years later the image of midwives was still tainted in some regions.

For example, Charles Dickens's 1843 serialized book *Martin Chuzzlewit*, written at the beginning of the Victorian period, includes the intriguing character Sairey Gamp, a midwife, nurse, "layer out" of the dead, and unrepentant alcoholic who is much more concerned with her own creature comforts than the health of her patients. Dickens's denigration of the image of the community midwife through the character of Sairey Gamp influenced social perception of the midwife as unreliable, a view with which the profession still contends today.[10]

The reputation of midwifery not only suffered from associations with witchcraft and unreliable characters but also lost popularity due to scientific and technological advances over time. We know from the biography of Hungarian physician Ignaz

Philipp Semmelweis (1818–1865) that while he was an assistant at the first obstetric clinic of Vienna's Allgemeines Krankenkhaus in 1847, he discovered a means of preventing puerperal fever, an infection of the female reproductive system after childbirth, or abortion that was deadly. His method of prevention was to have physicians and medical students wash their hands in a chlorinated solution before entering obstetric wards and again before examining each patient.[11]

Further contributing to the decline of midwifery is the fact that forces of modernization in technologically oriented societies worldwide conditioned women to fear natural childbirth, focusing on potential pain and medical complications. Images of laboring women screaming in agony cast doubt in the minds of even the most self-assured women who would otherwise opt to birth their babies naturally. Consequently, industrialized nations, such as European countries and the United States, eventually rejected natural childbirth and midwifery in favor of modern methods of childbirth, a position that developing countries are now adopting. For example, the People's Republic of China is currently witnessing a shift from birthing with a traditional midwife (*jie sheng po*) to relying on a professional (*zhu chan shi*).

Among traditional populations in largely unindustrialized countries, however, midwives are still employed in birthing. For example, midwives remain important in rural Thailand because childbirth practices there reflect the larger social system evident in Thai culture, which revolves around the birthing woman, her family and community, the society, and the supernatural world.[12]

In traditional cultures that have lost their birthing identity because of a policy that keeps women from having a community birthing experience, midwifery and natural childbirth practices have radically declined. One example of such a society is in northern Canada, where for many years there has been a policy of evacuating indigenous women from the region to give birth in hospitals in southern Canada. In an attempt to reverse this trend, Nunavik women are being trained as midwives, but despite regional recognition and wide acknowledgment of their success in developing and sustaining a model for remote maternity care for the past twenty years, the Nunavik midwives have not achieved formal recognition of their graduates under the Quebec Midwifery Act. Thus the airlifts continue.[13]

By contrast, other countries on the fast track of industrialization are once again embracing midwifery. In Brazil during the last decade nurse-midwifery has gone through positive changes. In the 1990s, Brazil's Ministry of Health generated policies to improve childbirth services, including legislation for the reimbursement of nurse-midwifery services and financing of nurse-midwifery schools throughout the country.[14]

Likewise, in Costa Rica, where for a while the rate of hospital births rose to 98 percent, like that of many industrialized countries, studies now correlate the hospital birthing practices with important in-hospital iatrogenic risks. Costa Rican women have expressed fear and distress about hospital births, claiming that the procedures are degrading and painful, and that they do not allow for participation in decision making.[15]

Similar views are frequently expressed in other industrialized countries, where midwives deliver high-quality, cost-effective care and young, educated women are opting for midwife-assisted natural childbirth.[16] The Netherlands, especially, is known for its high rate of home births and low rate of medical intervention. In addition, midwives in the Netherlands are seeing more younger women (ages twenty-nine and younger) than older women influencing the decision-making process.[17] Contrary to Dutch practices, home births in Belgium are uncommon and reliance on drugs is taken for granted. Nevertheless, in both countries women who plan a home birth are the most satisfied.[18]

In the United States, according to one study, a typical Connecticut midwife has an average full-time workweek consisting of two twenty-four-hour call days and three seven-hour office days, seeing nineteen to twenty-four patients per office day. Most hold a master of science degree in nursing, work in physician-owned practices, and attend births in hospitals or medical centers. Health insurance, paid sick time, and retirement plans are offered to the majority of such midwives, who have a mean annual salary of $79,554.[19]

In comparison with European countries, however, the number of midwife-attended births is very low in the United States—only 7 percent—a reflection, in part, of the influence of medical institutions and political-economic forces. In the words of one researcher: "It was found that institutions successfully altered maternity care and diminished midwifery services without accountability for their actions. These findings illuminate the larger political-economic forces that shape the marginalization of midwifery in the US."[20]

Current Views on Childbirth Practices

Despite these statistics, today in the United States and elsewhere in industrialized countries, many professionals are emphasizing the numerous advantages of natural childbirth and the effectiveness of midwifery. Birthing naturally, via vaginal delivery, is associated with far fewer delivery problems, requires less anesthesia, involves a shorter hospital stay, saves money, encourages earlier and better interaction between mother and infant, and poses less risk for both mother and child of death during childbirth.[21] Women who have had cesarean or assisted vaginal deliveries, on the other hand, are at increased risk for rehospitalization, especially with infectious illnesses.[22] Given these advantages of natural childbirth in the United States and other industrialized nations, it is difficult to understand why this form of birthing has become the exception rather than the rule.

Cesarean Births

In the United States, one out of every three babies is born by cesarean section, or C-section, an operation in which a surgical incision is made across the lower belly and uterus and the baby is taken from the mother's womb.[23] Traditionally it is thought that this operation received its name because of a belief that Julius Caesar was born this way. But the name could also have been derived from the *lex caesarea*, a law to have a baby cut out of a woman who dies in childbirth, or from the Latin *caedere*, whose past participle *caesum* means "to cut."[24]

Cesarean section can be a lifesaving operation when either the mother or baby faces certain problems before or during labor and delivery. The healthcare provider may suggest a C-section for one or more of the following reasons:

The mother has already had a cesarean section or another surgery on her uterus. Although many gynecologists want to repeat the operation after a woman has already delivered this way, such a decision should not be automatic. Today there is increasing acknowledgment that a repeat cesarean section is elective, a decision to be made jointly by physicians and well-informed birthing women.

The baby is too big to pass safely through the vagina. When the weight of the baby is five pounds or more—macrosomic—a caesarean operation will be recommended. However, "despite a one-third recurrence of macrosomia, first vaginal delivery of a macrosomic infant [is] associated with a high incidence of second vaginal delivery. Conversely, primiparous macrosomic cesarean delivery [conveys] a high risk (56 percent) for repeat intrapartum cesarean whether macrosomia recurred or not."[25]

The baby's buttocks or feet are positioned so they will enter the birth canal first, instead of the head—called a breech position. Women who are delivering their first child and carrying the baby in this position have a higher risk of the baby dying during vaginal birth compared with the fetus being delivered by cesarean section.[26]

The baby's shoulder is positioned so it will enter the birth canal first, instead of the head—called a transverse position.

There are problems with the placenta. Difficulties with the placenta, the organ that nourishes the baby in the womb, can cause dangerous bleeding during vaginal birth. Unfortunately, the incidence of *placenta accreta* is rising, primarily because of the increase in cesarean delivery rates.[27]

Labor is too slow or stops. If labor fails to progress, cesareans are often done to avoid complications. Unfortunately, many cesareans are done during the dormant phase of labor and also the second stage, when labor is not prolonged. These practices diverge from the documented criteria for lack of progress.[28]

The baby's umbilical cord slips into the vagina. If the baby's umbilical cord slips into the vagina, it could be flattened during vaginal delivery, a situation called "umbilical cord prolapse." About one-third of cesareans performed for emergency reasons, however, are begun more than thirty minutes after the decision has been made to operate,[29] when umbilical cord prolapse may already be in effect.

The mother has an infection such as HIV or genital herpes.

The mother is having twins, triplets, or more.

The baby has problems during labor that show it is under stress, such as a slow heart rate or fetal distress.

The mother has a serious medical condition that requires intensive or emergency treatment, such as diabetes or high blood pressure.

The baby has a certain type of birth defect.

The mother is more than 100 pounds (45 kg) over her ideal body weight, the definition of morbid obesity.

The baby is very small and has a very low birth weight. Babies with a very low birth weight do better when delivered by cesarean section.

It used to be assumed that if you previously had a cesarean section, you would birth future children also by cesarean. But this assumption has been challenged by many gynecologists who now believe that a vaginal birth after even multiple cesareans should remain an option for eligible birthing women.[30] Indeed, participating in this decision gives birthing women more power and control over their circumstances. Ultimately, the choice between a cesarean section and a trial of labor is best made jointly by an informed physician and expectant mother. However, documentation reveals that many hospitals are not providing sufficient information to expectant mothers who are facing this decision.[31]

Another problem is the tendency of some gynecologists to perform requested cesareans despite their own strong belief in natural birth. In Israel, 91 percent of all gynecologists realize that natural childbirth is the best option for mother and child, but many defer to women's decisions about birthing. In a study conducted in 2002, about 50 percent of responding gynecologists were willing to "perform cesarean delivery on request because of their support of women's autonomy, despite the fact that they believe that vaginal delivery is a better option."[32]

Such a stance is complicated by the fact that expectant mothers are not always making decisions for themselves but are influenced by cultural, political, and family pressures. In Aruba, women's decisions to birth at home, a reflection of the prevailing Dutch attitudes, are being thwarted by the concerns of expectant fathers and grandmothers. This problem is mirrored in other parts of the world where caregivers have a "low tolerance for fetal risk associated with vaginal birth."[33] In general, if expectant mothers, partners, and other family members know about the risks associated with cesarean sections, they will be better informed to make decisions about vaginal delivery versus cesarean section.

Adverse Effects of Cesarean Operations

Statistics seem to support the view that cesarean operations are not safer than vaginal delivery and potentially hurt both mother and child. Researchers believe that a rise in cesarean sections combined with increasing maternal obesity is partly to blame for the fact that the maternal mortality rate in the United States in 2004 was the highest in decades—13 deaths per 100,000 live births, according to statistics released by the National Center for Health Statistics. Studies also show that the maternal death rate among black women is at least three times greater than among white women, perhaps because black women are more susceptible to complications like high blood pressure and more likely to get inadequate prenatal care.[34]

Also, the rate of cesarean operations is far higher than is appropriate, given the potential risks involved. Like other surgeries, cesareans incur risks related to anesthesia, infections, blood clots, and excessive bleeding, one of the leading causes of pregnancy-related deaths. In addition, birthing women who have had several previous cesareans are at especially high risk for one or more of the following complications:

- Increased bleeding, which may require a blood transfusion
- Infection in the incision, the uterus, or other nearby organs

• Reactions to medications, including the drugs used for anesthesia
• Injuries to the bladder or bowel
• Blood clots in the legs, pelvic organs, or lungs
• Postpartum fever, associated with an increased risk of uterine rupture during subsequent labor

Cesarean sections may also contribute to the growing number of babies who are born late preterm, between thirty-four and thirty-six weeks' gestation. While babies born at this time are usually considered healthy, a baby's lungs and brain mature late in pregnancy, which explains why infants born between thirty-four and thirty-six weeks' gestation are more likely to have problems with:

• Breathing
• Feeding
• Maintaining body temperature
• Jaundice

Other potential difficulties associated with birthing by cesarean section are:

Adverse effects of drugs. Some babies are affected by drugs given to the mother for anesthesia during surgery, medications that cause numbness so she can't feel pain but that can also cause the baby to be inactive or sluggish.

Breathing problems. Even if they are full term, babies born by cesarean operations are more likely to have breathing problems than babies delivered vaginally.

Missing the benefits of breastfeeding and early bonding. Because of discomfort from the surgery, women who have cesareans are less likely to breastfeed than women who have vaginal births. Hence, they do not bond as well with their babies, due to the lack of oxytocin, the "mothering hormone" produced by lactation that bonds mother to child and child to mother.

Fetal injuries. Fetal injuries complicate 1.1 percent of cesarean operations.[35] Considering the reported fetal mortality rate of 6.9 deaths per 1,000 births of the 4,021,726 births in the United States in 2002, [36] more than 27,500 of them, a certain percentage of which followed cesarean operations, resulted in fetal death. The frequency of fetal injury at cesarean delivery varies with the indication for surgery, passage of time between the skin incision and delivery, and type of uterine incision.

Operative Vaginal Deliveries

A mother-to-be experiencing natural childbirth may have to undergo an operative delivery, which is generally defined as any obstetric procedure in which active measures are taken to accomplish delivery. Birth trauma, due in part to obstetric procedures, while underreported and often misdiagnosed, is estimated to be between the sixth and tenth leading cause of infant mortality in the United States.[37] Such procedures include the use of obstetric forceps, instruments resembling long tongs, utilized to speed up delivery or twist the baby's head into position for delivery, or a vacuum extractor, a specially designed cup that goes on the baby's head with a vacuum pump and a chain attached to pull the baby through the birth canal. The vacuum extractor, when used correctly, is safe but leaves a grotesque knot of skin on the top of baby's head. The use of forceps, on the other hand, is associated with injuries to both mother and baby, many of them serious and some fatal. Such injuries include torn nerves and spine structure, torn cartilage in the knees or elbows, and traction injuries resulting from trauma to the neck and shoulder. The primary symptom of traction injuries is burning pain radiating down one upper arm, sometimes accompanied by numbness or a skin sensation such as burning, prickling, itching, or tingling, with no apparent physical cause.[38]

Importance of Birth Posture

The position a woman assumes to birth her baby can have a significant effect on the outcome, minimizing potential risks. In many traditional societies, a woman's birth posture is squatting, with knees splayed and attendants holding the woman's arms, bent about 90 degrees at the elbows. When tired or between contractions, the woman may shift to a kneeling position. I have seen women around the world assume this position, and I have also witnessed women laboring in hospitals instinctively try to get up from a lying position in an effort to squat.

The traditional squatting or kneeling positions are the most efficient and least harmful birth postures. A cross-cultural evaluation of birthing in the squatting posture shows that it increases the diameter of the pelvic outlet, uses gravity to aid in delivery, frees the movement of the sacrum, and allows the mother to bear down using the thighs and legs for resistance and, with the aid of gravity, deliver with less trauma than those who lie in a supine or semi-recumbent position.[39]

By contrast, the lithotomy position—on the back with feet up in stirrups—although preferred in modern obstetric practice, is designed more for the convenience of the attending doctor than for the efficiency and safety of birthing. It closes the birth canal by as much as 30 percent,[40] causing obstetricians to sometimes pull so hard they damage the baby's spinal nerves, resulting in paralysis or even death.

Natural Childbirth

There is no better place to birth a child than at home, assisted by a midwife, surrounded by family or close friends, and in the squatting or kneeling posture. Women who decide on natural childbirth realize that any artificial interruption in birthing, even arising from the best intentions, can increase the risks to both the mother and child. Choosing natural childbirth is choosing to trust your body and knowing that you already possess all the tools you need to give birth. Trusting the body's innate ability to birth can lead to a good natural birth experience.

Home deliveries have been found to reduce newborn stress, make labor less difficult, lessen the possibility of maternal infection and bleeding after birth, and minimize the release of dark green intestinal substance into the amniotic fluid before birth, which can choke the baby.[41] Thus the best medical evidence suggests that home birth not only is safe but has distinct medical advantages women should know about in advance.

Deciding on a natural birth also imparts psychological and emotional advantages that add to the medical benefits. Having a natural birth, especially a home birth, surrounded by family and friends and using favorite relaxation techniques, can engender a good attitude. And having a good attitude about childbirth improves your chances for a successful outcome. In fact, research conducted recently in hospitals in Switzerland and Canada reveal the importance of birth philosophies in attaining successful births.[42]

Choosing a natural birth does not mean opting for a painful birth. Rather, it places the birthing woman in control of every aspect of her experience, from early labor to afterbirth, including the degree of discomfort she does or does not feel. A wide variety of natural comfort measures can be employed. For example, when a baby's positioning is not ideal for vaginal birth, an acupuncture procedure of repeatedly holding a glowing cylinder of smoldering mugwort herb close to an acupuncture point on the little toes of the birthing woman will rotate the baby into the correct birthing position.[43]

THE BIOCOMPATIBLE VIEW

Decisions you make about birthing should focus first and foremost on the safety and well-being of your baby. Ideally, preparation for birth would begin years in advance with detoxification of your body from heavy metals and fat-soluble toxins from insecticides, pesticides, and petroleum-based chemicals. In our clinic, where we use a hair test to determine the body burden of toxic heavy metals, we have found that in each successively born child of a detoxified woman, progressively lower levels of toxic metals have crossed the placenta.

WORDS OF ADVICE

• Detoxify at least a year before starting to conceive. This means removing amalgams to prevent infection from taking root in jaws or gums, and chelating heavy metals. It is also helpful to undergo colon cleansing before becoming pregnant, since the buildup of toxins, mucus, and waste in the intestines can inhibit the body's absorption of nutrients needed to nourish you and your baby. Then once pregnant, strive to empty your bowels at least twice a day.

• Nourish yourself during pregnancy by taking in about 300 extra calories a day. Eat well from your metabolic food list, and include plenty of fresh, organic fruits and vegetables. In addition, take vitamins and minerals, toning and healing herbs, and supplements such as red raspberry leaf tea, stinging nettle, yellow dock, alfalfa, red clover, and chlorella. Also, whether you are contemplating pregnancy or are already pregnant be sure to take 400 micrograms of folic acid daily to help prevent spina bifida and other birth defects; good sources of this B vitamin are leafy greens, dried beans, legumes, and natural prenatal vitamin supplements. In addition, it is well known that ginger root helps alleviate "morning sickness."

• Exercise during pregnancy, after first checking with your doctor or midwife to make sure it is not contraindicated. Exercise during pregnancy keeps the body healthy for birth and prepared to easily produce endorphins, which are natural painkillers, in labor and birth. If you were exercising before pregnancy, it is generally safe to continue a reasonable exercise program. If you have not been exercising but are healthy enough to exercise during pregnancy, begin moderately and gradually build up resistance and intensity. A good program is to do aerobic exercise (such as biking, walking, or running) for thirty minutes three times a week and strength training two to three times a week. While exercising during pregnancy, avoid getting out of breath or exhausting yourself. Also avoid soaking in a hot tub, which can cause a woman's body to overheat and harm the developing fetus.

- Learn as much as you can in preparation for birthing. In addition to taking a natural childbirth class, address emotional issues, including any fear of pain during birth or problems involved in becoming a parent.
- To minimize pain during labor, avoid artificially initiating labor through use of the pharmaceutical drug pitocin, which can cause contractions with two or more peaks and sometimes pain between contractions. Vaginal exams, monitors, and other needless interventions may also unnecessarily increase pain during labor.
- Stay active in labor and change positions frequently to minimize pain caused by any pressure on nerves, vertebrae, or tendons. If you are lying on your back, the baby may compress major blood vessels. If the baby is posterior or if you are experiencing back pain, try shifting your weight forward and applying counter-pressure to your lower back.
- Use the restroom often during labor. Pressure on a full bladder is always uncomfortable, all the more so when it is brought about by a baby at full term.
- Select a place to labor and birth where you will able to concentrate, remain undisturbed, and be supported by trusted friends. Plan on removing anyone who bothers you since such disturbances will make your body produce adrenaline, which causes more painful and less productive contractions, slowing down or even halting labor. Do anything that will relax you and inspire positive thoughts, such as laboring in water, lighting candles, filling the room with scented oils like lavender, listening to music, slow dancing with your husband, or visualizing scenes that make you happy.
- Use noninvasive techniques to minimize discomfort during labor and birth. Counterpressure, massage, hot or cold pads, birth balls, or herbal treatments help some women relax during labor and birth. Ginger root helps alleviate morning sickness, while red raspberry leaf tea, lobelia, blue cohosh, calcium, and B-vitamin complex often assist in easing labor pain. Use strong herbs such as blue cohosh and lobelia with caution.
- Remember that everything you do during labor and birth is preparing you for your wondrous first meeting with your child.

CHOLESTEROL

Imagine what would happen if the police force that protects your community were all fired. Cholesterol is the body's police officer in charge of protecting your brain, nerves, and organs from the deleterious effects of toxins. Under the stress of toxins, such as heavy metals, pesticides, and insecticides, the liver, the organ primarily responsible for converting toxins into harmless by-products, produces cholesterol. For example, mercury is sequestered into cholesterol then converted into bile that can be excreted through the gallbladder and intestines.

There are two types of cholesterol. One type, called HDL, is beneficial, and so it is desirable to have as much as possible, while the other kind, called LDL, is deemed harmful by many doctors, a conclusion that is both simplistic and physiologically incorrect. LDL cholesterol stimulates body cells to either produce or stop producing their own cholesterol. It also controls the thickness of the blood and carries valuable vitamin E and carotenoid antioxidants that dissolve in fat. LDL as fat globules comes in seven sizes—the bigger, the better. Oxidized LDL, at the small end of the spectrum, increases chronic inflammation, the foundation of arterial and heart disease.

Today, to treat high cholesterol most doctors tend to prescribe cholesterol-lowering drugs known as statins, which are proving to be killers. Before it was taken off the market, Baycol, a Bayer statin, produced a side effect called rhabdomyolysis that caused severe pain, muscle weakness, and had the potential to shut down the kidneys and trigger paralysis or death.[44] Suicide, too, is a stated risk from taking cholesterol-lowering medicine because as the cholesterol level falls, fewer lipoproteins are available for removing toxins, including heavy metals, solvent contaminants, pesticides, and petrochemicals, from the brain and nerves. Consequently, a knee-jerk reaction to prescribe cholesterol-lowering drugs is simplistic and dangerous.

The reason many physicians treat high cholesterol is that they regard it as a major predictor of cardiovascular problems. While it is true that if cholesterol becomes oxidized by free radicals, which develop from chronic inflammation, it can irritate tissues in the lining of the arteries, this is only one of numerous injuries to the lining of arteries. In fact, in the presence of toxic metals, the liver, a major detoxification organ, produces cholesterol to absorb them, thereby protecting more sensitive organs like the brain.

By contrast, biocompatible physicians do not view cholesterol as bad and point out that when cholesterol is naturally low or made low by drugs, the risk of cancer rises. This occurs because cholesterol, after being converted into bile acid, dissolves gallstones and carries lipoproteins in the bloodstream that have fat-soluble antioxidants, such as vitamin E, beta-carotene, and CoQ10, which help protect the body against cancer.

I, for one, view a high cholesterol level as a sign that the body is trying its best to protect the brain and nerves from toxicities, including those produced by continual fermentation in the colon. For example, excessive sugar, simple carbohydrates, alcohol, or overeating allows the yeast *Candida albicans* to grow out of control and sets up fermentation in the colon, producing extreme amounts of gas. And alcohol entering the bloodstream from the colon contributes to insulin resistance by converting to triglycerides. In our clinic, I have seen high triglycerides in laborers who did not drink alcohol but were exposed to organic solvents—especially those in paints, varnishes, lacquers, adhesives, glues, cleaning agents, plastics, or printing ink—or worked with pesticides. In such cases, the triglycerides were being produced to protect the liver from toxicities. My primary effort in these instances is to identify and remove the poisons, after which the cells stop making excess cholesterol for protection.

When fat-soluble poisons are present, the best way to remove them is by changing the diet.

Proper diet is the first line of defense against LDL, or "bad," cholesterol. To control this form of cholesterol, it is best not to consume sugar or alcohol; fried, salty, or refined foods; fatty dairy products; or fatty meats. When we tell patients this, many say we have just eliminated everything they eat—and indeed, these foods seem to epitomize the standard American or Aruban diet (SAD). Instead, it is helpful to eat fresh fruits and vegetables, lean meats, whole grains, and fish that swim constantly in deep water, which are loaded with HDL, or "good," cholesterol, needed to manufacture hormones such as sex hormones and help control LDL cholesterol. Medicinal oils packed with HDL cholesterol include olive, evening primrose, black currant, flax, and safflower. Herbs that lower LDL cholesterol are shiitake mushrooms, cayenne, ginger, cat's claw, fenugreek seed, garlic, and turmeric. It is also helpful to eat smaller meals, especially before bed, as food does not digest properly during sleep. Another good way to get cholesterol under control quickly is to eat only brown rice for three weeks, drink lots of water, and embark on an exercise program appropriate to you.

In our clinic, primary detoxification starts with colonics to "dilute" the pollution, followed by blood tests to indicate possible exposure to various types of toxins, such as organic solvents, pesticides, insecticides, or latex, and finally hair analysis to determine the presence of toxic metals in the body. Our clinic's second therapeutic response is composed of acupuncture and the following liver cleansing supplements:

Dandelion, or "teeth of the lion"—an important liver detoxification herb, clearing wastes and pollutants, and stimulating bile production. It helps treat gallstones and gallbladder inflammation, jaundice, and related liver conditions.

Fringe tree—a bile stimulant used in hepatitis, cirrhosis, enlarged liver, and jaundice, as well as for gallstones or inflammation. It can also help with liver detoxification in chronic illness. In traditional Chinese medicine, it is thought to be a tonic to strengthen the spleen, pancreas, and supporting organs, such as the small intestine, the liver, and the gallbladder.

Glutathione (g-glutamylcysteinylglycine, GSH)—a major aid in preventing and even reversing degenerative brain diseases, and one of the main antioxidants, antitoxins, and enzyme cofactors produced by a healthy liver. This peptide, present in all animals, plants, and microorganisms and found mainly in the fluid component of cells, can produce and repair DNA, participate in protein production, and help make prostaglandin, an unsaturated fatty acid that resembles hormones in its activity of controlling smooth muscle contractions, blood pressure, inflammation, and body temperature. Glutathione helps move amino acids around the body, enhances the immune system, and most importantly, metabolizes toxins and carcinogens, preventing oxidative cell damage.

Milk thistle—used since Greco-Roman times as an herbal remedy for a variety of ailments, particularly liver problems. In the late nineteenth and early twentieth centuries, physicians in the United States used milk thistle seeds to relieve congestion of the liver, spleen, and kidneys. Today, several scientific studies suggest that active substances in milk thistle (particularly silymarin) protect the liver from damage caused by viruses, toxins, alcohol, and certain drugs, such as acetaminophen, a common over-the-counter medication used for headaches and pain. Acetaminophen, or paracetamol, can cause liver damage if taken in large quantities or by people who drink alcohol regularly. Many professional herbalists recommend milk thistle extract for the prevention or treatment of various liver disorders, including viral hepatitis, fatty liver associated with long-term alcohol use, and liver damage from drugs or industrial toxins such as carbon tetrachloride.

SAMe (S-adenosylmethionine)—a substance produced constantly by all living cells that affects everything from fetal development to brain function. It regulates the expression of genes, preserves the fatty membranes that insulate cells, and helps control the action of various hormones and neurotransmitters, including serotonin, melatonin, dopamine, and adrenaline. In a dozen clinical trials involving more than 22,000 patients, researchers found SAMe as effective as pharmaceutical treatments for pain and inflammation.[45] Unlike these nonsteroidal anti-inflammatory drugs, however, SAMe shows no signs of damaging the digestive tract. Instead of speeding the breakdown of cartilage, SAMe may help restore it. As a result of SAMe, homocysteine can be broken down to form glutathione (the most important antioxidant produced by the body) or remethylated to form methionine (the precursor to SAMe).

Turmeric—a premier Ayurvedic herb for natural liver cleansing. Turmeric can increase bile production by over 100 percent, and curcumin, the most researched compound in turmeric, also increases bile solubility, helping with the treatment of gallstones. As a potent antioxidant, turmeric has the same liver protective effect as milk thistle.

THE BIOCOMPATIBLE VIEW

Biocompatible physicians view cholesterol levels not as a reliable indicator of disease but rather as the body's attempt to protect itself from toxic heavy metals, solvents, and petrochemicals. In addition, we consider that people whose cholesterol levels are low may have been poisoned by perflurocarbons, especially if HDL cholesterol is low. In older individuals, low cholesterol values can be a strong indicator of early death.[46]

WORDS OF ADVICE

- Avoid taking cholesterol-lowering drugs, which can have dangerous side effects and may short circuit the body's attempt to protect itself from poisons.
- If you have high cholesterol, ask a biocompatible doctor for a metabolic survey to establish why your body is producing increased cholesterol. Correcting the specific metabolic imbalance should stimulate your body to produce normal amounts of cholesterol.
- Eat according to your metabolic type as an important first step in getting your cholesterol values under control.

CHRONIC INFLAMMATION

The body's inflammatory response, like the "flight or fight" response, is an evolved protective mechanism to aid survival, but if constant it becomes destructive. Whether due to exercise, an accident, infection, or degenerative disease, inflammation is the body's response to injury. Affected tissue usually causes pain, heat, redness, and swelling because blood vessels in the area dilate to bring in extra white blood cells that eat the bacteria and other foreign particles gathering at the site. During its inflammatory response, the body becomes acidic.

Bacteria, viruses, pollens, molds, pesticides, toxic heavy metals, the wrong foods for your metabolic type, modern overprocessed convenience foods, and lack of water can all stimulate the immune system into responding with inflammation. Chronic inflammation has also been linked to every type of serious degenerative condition and premature aging. A person with blood test results showing ongoing inflammation may be at high risk for a heart attack, stroke, or cancer.

Pesticides and toxic heavy metals that make their way into the body produce free radicals, which irritate tissues and start the inflammatory response; the body then becomes acidic, producing more free radicals. This negative spiral continues until the individual feels sick and is prescribed anti-inflammatory drugs and antibiotics that relieve symptoms for a while but do not address the sources of the problem.

By contrast, in our clinic we look for the source of free radical production, which sometimes is the person's profession and at other times is their toxic mercury fillings, but most often a combination of many factors, including diet, has progressively contributed to the crisis. It has been found repeatedly, for example, that women confronted with emotional trauma are more apt than men to react strongly. Clinically I have seen women who have been affected for years by insulin resistance (see "Diabetes Type II," p. 97) develop type II diabetes after the death of a beloved husband or child. Such outcomes are usually attributed to the fact that stress traumas produce a cortisol spike that triggers the pancreas to release glucagon, a hormone that raises blood glucose levels.[47]

Another source of the body's inflammatory response is omega-6 essential fatty acids (EFAs), found in most cooking oils, including corn, safflower, peanut, and soy, and in processed foods made with these oils. By contrast, the omega-3 EFAs form the foundation of the body's anti-inflammatory response, chief among which are eicosapentaenoic acid (EPA) and docosahexaenoic acid (DHA), found in salmon and other cold-water fish. The omega-3s compete against omega-6s to reduce levels of compounds that cause inflammation.

Because chronic inflammation is basically a problem involving free radicals, we place our patients on antioxidant supplements. Vitamin E, vitamin C, and the B-complex vitamins, as well as many fresh vegetables and fruits have antioxidant properties. It is important to make sure, however, that the fruits and vegetables a person eats are beneficial for their metabolic type.

I prescribe natural, food-based antioxidant supplementation not to eliminate symptoms, as some practitioners do, but to treat the source of free radical activity and thus improve general health. Real health is found through a journey of removing toxins, consistently eating the best food for your metabolic type, and getting adequate exercise, relaxation, and rest.

THE BIOCOMPATIBLE VIEW

Biocompatible medicine assumes that the common denominator of all degenerative conditions is chronic inflammation, resulting from highly acidic conditions. The five factors contributing most to acidic conditions are eating the wrong food for metabolic type; infections in the body, including toxic material from the colon; a body burden of heavy metals; the presence of insecticides and pesticides in the body; and the detrimental effects of petroleum products on health.

WORDS OF ADVICE
• Eat the right foods for your metabolic type.
• Make sure there are no infections in your mouth, either in your gums or jaw-bones, and regularly remove toxic material from your colon.
• Have a hair test done to determine if you have a body burden of heavy metals.
• As much as possible, avoid coming into contact with insecticides and pesticides, and eating foods containing them.
• As much as possible, avoid coming into contact with petroleum products.

CLIMATE CONTROL

Climate control has become a major health hazard since numerous outbreaks of pneumonia, Legionnaire's disease, and other illnesses, as well as transmissions of viruses and bacteria, occur in airtight buildings, especially hospitals and hotels, many due to air-conditioning systems. For example, in February 2003, severe acute respiratory syndrome (SARS), an atypical pneumonia of unknown origin, was recognized as a worldwide health threat. After investigating, the World Health Organization concluded that based on the more than eight thousand people who developed the disease worldwide, it was likely that infectious water droplets, aerosolized by coughing and dried in air-conditioned spaces, contaminated the air in closed spaces long after the sick individuals had left them, infecting many more people.[48] The recent spread of tuberculosis (TB) is also, at least partly, the result of air-conditioning systems used in closed spaces.[49] Certainly, *mycobacterium tuberculosis,* the bacterium that causes most cases of TB, has been shown to survive well in cool, dark places and to be destroyed in fresh air and sunlight.

Twenty-five years ago, when I worked in public health in New York, I predicted that TB, which is spread by breathing in the tiny water droplets coughed or sneezed out by an infected person, would become a major health concern in the United States, but doctors scoffed and declared that they had eradicated the disease from the country years before. From my fieldwork, I knew tuberculosis continued to be a major health concern in Central America, and that eventually, because of the untreated immigrants from these countries, the United States geared up for a tuberculosis epidemic, worsened by low-key media attention and inappropriate antibiotic treatments. Today in the United States, 20,000 new cases and 1,800 deaths from TB are reported annually,[50] and when autopsied, most of these victims are shown to have had clinical TB infections in the past that were never adequately treated. Unless air-conditioning filters are cleaned daily, they are a breeding ground for molds and bacteria.[51] Children with constant colds and ear infections have improved dramatically when removed from sleeping in air conditioning or when the filter was cleaned daily.

In our clinic, because of these health risks, as well as the type of treatments we provide, our consultation room has no air conditioner, nor is it a closed environment. Indeed, traditional acupuncture cannot be performed in a closed room since it often calls for moxa herb to be ignited on the ends of needles, which fills the room with smoke. From a diagnostic standpoint, we have found that in this natural environment, patients who complain of feeling hot are most often either obese, sickly, or cocaine abusers. Menopause, too, can bring on problems of temperature regulation, amidst the changing levels of estrogen and progesterone. In effect, individuals who complain about the heat or perspire inappropriately are showing signs of physical or hormonal deficiencies.

On the other hand, a cold climate is a primary source of pathogenic stress, contracting blood vessels, constricting circulation, depressing metabolism, and eventually, over time, resulting in weariness and weakness. Alternating between hot and very cold environments, such as going in and out of air-conditioned settings, also shocks the body, overloading the regulatory system. For truly healthy climate control, open the windows to get fresh air.

THE BIOCOMPATIBLE VIEW

Air conditioners have a propensity to do more harm than good as their filters and ducts are a breeding ground for viruses, molds, and bacteria. Moreover, chilling the body contracts blood vessels, impedes circulation, depresses metabolism, and reduces oxygen delivery to the organs and tissues. In short, being in a closed air-conditioned room for a long time causes debilitation or illness.

WORDS OF ADVICE

- Clean air conditioner filters daily to prevent the spread of viruses, molds, and bacteria.
- Avoid spending long periods of time in air-conditioned environments.
- If you have a central air-conditioning unit at home or in the office, install an ultraviolet light sanitizer inside it.
- In warm weather, wear clothes made of natural fabric that "breathes," allowing evaporating perspiration to cool you down.

COLON HYDROTHERAPY

The value of cleaning items so they maintain efficient functioning became apparent to me when, as newlyweds, Phyllis and I moved into a new apartment before we had the usual domestic paraphernalia, and neighbors gave us an old vacuum cleaner that I had to clean before it worked well. The same is true of many body parts, including the colon. Natural physicians say that "old age starts in the colon." And according to health statistics, in 2006 an estimated 130,000 new cases of colon and rectal cancer were diagnosed in the United States, making it the fourth most common form of cancer among Americans and the third most prevalent malignant disease in industrialized countries.[52] The colon, together with the lungs, skin, and kidneys, is designed to keep us healthy by eliminating toxins from the intestines, blood, and lymph systems.

One good way to clean the large intestine is through colon hydrotherapy. A treatment often recommended by physicians in the 1930s and 1940s, and recently regaining popularity among natural physicians, colon hydrotherapy is of great value because serious health problems can develop if the colon is not properly cared for and because colon health care in developed countries has been neglected.[53] Colon toxicity can be the underlying cause of many commonly reported health problems, including constipation (see "Constipation," p. 88), backaches, diarrhea, skin problems, difficulty with weight loss, insomnia, hypertension, headaches, arthritis, bad breath, asthma, and allergies. Colon hydrotherapy is an enema designed to cleanse the area from the rectum to the cecum, which is the beginning of the large intestine, located on the lower right side of the abdomen and having the worm-shaped appendix branching off from it. The procedure involves a gentle infusion of warm filtered water into the rectum by the therapist, without the use of chemicals or drugs, as a natural solution to conditions that interfere with the normal functioning of the colon. The individual lies on his back, and the water is mechanically infused into and out of the intestine; the outflowing water removes excess gas, mucus, infectious material, and feces, while the incoming water helps hydrate the body.

Similar procedures were used in ancient times. Colon "lavage," first recorded in the Ebers Papyrus of 1550 BCE, which deals with ancient medical practices, was described as an infusion of aqueous substances into the large intestine through the anus. Hippocrates (ca. 460–377 BCE), the father of medicine, recorded using enemas as a therapy for the reduction of fevers, while in the second century the Greek physician Galen (AD 129–ca. 199) also advocated for the use of enemas. And in AD 1600, the French surgeon Ambroise Paré, whose practical skills and humaneness distinguished him from his contemporaries, offered the first differentiation between colon irrigation and the popular enema therapy of the times, which contained mercurial compounds used to treat syphilis.

Colon hydrotherapy is superior to other types of enemas for many reasons. Fleet-type enemas that can be purchased in drugstores have hydroscopic salts that pull water out of the body to increase the bulk in the colon and help expel fecal material, dehydrating the individual. And while the old-fashioned red bag type of enema with a white hose attached to an anal tip that allows the water to slowly enter the colon is an excellent first response to a fever—better than a fever-reducing over-the-counter medication—it cleans only the lowest one-fifth of the colon. Enemas should be used sparingly, if at all, as a laxative.

An alternate type of treatment, the ingestion of laxatives, is also inferior because they act as chemical irritants and stimulate the muscular walls of the colon to abnormally contract to expel irritating substances. Such drugs are a less effective method of cleaning the large intestine because they interfere with important digestive processes that occur high up in the alimentary tract (stomach and small intestine) and often dehydrate the body. By contrast, colon hydrotherapy alternately fills and empties the colon and improves the hydration status of the patient.

In addition to cleaning, good colon health depends on the quality of food eaten, based on blood type. The standard American and Aruban diet (SAD)—comprised of refined, processed foods high in saturated fats; containing preservatives, sugar, and flour; and limited in fiber—inevitably causes problems for the colon. Over time, the colon loses the ability to process vital nutrients, absorb water, and eliminate fecal matter from the body, a condition commonly known as constipation. With constipation comes toxicity. Toxins present in the unhealthy colon can be transported into the circulatory system, undermining the body's ability to metabolize food properly or provide vital energy for living.

As a traditional Chinese medicine physician, I believe that although from the colon we absorb water, electrolytes, and some vitamins, especially B-complex vitamins, the majority of bowel content is expelled from the body, and thus the emotional aspect of the organ is about "letting go." Certainly, at our clinic we have found that problems with the colon are also reflected in emotional resistance to releasing and letting go, which resolves when colon health is improved.

Colon hydrotherapy, as opposed to drug therapies that treat only symptoms, can address the source of many medical problems. It can clean and dilute the toxin load in the large intestine, reducing the burden on the liver, improving functioning of the eliminative organs, and minimizing the colon wall's exposure to carcinogenic agents. Moreover, the infusion of coffee during colon hydrotherapy has been shown to stimulate the liver to produce glutathione S-transferase, a peptide that picks up and removes a variety of free radicals, poisons, and cancer-producing elements. The combined effect may serve to rejuvenate the immune system while providing a pathway to overall better health.

THE BIOCOMPATIBLE VIEW
Biocompatible medicine maintains that degenerative medical conditions and accelerated aging, which reflect chronic inflammation, start in the colon. Removing the buildup of toxic material and supplementing with lactobacillus products helps promote good bowel health. In particular, lactobacillus acidophilus, a live culture of bacteria known as probiotics, is highly beneficial in this regard, often capable of reestablishing the health of the colon. Lactobacillus dietary supplements are readily available through pharmacies, health food stores, drugstores, and grocery stores.

WORDS OF ADVICE
• Eat the right foods for your metabolic type.
• Find a certified colon hydrotherapist and start a program of regular colon hydrotherapy treatments to remove toxic materials from the colon.
• Drink sufficient water for your weight.

• Take magnesium citrate supplements to stimulate the peristaltic waves of involuntary muscle contractions that transport food and waste through the colon.
• Replace beneficial bacteria by supplementing with lactobacillus products immediately after having colon hydrotherapy.

CONSTIPATION

Constipation is a medical condition in which fecal matter is so tightly packed together that bowel movements are infrequent and incomplete, causing much straining, producing dry, hardened feces and painful hemorrhoids, as well as bleeding varicose veins in the canal of the anus. The old feces stick to the walls of the colon, inhibiting its proper function of absorbing nutrients and instead forcing it to absorb toxins from the buildup and fight parasites that make this debris their breeding ground. The passage through which the feces are forced to travel is also greatly reduced in diameter, causing the stools to become much narrower, sometimes as thin as a pencil.

In Western society, bowel movements of the chronically constipated are often not considered a serious problem. Most doctors are taught that there is no evidence to support the theory that disease may arise when toxic substances from stools within the colon are absorbed and thus do not recognize connections between constipation and a host of other medical problems. But having a bowel movement once every few days, straining for half an hour, and passing black, hard "pebbles" that drop to the bottom of the toilet is an indication of potentially serious medical trouble.

In our clinic, we understand that the most common sign of a toxic colon is chronic constipation and that there can be metabolic, energetic, or emotional factors underlying this condition. We recognize that every cell of the body is affected by self-poisoning, and we view constipation as the body's reaction to diet. When the toxins accumulate in the nervous system, people feel irritable and depressed. If they reach the stomach, people feel bloated; if they reach the lungs, the breath is foul; if they escape through the skin, rashes and blotches develop, or people look pale and their skin appears wrinkly; if they make it to the glands, people feel fatigued, have reduced sex drive, or may appear much older than they actually are.

Constipation is caused by a disturbance in the normal functions of the colon, which are to remove water from the waste material that passes from the small intestine into the colon, to serve as a storage area for waste material, and to help move and expel stool from the body. In our clinic, we see constipation occurring because of dehydration that causes the colon to absorb water from food, producing dry or hard stools, and, as a result of not eating foods beneficial for metabolic type, causing stool to move too slowly through the colon, interfering with the person's ability to expel stool.

All these colon problems set the stage for hemorrhoids, abnormally swollen veins in the rectum and anus. Hemorrhoids occur when there is too much pressure in the rectum, forcing blood to stretch and bulge the walls of the veins, sometimes rupturing them. The most frequent causes of hemorrhoids are constant sitting, straining from constipation or hard stools, diarrhea, sitting on the toilet for a long time, severe coughing, childbirth, or incorrectly lifting heavy weights. When bulging hemorrhoidal veins are irritated, they cause surrounding membranes to swell, burn, itch, become painful, and bleed.

At our clinic, we start treatment of constipation with colon hydrotherapy, followed by nutritional recommendations that include eating according to blood type; adding brown rice to the daily diet, which cleanses the body while providing necessary B vitamins; and drinking adequate filtered water for weight (see "Dehydration," p. 93). If constipation is chronic, eating a cleansing diet of only brown rice and water is recommended for a day, a week, or longer until the desired level of cleansing is reached, under supervision of a clinical nutritionist.

We also recommend food-based supplements, such as magnesium (see "Energy Refinery," p. 106). The unique properties of magnesium oxide, when mixed with water and drunk, allow it to release large amounts of oxygen in the intestinal tract, which encourages healthy, oxygen-loving (aerobic) bacteria while inhibiting the growth of unhealthy bacteria and fungi (*Candida albicans*). Magnesium oxide's main cleansing benefits are derived from its ability to promote hydration. Once the oxygen is released from the magnesium oxide, it reacts with hydrogen to form water inside the intestinal tract, a process that helps soften the impacted fecal matter. Thus, the undigested and putrefying material that has stuck to the colon wall, blocking the absorption of nutrients and creating a source of toxicity, is eliminated safely, gently, and painlessly, unlike many laxatives, which are too aggressive, can be habit forming, and have been associated with bowel cancer. Even some herbal laxatives contain a form of mycotoxin, a mild poison that irritates the bowel wall, inducing the body to get rid of it by purging, often causing pain and, if used a long time, damaging the bowel lining.

In addition, we recommend taking probiotics, microorganisms consumed in specially designed foods that enhance digestion; aid in the absorption of protein, fat, calcium, and phosphorus; as well as produce their own lactase and help manage lactose intolerance. There are nine types of lactobacillus, which include lacto acidophilus, bifidus, rhamnosus, plantarum, salivarius, bulgaris, lactis, casei, and brevis. The most common forms for probiotics are dairy products and probiotic-fortified foods, such as live yogurt, which many people ingest to enhance their intestinal flora and aid digestion. Tablets and capsules containing the probiotic bacteria in freeze-dried form are also available, although capsules may be more effective because they protect the beneficial bacteria from stomach acids.

Today, such harmless bacteria colonies are being introduced into various environments to prevent harmful bacteria from multiplying, a technique known as competitive exclusion. For example, a recent concept in the maintenance of healthy teeth involves populating the mouth with harmless bacteria that prevent those that cause decay from gaining hold.[54]

Since another aspect of keeping the colon healthy is controlling yeast and *Candida albicans*, we recommend products for this according to metabolic type. For the sensitive stomachs of people with type A or AB blood, we advise using olive leaf extract, which has important antiviral, antifungal, antibacterial, antioxidant, hypoglycemic (blood sugar lowering), and vasodilatory effects. For individuals with type O or B blood, we recommend grapefruit seed extract synthesized from the seeds and pulp of grapefruits. Sometimes also called citrus seed extract, this supplement has strong antifungal properties that help control overgrowth of *Candida albicans* in the colon and vagina (see "Yeast Overgrowth," p. 205).

Finally, we recommend moderate exercise and, for chronic constipation, abdominal massage by trained massage therapists.

THE BIOCOMPATIBLE VIEW
Lack of a bowel movement every twelve hours after eating a meal indicates the colon is generating toxins such as putrescine and cadaverine, compounds or by-products of decaying flesh that acidify the body, stimulate the growth of yeast infections, and produce mucus and sinus infections.

WORDS OF ADVICE
• Eat the right foods for your metabolic type.
• Find a certified colon hydrotherapist and start a program of regular colon hydrotherapy treatments to remove toxic material from the colon.
• Drink sufficient water for your weight.
• Take magnesium supplements to stimulate the peristaltic waves of involuntary muscle contractions that transport food and waste.

CORAL CALCIUM
Coral calcium has been heavily promoted as a superior product that provides miraculous health benefits, including eliminating pain, increasing life span, and helping to build a healthy body. Advocates of coral calcium maintain it can make the body more alkaline, but in reality, since there are seven layers to the body's acid-alkaline buffering system, an excess of free calcium may actually lower the pH and make the body more acidic. Advocates also claim that a deficiency in calcium increases the chances of getting cancer; but while low calcium can be seen in cancer patients, the low calcium reading is more typically produced by a deficiency in the patient's protein, and an excess in calcium may actually increase cancer risk.

Moreover, proponents of coral calcium claim that people residing on the Japanese island of Okinawa live longer than many other populations because there is a lot of coral calcium in their drinking water.[55] But while Okinawa does have an abundance of calcium in the water, many other factors may account for the longevity of the community, including the fact that they eat a lot of soybean isoflavones, which, according to various experiments, have properties that help lower the risk of cancer, heart disease, osteoporosis, and offer relief from menopausal symptoms such as hot flashes.[56]

Coral calcium is primarily calcium carbonate, or limestone, a common component of Aruban beaches. It is not easy to absorb this form of calcium since calcium has to be bound to a different organic anion (negatively charged molecule) or to protein; and while the body's anions are chloride, uric acid salt, phosphate, sulfate, lactate from cultured dairy products, and citrate from lime and lemon juice, many people are deficient in organic anions, or they are not metabolizing protein correctly. If this form of calcium is not bound, it ends up as free calcium, which makes individuals more susceptible to developing arteriosclerosis, osteoarthritis, dental tartar (which causes tooth decay), cancer, and high blood pressure.

In addition to problems with intake of certain kinds of calcium, many people do not need calcium supplements because they have enough; they just need that calcium to be pushed into their bones, which requires increased protein intake or improved metabolism. For example, a man came into our clinic whose doctor had put him on calcium supplements when a broken bone in his elbow didn't heal quickly enough. Upon checking his urine, we found it contained calcium oxalate crystals, which could produce kidney stones, and after evaluating his blood test, we knew he had a protein deficiency. We corrected his protein assimilation problem, and within a week his elbow was pain free and gaining strength.

If your clinical nutritionist or heart specialist recommends calcium supplementation following blood tests showing a need for it, the best sources, according to metabolism, are: for people with type B or AB blood, cottage cheese, which contains magnesium and phosphate that helps them absorb the calcium and pushes it into their bones; and for people with type O or A blood, calcium citrate or malate and calcium bisglycinate, because it is easily absorbed and does not lead to free calcium excess.

THE BIOCOMPATIBLE VIEW
The hype surrounding coral calcium is not warranted since there is no benefit to this supplement. In fact, taking calcium supplements can result in an abundance of free calcium in the blood, which leads to increased acidity and a degenerative condition when the calcium is deposited in inflamed tissue, contributing to spurs and calcified joints.

WORDS OF ADVICE
• Do not believe the hype that coral calcium supplementation leads to miraculous health and longevity.
• If you have taken coral calcium in the recent past, supplement with magnesium and zinc to force any free calcium back into the bones.

D

DEHYDRATION

As a private pilot of a single-engine, four-seat airplane unequipped with a bathroom, the last thing I want while flying from Aruba to Curaçao is to be distracted by a call of nature just as I am communicating with an international airport. Although the easy solution is to limit my drinking before I fly, I realize that air travelers who do not drink enough water can become dehydrated and that dehydration can take a toll on the body.

Dehydration can be caused by not drinking enough water, losing too much fluid through perspiration, or having the body robbed of water reserves in joints and blood by drinking beverages containing caffeine such as coffee or tea, and all fruit juices except apple juice, which cause excess urine production yet gives the person an illusion of not being thirsty. Unfortunately, advertisements tell us we can quench our thirst with tea, coffee, soft drinks, sugary juices, or alcoholic beverages that not only taste much better than water but add sex appeal, and I am told by patients that they feel deprived by having to drink only water.

Because it's not well understood, dehydration frequently continues undetected. Research has shown that people do not become thirsty until they have already lost about 28 percent of their blood plasma, or two of the normal seven quarts of blood liquid—when it is essential to rehydrate or risk having the solids in the blood come out of solution and plug up the circulatory system.[1] Unfortunately, many people do not seem to understand the critical need for sufficient water and thus become chronically dehydrated, especially as they get older. Dehydration creates an imbalance in the inner chemistry of the body. Some cells can tolerate less water content and still carry out their functions, while others, such as brain and heart cells, cannot tolerate even the slightest reduction. In these instances, when the body becomes dehydrated water rationing takes place to ensure that the brain and heart cells continue to receive more blood (and hence water) supply while other cells become increasingly dehydrated.

Dehydration can have serious and even fatal consequences. There are three stages of dehydration, based on the percentage of body water weight lost:

Heat stress—mild dehydration, in which there is a slight rise in body temperature and a reduction in dexterity and coordination, visual capability, alertness, and the ability to make quick decisions.

Heat exhaustion—moderate dehydration, symptoms of which include fatigue, nausea and vomiting, giddiness, cramps, rapid breathing, and fainting.

Heat stroke—severe dehydration, a life-threatening emergency characterized by a rise in body temperature above 105°F (40°C), indicating that the body's heat control mechanism has stopped working, leading to mental confusion, disorientation, bizarre behavior, and finally coma.

Pain caused by dehydration can appear anywhere in the body. When one area becomes inflamed from an injury or weakness, the body produces chemicals referred to as P-factors, which send more blood, and thus water, to the area, taking away water from other areas and causing pain.

During severe dehydration, the fluid outside the cells has difficulty performing its two primary functions: providing cells with nutrients (blood) and removing the toxic by-products of cellular activity (blood and lymph). When the flow of blood and lymph slows down, the removal of toxins does, as well. Toxins that become trapped between the cells then contribute to more pressure on the capillaries, gradually reducing the blood supply at the cellular level. The decreased blood supply leads to serious nutritional insufficiencies and other problems, depending on the organs that are most affected. Thus, almost any disease or poor health condition can be caused or aggravated by severe dehydration.

Some of the medical conditions we see daily are signs of first-stage dehydration, including allergies, asthma, chronic back pain, constipation, migraines, obesity, and peptic ulcers. The medical problems associated with moderate dehydration include angina, arthritis, high cholesterol, high blood pressure, heart problems, diabetes, and water retention, or edema—a condition commonly treated with prescribed diuretics, which can make the problem worse—and bizarre behavior often misinterpreted as dementia. Another response to dehydration is hunger, which is why drinking more water results in eating less and losing weight.

Dehydration can be avoided by drinking sufficient water—and apple juice, if appropriate for your metabolic type—as well as eating fresh organic vegetables and fruits, according to your metabolic type. If you weigh yourself in pounds, you should drink half your body's weight in ounces of water per day. For example, if you weigh two hundred pounds, you should drink one hundred ounces, or a little more than three quarts of water daily. If you drink any beverage other than water or apple juice, add that amount of water to your daily intake. If you weigh yourself in kilos, you should drink one liter for every thirty kilos of weight. For example, if you weigh ninety kilos, you should drink three liters of water daily.

It is possible to eliminate many medical symptoms by drinking mineralized water instead of the fluids that rob the body of its precious water reserves. If you are older and have a history of not drinking sufficient amounts of water, see a medical professional first to assess your kidney, liver, and heart functions and determine your level of dehydration. If you are not used to drinking water and find it difficult to drink the proper amount for your body weight, squeezing the juice of half a lemon or lime into a quart or liter of water may make it easier to consume.

Finally, colon hydrotherapy can rehydrate an individual while eliminating dry, hard waste that obstructs proper functioning of the colon and other organs (see "Colon Hydrotherapy," p. 85).

THE BIOCOMPATIBLE VIEW
The usual approach to avoiding dehydration—by drinking lots of fluids, especially on hot, dry, windy days—is incorrect, since only water and apple juice hydrate the body, while other fluids act as diuretics, removing water from the body. Because water is heavily involved in every major bodily function and every metabolic process, the first aim of biocompatible physicians is to verify that an individual's body is sufficiently hydrated.

WORDS OF ADVICE
• Have your tap water tested at a lab to ensure that heavy metals and pathogens are filtered out of your water supply. The United States Council on Environmental Quality maintains that many illnesses are linked to toxins in our drinking water. It is also known that soft water can leach copper out of pipes and that aluminum salts and other substances used to purify water may have negative consequences on human health.
• Research types of bottled water or water filters that remove heavy metals. Many bottled waters are just tap water put in convenient containers; natural mineral water is far better for your health. In terms of filters, carbon filters are generally unsuccessful at removing dissolved inorganic contaminants and metal; instead, choose filters that are rated to remove heavy metals.
• Get in the habit of drinking more water and fewer artificially flavored sweet drinks and sodas.
• Refrigerate tap water to improve flavor.
• If your goal is to lose weight, drink lots of water to suppress your appetite. Many people who want to lose weight fail to do so because they eat in response to what is actually the body's thirst signal.
• To ease your consumption of water, add a squeeze of lemon or lime juice, especially if you have type A blood.
• Use a straw if you enjoy seeing your water disappear more quickly.

DEMENTIA
The word *dementia*, which is derived from the Latin stem *dement*, meaning "mind away," refers to the deterioration of intellectual functions, which can occur while other brain functions, such as those controlling movement and the senses, are retained. Impairment of memory, with short-term memory affected first, is often considered the only symptom of dementia, but the condition can also be characterized by other kinds of mental deterioration, as well as disorientation. Various factors contribute to dementia at any age, including alcoholism, thyroid metabolic disease, diabetes, AIDS, cancer chemotherapy treatments, "mad cow" or Creutzfeldt-Jakob disease, trauma to the head, exposure to toxic metals, and all degenerative brain diseases like Parkinson's and Alzheimer's.

When the condition occurs after age sixty-five, it is called senile dementia, from the Latin *senilis*, meaning "advanced in age." Senile dementia manifests in behaviors such as making rash and foolish decisions, difficulty grasping new ideas or accepting new situations (like developing a resistance to medical care), or becoming regressive and rigid—the stereotypical "silly old woman" or "stubborn old man." Senile dementia can be distressing for families: the affected individual may speak of the dead as if they were alive; their personality may change radically; emotional instability may produce anger, triggered by such trivial incidents such as inability to tie a shoelace; social inhibitions can be forgotten, resulting in aggressive or promiscuous behavior; and moral standards and personal hygiene can deteriorate.

Many doctors erroneously believe that dementia in older patients is a normal aspect of aging, but in fact dementia affects only about 1 percent of people aged sixty to sixty-four and about 30 to 50 percent of people over eighty-five.[2] Also, most people who suffer from dementia do not die from it but rather from a secondary condition such as pneumonia or complications from a fall. Even so, among both women and men in the United States, instances in which Alzheimer's disease or other dementia is listed as the primary cause of death are increasing.[3] Moreover, dementia is the foremost reason given for placing elderly people in institutions such as nursing homes.

The leading cause of dementia is chronic inflammation, which can develop after white blood cells are repeatedly activated to protect an individual against foreign substances, such as bacteria and viruses. Once chronic, the inflammation may become lodged in the muscles, joints, or tissues, permanently increasing the workload of the liver and interfering with its ability to produce glutathione. This enzyme, often referred to as the body's "master antioxidant," is so important to cellular health that its depletion leads to cell death as well as to the progression of dementia and other brain disorders. The brain generates more oxidative by-products per gram of tissue than any other organ, and without the full protection conferred by glutathione it is particularly susceptible to free radical attack.

Professionally, I believe the instigating chronic inflammation is related to diet, particularly the elevated level of fats and low level of antioxidants present in the modern diet of highly processed foods. Over the years, the amount of pro-inflammatory fats in the diet has increased substantially, while anti-inflammatory fats have decreased. Food-based antioxidants also are anti-inflammatory, suppressing free radicals that are involved in inflammatory reactions. The major dietary sources of antioxidants are fruits and vegetables, food groups that, according to studies, the majority of Westerners do not consume.[4]

Steps to ward off dementia include changing the diet to avoid highly processed foods, and instead consuming ingredients rich in antioxidants that are anti-inflammatory, as well as supplementing the diet with vitamin C, magnesium, zinc, lecithin, and ginkgo biloba, and avoiding exposure to toxic substances. It is also helpful to have a hair analysis done to identify heavy metals in the body, especially aluminum, which is found in high amounts in people with dementia. Because of the correlation between aluminum and dementia, to protect your brain from heavy metals it is wise to eliminate products containing trace amounts of aluminum that are likely to enter the body, including cooking pots,[5] most underarm deodorants,[6] toothpastes,[7] sliced American cheese,[8] and baking powder.[9]

THE BIOCOMPATIBLE VIEW

According to biocompatible medicine, dementia, as well as other degenerative brain diseases, is caused by chronic inflammation that affects the brain. It distresses the brain by impairing the liver's ability to produce glutathione. The inflammation is regarded as an outcome of elevated levels of certain dietary fats and decreased levels of antioxidants.

WORDS OF ADVICE

• Supplement your diet with glutathione. It was previously thought that this antioxidant could not be absorbed orally, or that what was absorbed through the gastrointestinal tract was made relatively inaccessible. Biocompatible doctors therefore introduced glutathione by either intravenous injection or rectal suppository. More recently, upon the discovery of glutathione receptors in the small intestine and the mouth, we have begun presenting troches of glutathione to be melted in the mouth, where it can be absorbed by the mucous membranes.
• Consume the substances your body uses to make more glutathione. One possibility might be animal protein that is beneficial for your metabolic type, since animal protein contains the amino acids L-cysteine, L-glycine, and L-glutamic acid, which the body uses to make glutathione. Supplementing with these amino acids themselves, however, has not been proven effective. Other sources of glutathione precursors include SAMe, melatonin, and alpha-lipoic acid.
• Exercise daily to maximize physical and mental functioning and to maintain a healthy weight.
• If you are already experiencing symptoms of dementia, maintain a familiar and safe environment to minimize confusion.
• Engage in as much mental activity as possible, such as puzzles, games, reading, and hobbies and crafts, since mental activity is believed to slow the progress of some types of dementia.
• Participate in social interaction for stimulation, such as activities at senior or community centers.

DIABETES TYPE II

The World Health Organization (WHO) estimates that by 2025 the number of people with diabetes will reach 300 million—a staggering 122 percent increase over less than thirty years, with the greatest increase projected to occur between 1995 and 2025 in North and South America.[10] Health departments the world over recognize the condition as a primary cause of kidney disease,[11] adult blindness,[12] limb amputations unrelated to trauma,[13] and cardiovascular diseases.[14] Diabetes is already one of the top causes of death in Aruba, the United States, and Europe.

Diabetes occurs more often among certain ethnic groups. Native Americans, Hispanic-Latino Americans, and African Americans show an increased suscep- tibility compared to the non-Hispanic white population. More specifically, when leading causes of death are examined by race, diabetes ranks as the seventh leading cause among whites, Chinese, and Filipinos; the sixth leading cause among blacks, Hispanics, and Japanese; the fifth leading cause among Hawaiians; and the fourth leading cause among American Indians.[15] In Aruba, type II diabetes is a major epidemic exacerbated by Native American genes that are highly sus- ceptible to insulin resistance, high alcohol consumption, smoking, and a diet overloaded with white bread.

Today, more than eighty years after the discovery of insulin, we are just beginning to understand the complexity of a disease process in which almost every aspect of the body's metabolism malfunctions. Diabetes is misunderstood as a simple sugar imbalance that can be readily corrected through medical inter- vention, when in fact it is a complex metabolic disorder with serious implications for vision, cardiovascular health, kidney, and neural functions. Its expression largely depends on lifestyle issues such as diet, weight management, and physical exercise that add to an underlying genetic susceptibility.

Type II diabetes, the most common form of this condition, is also known as adult-onset diabetes. Everyone who develops type II diabetes initially has insulin resistance. The preclinical stage of type II diabetes is Insulin Resistance, previously called metabolic syndrome, or syndrome X—identified by metabolic changes that progress over years, characterized by increased resistance to insulin, the regulatory hormone that suppresses liver glucose output and removes excess glucose from the blood. During this preclinical stage the body is making insulin, but the insulin is not available to the cells to convert glucose to energy.

The risk of developing type II diabetes is highest among obese people with excess body weight around the waist. Among such individuals, the liver becomes resistant to the hormone insulin and its ability to suppress liver glucose production. Under these conditions, the excess insulin turns the liver into a "fat-producing factory," causing disturbances in metabolism that are devastating to blood sugar balance and weight management. It is the acceleration of this negative cycle, including the decline of pancreatic insulin production, that heralds type II diabetes.

In our clinic, we manage type II diabetes by examining the diet to discover which foods are most responsible for insulin resistance. Specific foods for each metabolic type result in abnormal blood reactions and insulin resistance. For example, gluten in wheat provokes a reaction in the blood, causing insulin to become trapped and thus unavailable to transport glucose into the cells. Nicotine also causes abnormal blood reactions, and consequently smokers and individuals who chew tobacco are more insulin resistant than those who have stopped using tobacco products. Grain alcohol consumption causes a similar blood reaction.

THE BIOCOMPATIBLE VIEW

Biocompatible medicine considers type II diabetes a metabolic disorder and corrects dietary and metal imbalances. Hair tests generally show that diabetic individuals have low nickel, high selenium, high sodium, either high or very low magnesium, low chromium, low sulfur, and low potassium levels, reflecting difficulty in regulating blood sugar.

WORDS OF ADVICE
- Do not let your doctor check your blood glucose levels without also checking your blood insulin levels, since a high blood glucose level with a high insulin level means you are not utilizing insulin efficiently but does not mean you have type II diabetes.
- If you are overweight and have a family history of type II diabetes, get professional help for possible carbohydrate addiction.

DIETING
Dieting can seem like walking briskly in the direction of a goal while watching it recede in the distance, since many people who diet to lose weight or drop clothing sizes end up getting fatter—that is, increasing their total percentage of body fat. Some individuals who say they have lost weight have in fact lost muscle (which weighs more than fat) or water (which weighs more than muscle). Then as soon as they stop dieting, the weight comes right back, often with extra fat.

Another problem with dieting is that many people believe losing weight merely involves reducing food intake, following a fad diet, taking pills that burn fat, or worse, having injections or fly-by-night acupuncture treatments that endanger the tenth cranial vagus nerve, which controls not only appetite but other functions of the digestive tract, as well as the larynx and the heart.

For a healthy perspective on dieting, it is first necessary to consider the logic of body mass index (BMI). BMI is a measurement of the ratio of weight (in kilograms) divided by the square of height (in meters): BMI = kg/m2. To figure out your BMI, using a calculator divide your weight by your height squared. For instance, if you weigh 70.5 kilograms and are 1.82 meters tall, dividing 70.5 by 3.3124 (the square of your height) results in a BMI 21.3. (See "http://nhlbisupport.com/bmi/" http://nhlbisupport.com/bmi/ or other Web sites offering BMI calculators.) If you know your measurements in pounds and inches the steps to calculate your BMI is:

- Multiply your weight in pounds by 703.
- Divide that number by your height in inches.
- Divide that number by your height in inches again.

Among adults, a BMI greater than 30 is considered obese; between 25 and 29.9 is overweight; between 18.4 and 24.9 is healthy; and less than 18.5 is underweight. So while a wide range of weights is compatible with good health, only a defined spectrum of BMI values is. A BMI greater than 25 increases the risk of cancer, diabetes, and even death. A BMI less than 18.5 indicates the need to consult a clinical nutritionist to start putting on some fat; individuals lacking sufficient fat reserves to carry them through a medical crisis are at increased risk of dying spontaneously, especially if cholesterol levels are also low. People with BMIs between 19 and 22, a minority, live longest, although recently the United States government changed the optimum range to between 20 and 24, most likely to account for the increased incidence of obesity in the population.

Losing weight effectively requires planning, understanding, and the self-discipline needed to prevent muscles from being cannibalized by the body. The body continually breaks down and rebuilds muscles to match physical activity; so when a person greatly reduces their caloric intake without engaging in increased physical activity, especially weight-bearing exercise, the body converts muscle rather than fat stores into energy. As a result, the person will lose muscle and end up with proportionately more fat than muscle. To preserve muscle and force the body to use fat reserves instead, it is essential to increase physical activity. Acupuncture treatment that does not endanger the function of the vagus, or pneumogastric, nerve can help restore the body's energetic balance and significantly enhance a realistic weight loss program.

THE BIOCOMPATIBLE VIEW

Because one of the body's defenses is to sequester heavy metals, solvents, insecticides, pesticides, and petrochemical product contaminants in fat cells, including those of the brain, which is 80 percent fat, rapid loss of fat can expose individuals to a host of toxins that could negatively affect health. In dieting it is important to lose belly and hip fat, not brain cells or muscle.

WORDS OF ADVICE

• Detoxify before losing weight.
• While dieting, consume the ideal protein source for your metabolic type and drink plenty of water.
• During dieting, exercise to protect muscle while burning fat.

DIVERTICULITIS

Diverticulitis is a condition in which intestinal inflammation causes the colon walls to collapse into pockets of infected material, resulting in severe abdominal pain, often with fever and constipation. Each individual pocket is called a diverticulum and viewed as a pouch or sac formed in the lining of the mucous membrane where the bowel wall was ruptured. The toxins released from food trapped within the each pocket contribute to further infection, to which the body responds by becoming more acidic, thereby increasing the inflammation.

Doctors report that over 50 percent of Westerners possess diverticuli, which can be a serious problem if they forge a passageway between the colon and the bladder.[16] The presence of diverticuli is also dangerous for people who have had residual fecal material trapped in these pockets for a long time, possibly for decades, since the poisons consistently leak into the blood and lymphatic systems.

A major cause of diverticulitis is poor digestion, which results in two major problems: food is not broken down into the elemental building blocks necessary for the body to restore itself and generate energy, and remnants of food remain in the gut, leading to any of several pathological reactions. Poor digestion irritates the intestines, increasing the rate at which material crosses the cells in the intestinal wall. Undigested protein that leaks into the lymph system—a condition known as "leaky gut syndrome"—can then enter the general circulation. The immune reaction system reacts to the foreign invaders, becomes overtaxed, and deteriorates. With depleted oxygen and fuel, the immune cells wear out faster and do not reproduce properly.

Undigested food can also become a breeding ground for parasites and *Candida albicans*, yeast cells that produce toxins capable of increasing digestion dysfunction, food allergies, and fatigue, further depressing the immune system. The resulting inflammation produces free radicals as waste by-products. These negatively charged oxygen molecules then begin chopping holes in cell membranes in an attempt to grab a positive charge, resulting in further damage to the intestinal walls and ever-increasing permeability. The longer the "leaky gut syndrome" continues, the more food particles enter the bloodstream.

Many doctors prescribe increased fiber for this condition. But such treatment must be undertaken with caution, since people with different blood types react differently to various types of fiber, leading to particular bacteria and blood group antigens in the colon. For example, individuals with type O blood who use an over-the-counter wheat product to increase fiber will feel worse because wheat husks thicken their blood and produce gas. Brown rice, however, works well for all blood types.

An excellent treatment for diverticulitis recommended by our clinic is colon hydrotherapy, a safe medical procedure that detoxifies the colon with clean water and is a healing technique for irritable bowel syndrome with gas and bloating, chronic constipation, and abdominal discomfort (see "Colon Hydrotherapy," p. 85). In addition to administering colon hydrotherapy, we replace the beneficial bacteria in the colon. *Lactobacilli,* one of the most important types of friendly bacteria, inhibit the growth of unfriendly bacteria by producing lactic acid, increasing the acidity of the digestive tract. *Lactobacilli* also help normalize cholesterol levels, control *Candida albicans*, and relieve anxiety and depression by releasing the amino acid tryptophan, the precursor to 5-hydroxythyrtophan that metabolizes into serotonin and dopamine. After these procedures and cleansing with a brown rice diet for a short-term return to health, we advise slowly adding the vegetables, fruits, and lean proteins for the individual's metabolic type.

THE BIOCOMPATIBLE VIEW
Toxins produced from food trapped in pockets of the colon contribute to infection. The body responds to such infection by becoming more acidic, in turn stepping up chronic inflammation.

WORDS OF ADVICE
• Eat according to your metabolic type to avoid poor digestion.
• Start a program of colon hydrotherapy to remove toxins from the colon.
• Drink plenty of water, or apple juice if it is appropriate for your metabolic type.

• Avoid processed or refined foods, such as white flour and white rice.
• Supplement with magnesium to soften your stool.
• Exercise regularly to help the muscles in your intestine retain tone, which encourages regular bowel movements.
• When constipated, do not use suppositories or strong herbal laxatives containing senna (*Cassia senna*), because your system may become addicted to them.

E

EDTA CHELATION

EDTA (ethylenediaminetetraacetic acid) is a synthetic amino acid developed between 1934 and 1935 by Ferdinand Munz in Germany's I.G. Farbenindustrie laboratories as a substitute for amino acids in textile processing. Introduced in the United States in 1948, EDTA became recognized by the medical community in the 1950s as a treatment for snake venom poisoning, digitalis intoxication, cardiac arrhythmia, and heavy metal and radiation toxicity. Today, because EDTA has an ability to bind with most metal ions, the food industry uses it as an additive since it reacts with unwanted metals that spoil food and removes the metallic taste that comes from metals included during processing. EDTA is added to many commercial beers to stabilize foaming; to typical iron fortification compounds in cereals to increase adults' absorption of iron; and to many shampoos and cosmetics for the blue color of the copper-EDTA complex.

In biocompatible medicine, EDTA's ability to bind with, or grab, metal ions is called chelation, from the Greek word *chelè*, meaning "claw." It is used by biocompatible doctors to remove undesirable metals from the body and thereby reverse the detrimental effects of heavy metal toxicity. Removing heavy metals from the body can ultimately reverse the development of arteriosclerosis; alleviate cerebrovascular arterial occlusion; improve memory, concentration, and vision; ameliorate gangrene; and prevent or reverse problems associated with degenerative diseases.

The presence of heavy metal, detected by physicians who use blood, urine, or hair diagnostics, can be found in the bodies of most people today. For example, in a study conducted by the Mount Sinai School of Medicine in New York, in collaboration with the Environmental Working Group and Commonwealth, researchers found an average of ninety-one industrial compounds, pollutants, and other chemicals in the blood and urine of nine volunteers who did not work with chemicals on the job or live near an industrial facility.[1] Worse, in a study organized by the Environmental Working Group in collaboration with Commonweal, researchers discovered an average of two hundred industrial chemicals and pollutants in umbilical cord blood from ten babies born in United States hospitals in August and September of 2004. Their umbilical cord blood, collected after the cord was cut, harbored pesticides, consumer product ingredients, and wastes from burning coal, gasoline, and garbage.[2]

These findings are not surprising given the fact that the United States annually manufactures over one million pounds of the more than three thousand chemicals toxic to the human body, classified as the following:

Dioxins—By-products of PVC (polyvinyl chloride) production, industrial bleaching, and incineration, these persist for decades in the environment, are very toxic to the developing endocrine (hormone) system, and cause cancer.

Furans—By-products of plastics production, industrial bleaching, and incineration, furans persist for decades in the environment, are very toxic to the developing endocrine (hormone) system, and are likely to cause cancer.

Metals—Lead, mercury, arsenic, and cadmium, at doses found in the environment, can cause lowered IQ, developmental delays, behavioral disorders, and cancer. Most exposures to lead are from lead paint. Occupational exposure occurs in relation to other sources as well, affecting construction workers, steel welders, bridge reconstruction workers, firing range instructors and cleaners, remodelers and refinishers, foundry workers, plumbers, scrap metal recyclers, auto repairers, and cable splicers. These laborers also expose their families due to the "take-home lead" on their work clothes. Hobbyists, too, may be exposed to lead, from casting bullets or fishing sinkers, remodeling homes, shooting targets at firing ranges, soldering, repairing autos, and making stained glass or glazed pottery. Additionally, individuals who use certain folk remedies, especially from India or Vietnam, or who consume moonshine whiskey or eat from ceramic ware, are at risk.

Exposures to mercury arise primarily from canned tuna. For arsenic, most exposures are from treated lumber and contaminated drinking water. For cadmium, major sources of exposure include cigarette smoke, nickel-cadmium batteries that are opened, plastic bottles and bottle caps, pigments, and bakeware.

Organochlorine insecticides—These pesticides (DDT, chlordane, and others) are largely banned in the United States, but they persist for decades in the environment, accumulate up the food chain to humans, and cause cancer and numerous reproductive effects.

Organophosphate insecticide metabolites—Breakdown products of chlorpyrifos, Malathion, and other substances, these are potent nervous system toxicants. Recently banned for indoor uses, the most common remaining source of exposure is residues in food.

PCBs—Industrial insulators and lubricants, although banned in the United States in 1976, persist for decades in the environment, accumulate up the food chain to humans, and cause cancer and nervous system problems.

Phthalates—Plasticizers that cause birth defects of male reproductive organs, phthalates, some of which have been banned in Europe, are found in a wide range of cosmetic and personal care products.

Volatile and semivolatile organic chemicals (SVOCs)—These industrial solvents and gasoline ingredients, especially xylene and ethyl benzene are toxic to the nervous system. Some heavily used SVOCs, such as ethyl benzene, can cause cancer.

Scientists refer to the total amount of a person's poisonous contamination as their body burden. "Sam" Queen, of the Institute for Health Realities, teaches professionals how to find the "toxic footprints" of various poisons in blood test results. He has found that the presence of toxic heavy metals may be up to several hundred times more highly concentrated in hair than in blood or urine, because hair levels, unlike those in blood or urine, are not regulated by body activity to stay in balance. Hair is therefore the tissue of choice for detection of recent exposure to elements such as arsenic, aluminum, cadmium, lead, antimony, and mercury. During the last fifteen years, I have successfully used hair tests to identify people's body burden of toxic heavy metals and to screen for physiological excess, deficiency, or maldistribution of elements.

Once the presence of toxic heavy metals has been identified, detoxification is used to remove the contamination and lower the body burden of these metals. First, toxic metals and bone infections are removed from the mouth by a trained biocompatible dentist. Then blood tests are used to verify that the kidneys, liver, and red blood cells are capable of managing the heavy metal detoxification. Finally, EDTA, the best-known heavy metal remover, or chelator, can be used.

Intravenous (IV) EDTA therapy has been cited by mainstream medicine as dangerous due to potential seizures from excessively low calcium; however, properly trained technicians can manage any situation involving low calcium, and despite mainstream medical criticism, IV EDTA mini-clinics have been established, mainly in shopping malls, where a maximum of three grams of EDTA is administered from a one-liter bag over a six-hour period. Recently, chelation technicians in EDTA mall clinics have begun using smaller IV bags, shortening the time needed per treatment, and making treatments more convenient and less expensive. It is important to remember, however, that IV treatments using calcium-EDTA can be dangerous unless administered slowly, allowing the EDTA to chelate before being excreted by the body.

My own method of using EDTA chelation detoxification evolved over a period of time. When I first began, I noticed that our EDTA patients were losing their amalgam fillings, and follow-up hair tests showed a reduction in all heavy metals except mercury. Since mercury is the second most toxic element in the world (see "Biocompatible Dentistry," p. 59), I found these results unacceptable. After trying DMPS (2,3-dimercapto-1-propanesulfonic acid) and DMSA (2,3-dimercaptosuccinic acid) with the same results, I stopped our chelation treatments. I knew the solution was to remove the toxic metals before chelation; but from a toxicologist's point of view, subjecting patients to mercury gas exposure during the removal of amalgams did not warrant the risks. Fortunately, I found in the book *Whole Body Dentistry* by Mark A. Breiner, DDS a safe way to remove amalgams in preparation for chelation detoxification. But I still needed a slower, better mechanism to administer a chelating agent.

Then, while attending a seminar of the Cancer Control Society, I saw a calcium-EDTA suppository and realized the benefits of having these melt slowly into the descending colon, the contracted and crooked part of the large intestine immediately above the rectum. As a certified colon therapist, I knew that absorption of water, minerals, and some nutrients from the stool takes place in this part of the colon and that it would be a perfect place for absorbing calcium-EDTA.

As a result of this knowledge, I started clinical trials of calcium-EDTA suppositories, and within weeks we were verifying that low-dose suppositories were as efficacious as larger IV chelation treatments. Immediately, we began seeing positive changes in patients whose legs had been darkened by lack of blood circulation, as the development of arteriosclerosis had been reversed; improvement in memory, concentration, and vision; and reversal of gangrene in the legs of type II diabetic patients. We concluded that the low-dose calcium-EDTA suppositories had prevented and reversed problems of degenerative diseases.

As calcium-EDTA suppositories gained popularity, they became cheaper and safer, offering a lower amount of EDTA. But the staffs at IV chelation clinics, intent on maintaining the status quo for economic and professional reasons, have claimed that calcium-EDTA has never been shown to provide the benefit of disodium EDTA, that the suppositories are not safe, and that the EDTA in the suppositories does not penetrate cell walls in arteries and therefore cannot get access to the calcium, thus discouraging patients from using this type of detoxification for regaining health. Nevertheless, our success continues: our patients who have used EDTA suppositories for the last fifteen years report vast improvements in the way they feel, an outcome substantiated by their greatly improved blood test results.

THE BIOCOMPATIBLE VIEW

The removal of toxic heavy metals with EDTA and the regaining of healthy ratios between the minerals of the body is a key element of biocompatible medicine, which focuses on the body's metabolic reactions, the assembly of new body cells, and the efficient elimination of waste.

WORDS OF ADVICE

• Have a qualified physician order a hair test before detoxification, to provide a baseline measurement of toxic chemicals in your body.
• Before using EDTA suppositories, have a physician knowledgeable about EDTA chelation test your blood creatinine levels to verify how much EDTA is safe for your kidneys.
• Before using EDTA, either via suppositories or IV, have your blood tested to verify that your liver is functioning normally.
• Before using EDTA, either via suppositories or IV, have a blood test to screen for G6PD deficiency, since EDTA is contraindicated for individuals with this deficiency.

ENERGY REFINERY

To operate efficiently, the body must synthesize approximately thirty different kinds of chemical energy for its various organs and cells, and if even one of these functions becomes impaired the person will lack vitality and feel tired. For optimal energy refinery, sufficient oxygen (see "Oxygen," p. 107) is required, meaning the body cannot be suffering from chronic inflammation (see "Chronic Inflammation," p. 83).

There are two ways for the body to produce energy in cells—one efficient, the other inefficient. The most efficient form of energy production takes place in the mitochondria, special structures in every cell that generate fuel for cellular respiration, according to two processes that both require oxygen: the Krebs cycle (the citric acid cycle or the tricarboxylic acid cycle) and the electron transport chain (ETC). The Krebs cycle was named for Sir Hans Adolf Krebs (1900–1981), the son of a Jewish physician who was forced to leave Nazi Germany in 1933 for England, where he was subsequently awarded the Nobel Prize in medicine for his discovery of the series of reactions that synthesizes 5 percent of biochemical energy while the rest is manufactured by the ETC. Both processes convert the chemical bonds of energy-rich molecules, such as glucose, into energy the body can use, breaking down carbohydrates, fats, and proteins into carbon dioxide and water to generate it.

By contrast, the body is forced to produce energy in an inefficient manner when suffering from acid stress (see "Oxidative Stress," p. 160), which causes the cells to convert glucose to pyruvate then ferment the pyruvate to lactate or ethanol alcohol and carbon dioxide, an enzymatic breakdown called glycolysis, a form of anaerobic metabolism. If most of the material is not recycled back to converting glucose to pyruvate, glycolysis will stop, resulting in death.

The Body's Raw Materials

The fundamental fuel for all bodily functions is adenosine triphosphate (ATP), which has been described as a miniature warehouse of energy because it is made up of three phosphate groups: oxygen, phosphorous, and adenosine. To make this ATP fuel, the body needs to convert raw materials, the most important of which are oxygen, magnesium, zinc, vitamin C, and the B-complex vitamins.

Oxygen

Oxygen plays a major role in the body's energy production. Unfortunately, many people are surviving on a bare minimum of oxygen in their bodies and consequently lack energy. One reason for an oxygen deficit is that, although the air we breathe is almost 20 percent oxygen, most people do not know how to effectively exchange it in the lungs for carbon dioxide. To further understand the process, imagine the nucleus of each cell in your body as a "city" surrounded by "countryside," or cytoplasm, that includes many "refineries," or mitochondria, where the Krebs cycle and the electron transport chain synthesize ATP—provided they have oxygen. Without oxygen, the mitochondria cannot make ATP but instead must convert glucose to pyruvate by fermenting the pyruvate to lactate or ethanol alcohol and carbon dioxide. Moreover, mitochondria made dysfunctional by chronic oxygen insufficiency stimulate inordinate amounts of lactic acid and allow for the growth of cancer cells.

In our clinic, an improvement in health is noted after people have enhanced the amount of oxygen in the body and corrected acidic stress. Aware that breathing efficiently helps maximize the use of oxygen, Phyllis and I, both professional scuba diving instructors, advocate learning how to breathe from the abdomen and also recommend a technique developed by "Sam" Queen of the Institute for Health Realities, who encourages clients to "flap their wings" in the following manner: stand upright; breathe in deeply while raising your arms above your head; hold your breath for a count of three; and lower your arms while breathing out completely. Repeat five times in the morning and before going to bed.

In addition, we educate clients about the need for acclimatizing the body to the decreasing availability of oxygen and understanding physiologic changes that occur when traveling to high altitudes, which include hyperventilation (breathing fast) leading to anxiety, shortness of breath during exertion, increased urination, changed breathing patterns at night, frequent night waking, and weird dreams. Unfortunately, when such symptoms are reported to customary doctors, many miss the fundamental cause—lack of oxygen in the body—and treat the symptoms with pharmaceutical drugs. For example, to treat anxiety, especially in older patients, they may prescribe antidepressants (rather than anti-anxiety medication) and psychosocial therapies, although clinical research findings on their effectiveness is still limited. On the other hand, biocompatible practitioners have found that many times all we have to do to treat a patient's anxiety attacks is teach them deep breathing techniques, which effectively produce the needed oxygen exchange.

Mainstream physicians may also disregard the fact that diminished oxygen in the blood might have been induced by acidic stress, or a drop in the pH level (see "pH Balance," p. 163). "Sam" Queen points out that a drop of a mere fifteen-hundredths of a point (from the ideal pH of 7.45 to a more acidic pH of 7.3) means the blood is carrying 64.9 percent less oxygen, a substantial reduction that creates many medical problems.[3] Again, the biocompatible solution is to treat the underlying cause by effectively moving oxygenated air into the deep lungs, where it can be absorbed.

Magnesium

Magnesium is involved in more than three hundred essential metabolic reactions, including the conversion of creatine into the ATP it synthesizes (MgATP). Magnesium deficiency causes increased levels of adrenaline, which can lead to anxiety and the development of dysfunctional mitochondria. Magnesium deficiency has also been linked to a constellation of conditions including mitral valve prolapse, migraines, attention deficit disorder, fibromyalgia, asthma, and allergies.

Today, many people in Aruba and the United States do not consume the recommended daily amounts of magnesium, due to water type or diet. For example, "soft" water low in mineral content can contribute to magnesium deficiency and other medical problems, such as susceptibility to heart disease. According to the U.S. National Academy of Sciences, more than fifty studies in nine countries point to an inverse relationship between water hardness and mortality from cardiovascular disease. In terms of dietary aspects, one major cause of magnesium depletion is the excessive consumption of soft drinks high in phosphorous.

To evaluate your magnesium intake, consider the following:

Best Food Sources—Berries, greens, nuts, wheat germ, whole grains, yellow cornmeal

Other Good Sources—Apples, apricots (dried), avocados, bananas (dried), beans, beet greens, black walnuts, Brazil nuts, cabbage, cashews, coconuts, comfrey leaves, dates, dulse, endive, figs (dried), filberts, fish, gelatin, grapes, green pepper, goat milk, hickory nuts, honey, lentils, mint, spinach, oats, okra, onion tops, parsley, peas (dried), peaches, pears (dried), peanuts, pecans, pistachio nuts, prunes, rice (wild or brown), rye, sorrel, soybeans (dried), soy milk, spinach, sunflower seeds, Swiss chard, tofu, turnip greens, watercress

If you believe you are not getting enough magnesium from your water and diet, it may be advisable to take a magnesium citrate supplement.

Recommended Supplementation—One capsule of powdered magnesium containing 500 mg of magnesium as citrate oxide daily

Zinc

Zinc, an essential mineral found in almost every cell, stimulates the activity of approximately one hundred enzymes, setting off biochemical reactions. Zinc is synergistic with magnesium, so they work very well together. On its own, zinc promotes a healthy immune system; helps maintain the senses of taste and smell; is needed for DNA synthesis and wound healing; supports normal development in utero and during childhood and adolescence; and facilitates healthy sexual functioning.

The highest concentration of zinc is in the male prostate gland, prostatic secretions, and spermatozoa, amounting to about 860 mcg per gram in normal tissue. Further, there is twenty-five times more zinc found in white blood cells than in red, indicating zinc's importance in resisting disease. Serum zinc levels decrease during pregnancy and following postmenopausal estrogen hormone therapy, indicating an increased need for zinc at such times. In addition, stress, which depletes the adrenal glands, lowers zinc levels. Zinc is excreted primarily in gastrointestinal and pancreatic secretions. Urine, an excretory secretion, contains 0.5 mg of zinc per day independent of dietary intake and urinary volume, indicating that 0.5 mg of zinc is lost daily, unable to be reabsorbed into the body.

Because body stores of zinc (held in bone, the prostate gland, and blood cells) are not easily released for use, dietary supplies are essential, although only about one-third of zinc intake from food is absorbed and delivered to tissues. It is important to remember as well that refined sugar, white rice, and white flour have been stripped of zinc. Also phytates, found in whole grain breads, cereals, legumes, and other products that are not good for metabolic types O and A, can decrease zinc absorption.

Best Food Sources—Zinc is found in a wide variety of foods. Oysters contain more zinc per serving than any other food, although red meat and poultry provide the most zinc in the Aruban and North American diet. Because zinc absorption is greater from a diet high in animal protein than one rich in plant proteins, vegetarians can lack sufficient zinc intake.

Other Good Sources—Beans, nuts, certain seafood, whole grains, fortified breakfast cereals, and dairy products.

Recommended Supplementation—One capsule of powdered zinc citrate containing 30 mg of zinc amino acid chelate daily.

Vitamin C

Vitamin C, or ascorbic acid, is instrumental in enhancing absorption of nutrients; has a vital role in the Krebs cycle and the electron transport chain on the cellular level; and is a chelating agent that helps remove heavy metals. Albert Szent-Györgyi isolated this vitamin in 1937, winning the Nobel Prize in medicine for his research.

Most animals produce their own vitamin C in the form of ascorbic acid, but humans, primates, and guinea pigs have lost this ability. Vitamin C helps protect the fat-soluble vitamins A and E as well as fatty acids from oxidation, can be beneficial in the treatment of iron-deficiency anemia, and is vital to the production of collagen, proteins that make up connective tissue. A deficiency in vitamin C causes the walls of blood capillaries to break down and bleeding to occur in cells throughout the body, producing symptoms of scurvy, including weakness, joint pain, and internal hemorrhaging that causes black-and-blue marks to appear on the skin and red spots around the hair follicles of the legs, buttocks, arms, and back. When the tiny capillaries of the hair follicles hemorrhage, the hair-producing cells do not receive the nourishment needed for the hairs to grow normally; and when gums hemorrhage and their tissue becomes weak and spongy, the condition contributes to periodontal disease.

Best Food Sources—Vitamin C is found in citrus fruits such as oranges, limes, and grapefruit, and in vegetables like tomatoes, green peppers, and potatoes.

Recommended Supplementation—2,000 mg for adults daily. Metabolic types O and B can take regular ascorbic acid supplementation, but metabolic types A and AB do best with Ester-C vitamin C to help protect delicate stomachs.

B-Complex Vitamins

The eight B vitamins that make up what we call the "B complex" are absolutely essential to the body, playing important roles in thousands of different molecular conversions. For one, the B vitamins help in the metabolic processes that release energy from the foods we eat—in carbohydrate, fat, and protein metabolism—and assist in the synthesis of new cells and tissues. Further, pantothenic acid (B5) combines with adenine (part of DNA) and ribose (a constituent of RNA and many other metabolically important compounds) to form coenzyme A, which participates in a variety of biochemical reactions and is instrumental in the pivotal first step of the Krebs cycle.

The discovery of B vitamins occurred in the 1870s, when the disease beri-beri—a term that in Sinhalese means "I cannot, I cannot," the repetitive emphasis suggesting severe weakness—was common in many parts of Southeast Asia. Previously, Europeans had introduced steam-driven mills to Asia and the rice-processing machines hulled and polished rice, removing the B vitamins; the processed rice was touted by promoters as tasting better and having a longer shelf life than the unpolished variety, which they called "dirty rice." With only polished rice available, millions of Asians died of beri-beri, found to be a simple deficiency of thiamine (B_1). In the 1940s, food items such as rice, white flour, pasta, and cereals became "enriched" with vitamin B_1, decreasing the incidence of beri-beri. Eating whole brown rice, with its B vitamins intact, on the other hand, effects a remarkable cure for fatigue that no drug can achieve.

Early symptoms of beri-beri include irritability, fatigue, restlessness, and decreased appetite, while later symptoms are tingling or burning in the extremities; numbness in the extremities; shortness of breath (dyspnea); bluish coloration to the skin (cyanosis); decreased mental ability; unusual behavior; seizures; and loss of consciousness. All these symptoms quickly disappear with vitamin B-complex supplementation.

Another condition caused by B-complex vitamin deficiency is pellagra (Italian for "skin that is rough"), brought about by a shortage of vitamin B_3, or niacin. For a long time pellagra was potentially fatal, characterized as the disease of the three Ds: dermatitis, diarrhea, and dementia. One of the first signs of pellagra is rough, thick, dry skin that is highly sensitive to sunlight and verging toward extreme redness in exposed areas. The skin then becomes darkly pigmented, especially in areas of the body prone to be hot and sweaty or exposed to sun. These symptoms are followed by diarrhea, weakness and lassitude, dementia, and finally the fourth D—death. Classic niacin deficiency occurs mainly in cultures relying heavily on corn but not preparing it in a way that releases its niacin reserves. In Costa Rica, my Native American grandmother would toss a bit of ash from the wood fire into her corn dishes since such ash contains alkaline potash, which makes the B vitamins in corn available for assimilation.

Despite today's increased knowledge about B-complex vitamins, many people are still deficient in them due to physical, emotional, or spiritual stress; eating processed foods that tax the body; ingesting refined sugar that robs the body of its vitamin B stores; the use of recreational and prescription drugs that deplete vitamin B; toxins in the environment and personal care products that deplete vitamin B; malnutrition as a result of not eating the right kinds of foods; and cooking, which depletes or kills the vitamin B present in raw foods.

One of the B-complex vitamins that deserves special attention is vitamin B_4, or choline, which, as a component of the neurotransmitter acetylcholine, supports brain, liver, cardiovascular, and reproductive health, while helping the body absorb fat-soluble nutrients. Choline is fast becoming a desirable part of any health-conscious diet, due in part to a report from the Food and Nutrition Board of the Institute of Medicine that links it to benefits in memory, heart function, liver function, and brain development.[4]

This rich source of essential fatty acids is very important because it helps the body utilize vitamins A, B, E, and K. As such, choline is integral to controlling fat and regulating the kidneys, liver, and gallbladder. Since it naturally disperses fat and cholesterol into smaller particles, choline prevents cholesterol from collecting on the arterial walls and thus keeps food moving through the body efficiently, helping with weight control efforts. Choline also helps produce good-quality bile and resist conversion to secondary bile acids; poor-quality bile, on the other hand, coagulates into gallstones, and when primary bile acids are metabolized by bacteria in the colon, they produce secondary bile acids, some of which promote the growth of colon cancer. In addition, this underrated supplement increases the release of acetylcholine, a neurotransmitter that helps the brain store and recall information.

Choline found in lecithin, a natural derivative of soybeans, is vital for expectant mothers and newborns. Choline will readily travel through the placenta to the fetus, where it plays a crucial part in brain and proper organ development. The latest medical data on choline suggest that augmenting the diets of pregnant women with this one nutrient could affect their children's lifelong learning and memory. Indeed, intake early in life diminishes severity of memory deficits in older age; we also have seen choline supplementation improve functioning in Alzheimer's patients. Lecithin supplementation benefits athletes as well, because it has been shown to increase stamina while minimizing fatigue.

Choline supplementation in general helps prevent liver damage and fatty liver, a condition associated with obesity, diabetes, and heavy alcohol consumption that often leads to cirrhosis of the liver or liver failure in those who drink too much alcohol or have it fermenting in their colons. Researchers, aware that alcohol increases choline metabolism, are investigating the use of choline among alcoholics to assess whether supplementation may prevent cirrhosis.

Choline supplementation is often necessary if the body is deficient in it, because the body cannot make enough on its own. Some medical researchers suspect that dietary supplementation of choline can even change the balance of chemicals that boost intelligence.[5]

Best Food Sources—Brown rice, butter, fish, green vegetables, meats (especially organ meats), nuts, peas, soybeans, whole-grain cereals.
Other Good Sources—Bread, cereal, corn, cheese, grains, legumes, milk, potatoes.
Recommended Supplementation—Since the B-complex vitamins are most effective working together, I do not recommend taking one B vitamin by itself. Further, natural, food-based supplements are superior. I recommend 50 mg for every 75 pounds (35 kilos) of weight daily to start, later reducing the dose to 25mg per 75 pounds (35 kilos).

D-Ribose
From the perspective of traditional Chinese medicine, which views humans as microcosms of the universe, the energy resources of our bodies can be depleted without sufficient d-ribose just as the earth's energy resources can be limited due to overuse. To carry the analogy further, just as raw petroleum is refined and converted to gasoline that can be used by vehicles for transportation, so are glucose, amino acids, and fats refined by the body so they can be used for human activity. The body's primary gasoline, or "energy molecule," is adenosine triphosphate (ATP). The raw material the body needs to make ATP from glucose is d-ribose, a simple sugar. As the exclusive sugar component of ATP, d-ribose is

crucial for preserving and restoring cardiac energy. It also protects tissues from oxygen deprivation, stimulates recovery following a hypoxic or ischemic event, and assists in cellular repair by promoting the synthesis of RNA and DNA. This sugar is the primary ingredient of ribonucleic acid (RNA) and deoxyribonucleic acid (DNA), the genetic materials used to pass on genetic code from one generation to the next to correctly repair the body. With sufficient amounts of d-ribose in the body, ATP moves raw material into and out of cells, both making the muscles function and relaxing them. In addition, ATP produces signals that stimulate hormones, helps detoxify the body, and combines with sulfate to renew and repair the body.

A healthy body can manufacture its own d-ribose from glucose, although this process is slow and requires considerable energy. Individuals with diabetes or a chronic degenerative disease, in particular, do not produce sufficient quantities of d-ribose; and people who engage in strenuous activity can quickly deplete their supplies of ATP. Just as a car without gasoline does not move, a body lacking an abundant supply of ATP becomes stiff and joints become sore, as with arthritis. Lupus, with its characteristic wasting muscles, chronic fatigue syndrome, cataracts, and autoimmune disorders like fibromyalgia, reflects an ATP deficiency that develops because of a chronic lack of d-ribose.

D-ribose supplementation can generate ATP recovery in the heart and muscles, increasing energy and leading to improved health and fitness even for people with cardiovascular problems, athletes who deplete their energy reserves, and individuals with fibromyalgia, or chronic fatigue syndrome. Other reports have shown that d-ribose can also lower blood sugar levels and alleviate altitude sickness and PMS cramping. In our clinic, among people who have been prescribed d-ribose supplements some have experienced a reduction in muscle soreness and cramping resulting from fibromyalgia or chronic fatigue syndrome; older individuals have shown an improvement in muscle health; and all groups have noticed a reduction in fatigue.

I have prescribed d-ribose to patients with heart problems who could not climb more than a few steps. After a week on d-ribose supplementation, such patients reported being able to climb a flight of stairs again.

Further, studies have shown that d-ribose supplementation can shorten post-ischemic recovery time for patients with partially blocked heart blood flow, or ischemia. During an ischemic event, such patients can lose as much as 50 percent of the heart's available ATP, and even after the heart's normal blood flow and oxygen levels are restored, it can normally take as long as ten days for ATP levels to rebound. D-ribose supplementation can cut this time to less than two days.

D-ribose supplementation can also assist in recovery from overexertion. Consequently, I recommend athletes take d-ribose after a workout, to lessen cramping, reduce swelling of joints, and help regain energy.

In general, supplementing with d-ribose can help you experience more energy and less fatigue. Because this supplement is mildly sweet and soluble, it can easily be mixed with water or juice. It should be ingested just before and immediately after exercise or less strenuous activity.

Recommended Supplementation—D-ribose should be taken in doses of up to 5 grams (approximately 1 rounded teaspoon) at a time. Multiple 5-gram doses, separated by 30 to 45 minutes, can be taken without side effects. In doses of 10 grams or more taken on an empty stomach, there are two known side effects. The first side effect is a temporary drop in blood sugar, which can be prevented by taking the supplement with juice. The second side effect is loose stools, which has been reported only by people taking doses greater than 10 grams.

Total daily intake of d-ribose should not exceed 20 grams, or approximately 4 rounded teaspoons. For energy enhancement, I recommend doses of $1/2$ to 1 teaspoon (about 2 to 5 grams). To maximize athletic performance or maintain energy reserves during strenuous activity, slightly higher doses may be required. In times of extended exercise, an additional 1 to 2 grams per hour of physical activity may be helpful. For this purpose, it can be convenient to mix the supplement with water and keep it in a water bottle. If you are under a physician's care or taking medication, or if you are pregnant or nursing, consult with a clinical nutritionist before using this product.

THE BIOCOMPATIBLE VIEW

From a biocompatible perspective, imbalances in the body are inefficient. In particular, an overabundance of calcium, sodium, iron, or toxic heavy metal can disrupt the metabolic processes. The body works best when a stable ratio of minerals is established that optimizes physical functioning. For example, adequate amounts of magnesium in the diet or magnesium supplementation can greatly reduce lead absorption from the intestinal tract and facilitate the formation of magnesium-dependent enzymes that appear in virtually every metabolic pathway in the body, so that binding of magnesium to biological membranes is frequently observed; magnesium is used as a signaling molecule; and much of nucleic acid biochemistry relies on magnesium, including all reactions that require release of energy from ATP. EDTA chelation treatments for removal of toxic heavy metals and the restoration of healthy ratios among the minerals of the body is integral to biocompatible medicine. Equally important is the use of d-ribose supplementation to improve the quality of the body's energy source.

WORDS OF ADVICE

• Supplement daily with magnesium, zinc, vitamin C, lecithin, and B-complex vitamins to comply with the requirements of the Krebs cycle so your body can easily produce energy.
• Make sure you are helping your body convert glucose to ATP so that you are able to process carbohydrates (sugars, starches, and celluloses) efficiently and do not experience insulin resistance. To do this, eat correctly for your metabolic type, supplement with d-ribose to help insulin transport glucose to the cells, and exercise to oxygenate your cells and convert the glucose to ATP.
• When a doctor checks your fasting blood glucose level, make sure your insulin level is checked at the same time, as a high insulin level indicates that you are suffering from insulin resistance. If your insulin level is high, supplementing

with d-ribose can generate ATP recovery leading to improved health and fitness even if you have cardiovascular problems, are an athlete accustomed to depleting energy reserves, or suffer with fibromyalgia or chronic fatigue syndrome.

ENVIRONMENTAL TOXINS

Modern conveniences have a dark side—they can poison the environment and everyone in it. These environmental toxins run the gamut from chemicals and heavy metals to pesticides and petrochemicals.

Chemical Compounds

More than three thousand new chemicals are introduced into the world annually, with over three hundred of them now known to be toxic to the environment. These toxic elements, all contributing to the accumulation of heavy metals in the body, include primary and secondhand cigarette smoke, which increases the amount of cadmium in the body;[6] refined carbohydrates of processed foods, which adversely affect blood pressure, the kidneys, lungs, testes, arterial walls, and bones;[7] and prescription drugs, adverse reactions to which cause the deaths of approximately 32,000 hospitalized patients (and possibly as many as 106,000) each year in the United States.[8]

In addition, chemical pollutants that poison people include PCBs (polychlorinated biphenyls), industrial chemicals that have been banned but are still present in the environment; VOCs (volatile organic compounds), chemicals found in many household products such as drinking water, carpet, paints, deodorants, cleaning fluids, varnishes, cosmetics, dry-cleaned clothing, moth repellants, and air fresheners; dioxins, compounds formed from burning coal, oil, or other fuels; asbestos or any of the other five naturally occurring minerals used widely as insulating material from the 1950s to 1970s and still present in measurable amounts; chlorine, a nonmetallic element, that is a highly toxic, yellow-green gas frequently found in household cleaners, drinking water, and air near industrial sites, such as paper plants; and chloroform, a colorless liquid with an ether-like odor, used chiefly as a solvent.

Heavy Metals

Heavy metals in the environment, such as aluminum, mercury, arsenic, lead, and cadmium, can accumulate in soft tissues of the body and increase risk for a range of medical problems, including cancer, neurological disorders, Alzheimer's disease, foggy headedness, fatigue, nausea, decreased production of red and white blood cells, abnormal heart rhythm, damage to blood vessels, clogged arteries, high blood pressure, diabetes, and inefficient elimination of toxins by the kidneys and liver. The major sources of toxic heavy metals are drinking water, vaccines, pesticides, preserved wood, antiperspirant, building materials, dental amalgams, and emissions from factories and refineries. Aluminum, one such metal, implicated in Alzheimer's disease, is widely used in personal care products and is even found in American cheese. Mercury, another metal and the most lethal nonradioactive element, is still being used by 90 percent of dentists as fillings and is also utilized as a preservative, called thimerosal, in flu shots, children's vaccinations, and B-complex injections.

Infections

Infections that lead to serious health problems can be caused by aspects of our modern-day environment and lifestyle, especially the improper preparation or storage of fast foods, sanitation conditions in crowded urban areas, lack of dental health, and close contact with people or sexual activity. Primary agents of infection are aerobic bacteria, anaerobic bacteria, fungal toxins, and parasites.

Aerobic bacteria, which grow in the presence of oxygen and are vital for health, can also cause a wide variety of diseases. The various types of aerobic bacteria, such as salmonella, shigella, staphylococcus, Campylobacter jejuni, clostridium, *E. coli*, and yersinia, produce slightly different symptoms, but all result in diarrhea and, perhaps, chronic inflammation of the large intestine. Some sources of infection are improperly prepared food, reheated meat dishes, seafood, dairy, and bakery products. In addition to the aspects of modern society that contribute to such infections, many over-the-counter treatments for diarrhea, although designed to congeal the contents of the colon, actually allow the bacteria to grow and invade the body more deeply.

H. pylori, spiral-shaped gram-negative bacteria that live in the stomach and duodenum, the section of intestine just below the stomach, cause duodenal ulcers, stomach ulcers, and stomach cancer. Often the source of the infection is periodontal disease, in which oral bacterial components enter the bloodstream and trigger the liver to make C-reactive proteins, a predictor for increased risk of cardiovascular disease.

Anaerobic bacteria, which grow in environments with deficient oxygen, can inflict serious and occasionally life-threatening disease, most often due to trauma, injury, surgery, or exposure to dirt or feces. Anaerobic bacteria are not present in healthy human tissues because blood replaces oxygen as it gets consumed, but impairment of blood supply due to vascular disease, acute trauma, or acid stress is associated with decreased oxygen in tissues and increased risk of anaerobic bacteria. Also, infection with aerobic bacteria can use up available oxygen, thus making the environment more suitable for growth of anaerobic bacteria. Sites commonly involved in anaerobic infection include the abdomen, lungs, pelvic region, brain, skin and soft tissue, blood, the lining of the heart and its valves, and the gums.

Fungal toxins, or mycotoxins, can cause a wide range of health problems, such as cancer, heart disease, asthma, multiple sclerosis, and diabetes. Major sources of these toxins are peanuts, wheat, corn, alcoholic beverages, and contaminated buildings, especially those that have been flooded and contain mold, to which one in three people has an allergic reaction.[9]

Parasites, which infect more than 80 percent of people in the world, can adversely impact health in numerous ways, including causing diarrhea.[10] The multitude of different symptoms caused by parasites can be baffling to doctors who have received little training in diagnosing and treating them. Many physicians in developed countries do not look for parasites, because automatically treating diarrhea with a broad-spectrum antibiotic is much easier, although antibiotics do not affect most parasites. Parasites are everywhere and can be easily spread through physical contact, including sexual activity or even a simple handshake, lack of sanitation, and colons clogged due to neglect.

Pesticides

According to the Environmental Protection Agency, of the various types of pesticides 60 percent of herbicides, 90 percent of fungicides, and 30 percent of insecticides are known to be carcinogenic.[11] Most health experts maintain, however, that allowed pesticides are low on the list of health hazards and that studies indicate pesticide residues are unlikely to be an important risk factor for cancer compared with smoking, alcohol consumption, asbestos, occupational chemicals, and hormonal and dietary imbalances. Such individuals tend to be looking at the one-time impact of such chemicals on our fruits and vegetables, while those sounding the alarm are looking at the *accumulated* PCB congeners, hexachlorobenzene, and organochlorine insecticides in human fat. The major sources of these chemicals are nonorganic fruits and vegetables, commercially raised meats, and bug sprays.

Of all pesticides in use throughout the world, 38 percent are organophosphates, which kill insects by disrupting their brains and nervous systems. These pesticides, also used in nerve gas and other weapons, can harm the brains and nervous systems of animals and humans, as well.

Pesticide poisoning is well documented. The accumulation of these chemicals in the human body blocks the absorption of food nutrients and increases the risk of cancer, Parkinson's disease, miscarriage, nerve damage, and birth defects. Parkinson's patients alone are more than two times as likely to have been exposed to insecticides in the home. Alarmingly, pesticide residues have been detected in over 50 percent of foods in the United States, and each year residues from intensive use of soil insecticides are found to be increasingly present in mother's milk and human fat.[12]

Latex and Petrochemicals

People exposed to natural rubber latex products can develop reactions ranging from a mild dermatologic rash to anaphylactic shock. Latex toxicity is associated with a severe allergic reaction to proteins found in natural rubber, which come from the white milky sap of the rubber tree. The amount of such proteins in the final product depends on how the latex was processed and how well the products were leached and washed.

Petrochemicals, which are derived from petroleum or natural gas, can be found in such products as pesticides, herbicides, perfumes, fragrances, paints, wood treatments, glues, carpets, furniture, shampoo, soap, detergents, cleaners, plastics, solvents, markers, raw fuels, engine exhaust, alcohol, medications, caffeine, and food additives. Manufacturers of most consumer soaps use a type of ingredient similar to brake fluid called diethylene glycol or triethylene glycol to give the skin a smooth, moist appearance, all the while they are removing the essential skin lipids.

Petrochemicals enlarge the holes in body membranes so that substances inside the cells that could not fit through those holes before can now travel out of the cells and into the general circulation. Similarly, substances outside the cells can now get inside them, causing allergies and neurological symptoms similar to multiple sclerosis.

Latex and petrochemical toxicities are difficult for many physicians to diagnose, and because of the symptoms they produce, none fit together as a syndrome. Symptoms of latex and petrochemical toxicity can be similar to those of traditional allergies, such as headaches, migraines, dizziness, nausea, anaphylactic shock, breathing difficulty, rashes and other skin eruptions, acute abdominal pain, prolonged fatigue, insomnia, neurological influences, loss of concentration, loss of memory, body pains, and even progressive coordination impairment. A further complication is that no single diagnostic test will detect every manifestation of the disorder. Fortunately, a protocol developed by "Sam" Queen, of the Institute for Health Realities, can detect the presence of these toxicities in the body from blood test interpretations.

THE BIOCOMPATIBLE VIEW

When assessing health issues, toxicological perspectives can no longer be ignored, as research points to ever more evidence of structural and genetic damage to the body potentially caused by industrial and agricultural toxins found in the air, soil, and water of today's world. Methods of detoxification have likewise become increasingly important for both preventing disease and regaining health.

WORDS OF ADVICE

• Identify types and sources of toxins in your immediate environment so you can avoid them as much as possible.
• Eat unprocessed, organic, or pasture-raised meat, fruits, and vegetables selected according to your metabolic type.
• Drink and cook with water filtered through units certified to remove heavy metals.
• Avoid vaccines containing the preservative thimerosal, and insist on amalgam-free fillings if you are not working with a biocompatible physician and dentist.
• Avoid pesticides contained in products used for care of homes and gardens.
• Identify and reduce your exposure to the more than 300,000 petrochemicals in today's homes, schools, and workplaces.

EYESIGHT

In the coming years, the number of people affected by eye problems leading to blindness is expected to double.[13] Like the mouth, the eyes reflect general body health, and diseases of the eyes are connected with general health problems. For example, retinopathy, a disease of the retina, the light-sensitive membrane in the back of the eye, in which there is damage to the blood vessels, is a risk factor for heart failure, even in the absence of preexisting heart disease, high blood pressure, or diabetes. Evidence of retinopathy is present in almost all patients with type I diabetes and up to 80 percent with type II. Diabetic retinopathy, the leading cause of blindness among adults aged twenty to seventy-four, is the retinal manifestation of diabetes mellitus, a sight-threatening chronic ocular disorder.

In addition to diabetic retinopathy, diabetics also develop two other eye diseases: glaucoma and macular degeneration. Glaucoma is caused when a fluid called aqueous humor does not drain correctly through the channels at the front of the eye and the buildup increases pressure on the optic nerve, causing damage. Glaucoma can be genetic, with people of African heritage being four to five times more likely to develop it and six to fifteen times more likely to go blind from it, compared with other groups. Glaucoma presents very few symptoms in the early stages, and by the time people notice symptoms, a large part of their vision may already have been lost. Individuals of African heritage can show signs of glaucoma by age thirty-five; Hispanics, Native Americans, and Asians, after age forty; and Caucasians, at age fifty and older. At present, standard medicine has no cure for glaucoma, which doctors control by using eyedrops, pills, or surgery.

Macular degeneration, the leading cause of adult blindness in the developed world, is the breakdown of a small yellowish spot in the middle of the retina that provides the greatest visual sharpness and color perception. Because so many of the activities that define us as productive members of society depend on good central vision, macular degeneration can have an extremely negative impact on quality of life. While many people accept eye problems as part of the aging process, this need not be the case. The National Institutes of Health states conclusively that supplements containing vitamins C and E, dietary lutein, and high concentrations of antioxidants and zinc may reduce the likelihood of progression to intermediate and advanced degrees of macular degeneration.[14]

I look for the underlying cause of eye problems in the body while keeping in mind the disorders and treatments for them that were described in traditional Chinese medical texts in great detail over five hundred years ago. For example, these texts describe the acute form of closed-angle glaucoma manifesting as "dim vision with eye pain resulting from liver wind," noting it causes depletion of the liver and exhaustion of the kidneys, insufficiency of liver chi, and depletion of blood. Age-related macular degeneration is described as the deterioration of vision gradually toward sunset, caused by depletion of the kidneys.

According to traditional Chinese medicine, the eyes are under the control of the liver, so in our clinic we treat numerous eye conditions with herbs such as milk thistle and Rhodiola, as well as dietary supplements like lecithin, SAMe, glutathione—all of which detoxify the liver. Acupuncture also yields excellent results in many people with eye conditions.

Ways to avoid eye problems and to care for the eyes in general are the following:

- If you spend a lot of time using your eyes, such as reading or working on a computer, take frequent breaks, looking at distant objects and circling the eyes clockwise and counterclockwise several times, then relaxing them by covering them with the palms of your hands.
- Avoid or minimize time spent in fluorescent lighting, which contributes to vision problems because it does not contain the full spectrum of light.
- For red, irritated eyes, wash them in the sea or with one teaspoon of sea salt dissolved in a quart of warm water.
- If you are over fifty-five years of age, get an eye exam at least every two years; if you have diabetes, make sure your exams include dilation of the pupils.

THE BIOCOMPATIBLE VIEW

Taking care of the eyes is a first step to preventing vision loss from common eye problems. Since the incredibly small arteries and veins in the eyes are susceptible to being clogged from free calcium, correction of the mineral ratios of the body is a strong tool to help maintain health of the eyes.

WORDS OF ADVICE

- Be aware that eye pain or redness and loss of vision require immediate medical attention.
- Get periodic eye exams that include dilation of the pupils, whether or not you experience any noticeable problems.
- When working with tools, use proper safety eyewear to protect your eyes.
- Consider getting rejuvenating cell injections of undifferentiated ribonucleic acid (RNA) to give your body the raw materials needed for improving eyesight.
- Minimize time spent in fluorescent lighting conditions.
- Take frequent breaks from extensive use of the eyes.

F

FASTING

Every major world religion and many indigenous belief systems incorporate fasting as a means of purification and becoming more receptive to the spiritual dimension. The Bible has thirty-three passages about fasting during Lent, and Pope John Paul II stated that fasting is therapy for the soul, while fasting during the sacred month of Ramadan is the fourth pillar of Islam. Many traditional cultures, including Asian, East Indian, and Native American, have long regarded abstaining from food as a dependable curative and revitalizing method. Hippocrates and Galen prescribed fasting, and it was practiced by Plato, Socrates, and Mahatma Gandhi. In modern Europe as well, many clinics support therapeutic fasting, stressing its ability to bring the body, mind, and spirit into harmony.

Fasting can be a healthy first response to illness, except in the event of a serious condition like tuberculosis, ulcers, diabetes, hypoglycemia, or blood, liver, kidney, or heart disease. Proponents of fasting offer thousands of testimonials from people who say it has helped asthma, arthritis, insomnia, migraines, skin and digestive disorders, and other ailments. Dr. Bernard Jensen, author of *Tissue Cleansing through Bowel Management*, has supervised over fifty thousand fasts at his center in Escondido, California.

There are several popular types of fasting. One is a water fast, which induces rapid internal purification but shocks the system. Another is a juice fast, as advised by Dr. Rudolph Ballentine, MD, author of *Diet & Nutrition: A Holistic Approach*, who says that the average American lacks the reserve nutrients necessary for a healthy water fast and instead recommends using natural vegetable and fruit juices that provide essential vitamins to sustain metabolism and minerals necessary for neutralizing toxins and removing pollutants.

Yet another type of fast is a brown rice fast lasting two weeks, a regimen we routinely supervise for patients at our clinic. With no intake of proteins or fats, the body quickly begins to break down its own excess deposits. For many of our patients we recommend a combination of a brown rice fast and periods of eating light, natural foods, almost exclusively vegetables. Celery, watercress, and alfalfa are all good cleansers, if appropriate for metabolic type.

The timing and duration of a fast depend on a person's medical condition, body weight, lifestyle, and other individual factors. Fasting is not recommended in times of high stress and is done most safely under medical supervision. In preparation for fasting, reduce quantity and complexity of food types several days before all solid food is eliminated. Also consider colon hydrotherapy before the fast, to rid the body of toxins. While fasting, drink at least three liters of water per day to wash your system internally. During the first two days of fasting, when you may feel weak and out of sorts, it is helpful to be alone or with supportive loved ones, and to rest.

THE BIOCOMPATIBLE VIEW

Today, the self-interest of the food and drug industries, combined with the inclination of most individuals to choose immediate gratification over long-term well-being, prevents most people from achieving optimal health. Fasting can help maintain health because within twenty-four hours of cutting back food, intake enzymes stop entering the stomach and travel instead into the intestines and bloodstream, where they circulate and break down waste matter, including dead and damaged cells, unwelcome microbes, and pollutants. As proteins they also cause the body's chemical processes to advance rapidly. At the same time, the tissues of all organs and glands are purified and their functions balanced, the entire alimentary canal is swept clean, and immunity is strengthened, resulting in the restoration of health and the disappearance of disease.

WORDS OF ADVICE

• If you are new to fasting, begin slowly, choose a restful time in your life, and preferably request medical supervision.
• Before starting a fast, have a colon hydrotherapy treatment to cleanse your bowels of pathogens.
• When not under stressful conditions, precede the fast with a cleansing fast, ingesting celery, watercress, and alfalfa if they are on the food list for your metabolic type, and drinking only pure, noncarbonated mineral water for one or two days.
• Practice dry skin brushing daily, unless you have varicose or thread veins, also known as spider veins.
• During your fast, practice deep breathing exercises and take short walks in the fresh air every day; also stimulate your senses with beautiful music and enjoy quiet reflection.
• During your fast, get plenty of rest.
• While fasting, drink at least three liters of water per day.

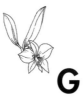

G

GALLBLADDER AND LIVER PROBLEMS

Common gallbladder and liver problems include gallstones and primary biliary cirrhosis of the liver. To understand the importance of liver health, it helps to comprehend the liver's functions. The liver plays a major role in metabolism and has a number of functions in the body, including warehousing the principal storage form of glucose, called glycogen; making blood plasma proteins that carry cholesterol, hormones, vitamins, and minerals and help regulate body tissue that lacks distinct cells; aiding the functioning of the immune system; producing bile, which is stored in the gallbladder, is important in digestion, and acts to break open fats so they can be digested by enzymes, as well as aiding in the absorption of fat-soluble vitamins D, E, K, and A; and detoxifying the body by neutralizing harmful chemicals that are then excreted through the gallbladder, bile, bowel movements, kidneys, and urine. When the liver's detoxification system is overloaded, toxins accumulate in the body, undermining many essential functions, particularly those of the immune system, and therefore causing chronic health problems. An over-burdened and also undernourished liver can be a root cause of many diseases.

There are two main types of liver damage: gallstones developed from retained bile salts in the liver and primary biliary cirrhosis. Conventional medicine maintains that gallstones occur in people with "5F" characteristics—female, fat, forty, fertile, and flatulent—and are most common among Native Americans and both males and females over age forty. Other risk factors include ethnic and hereditary predispositions, such as diabetes or liver cirrhosis. In our clinic, patients' symptoms have included abdominal fullness or gas, or severe belly pain on the right side or upper middle of the abdomen. In uncomplicated cases, the pain can occur after eating or drinking fatty substances, worsen during deep breathing, and radiate to the back or below the right shoulder blade. Other symptoms include fever, nausea and vomiting, heartburn, chills and shaking, or chest pain under the breastbone.

Doctors tend to believe that in most cases prevention of gallstones is not possible although reducing the intake of fatty foods and losing weight might lessen symptoms in people with gallbladder disease. In fact, surgeons in the United States remove nearly one million gallbladders per year, yet gallbladder removal does not correct the underlying problem. As a biocompatible physician, I believe prevention of gallstones is possible after taking into account their known causes. For example, women with higher blood levels of vitamin C and zinc are less likely to develop gallstones. In addition, physical activity, dietary monounsaturated fats, dietary cholesterol, and dietary fibers from cellulose are inversely associated with the risk of gallstone formation. Researchers report that a high body mass index (BMI) and intake of refined sugars and saturated fats are directly associated with a risk of gallstone formation.[1] Gallstones and other gallbladder problems are also linked to the use of oral contraceptives or having too much copper or estrogen in the body.

The generic medicine ursodiol, a naturally occurring bile salt, may shrink gallstones. Bile salts are made in the liver and flow down the bile ducts to the intestine, where they help individuals digest the fats in foods. Although some bile salts are toxic if retained in the liver, ursodiol, when taken as a medication, replaces them. The resulting bile may be superior enough to dissolve gallstones.

In our clinic, we also put everyone on a diet according to blood type and start them on food-based supplements. If, among those with gallbladder disease, we do not see dramatic results quickly, we include the amino acid taurine, available at health food stores. An adult of average size should take 1,000 mg daily with meals to thin the bile in the gallbladder. This thinned bile dissolves the sludge and allows it to exit the gallbladder so it can perform its main function, which is to emulsify fats so they can be absorbed.

As a certified clinical nutritionist, I know that certain nutrients taken as supplements will help produce good-quality bile and be beneficial to overall gallbladder and liver health. For example, zinc supplementation (30 mg) and the right ratio (1:1) of omega-3 and -6 oils will release sequestered bile salts from the liver and start the production of good-quality bile, which dissolves cholesterol gallstones and prevents gallstone formation during rapid weight loss.

In addition, it is very important to increase the intake of the omega-3 fats found in fish oil and cod liver oil and reduce the intake of omega-6 fats. Although both types of fat are essential for human health, the typical Aruban and American consumes far too many omega-6 fats in their diet from corn, soy, canola, safflower, and sunflower oil, while consuming very low levels of omega-3, typically found in flaxseed oil, walnut oil, and fish.

Olive oil also can also be beneficial for secretion of bile and lowering the risk of gallstone formation. Olive oil assists every metabolic type and does not upset the critical omega-6 to omega-3 ratio since most of the fatty acids in olive oil are actually a monounsaturated omega-9 compound. Olive oil activates the secretion of bile and pancreatic hormones much more naturally than prescribed drugs and consequently lowers the incidence of gallstone formation. It also protects against the development of ulcers and gastritis. The only problem is that sunlight, air, and even fluorescent light oxidize olive oil, turning it rancid and detrimental to health, and therefore olive oil in a clear bottle should be avoided, as the process of oxidation may have already begun.

Primary biliary cirrhosis, the second most frequently occurring type of liver damage after gallstones, slowly destroys the bile ducts in the liver, allowing bile to accumulate. Over time, this disease can cause fibrosis and the formation of nodules in the liver and may ultimately make the liver stop working. The most common symptoms are itchy skin and fatigue. Other symptoms include jaundice (yellowing of the eyes and skin), cholesterol deposits on the skin, fluid retention, and dry eyes or mouth. Some people with primary biliary cirrhosis also have osteoporosis, arthritis, or thyroid problems.

THE BIOCOMPATIBLE VIEW

In traditional Chinese medicine, the wood element represents the gallbladder (yang) and the liver (yin). While the gallbladder is responsible for storing and excreting bile, the liver stores blood and regulates the smooth flow of vital energy known as qi. And whereas the gallbladder is associated with indecisiveness, the emotion that creates imbalance in the liver is anger. Biocompatible medicine focuses on the body's metabolic reactions, which convert food into energy, assemble new cells within the body, and contribute to the efficient elimination of waste products—all functions of the liver. When the liver's detoxification system is overloaded, the organ does not function properly and toxins accumulate in the body, negatively affecting the immune system and causing chronic health problems.

WORDS OF ADVICE

- Learn about the possible toxic chemicals in your food and water and how to avoid exposures to them.
- Beware of nutritional deficiencies stemming from unhealthy eating habits that contribute to the production of toxins and stress the liver.
- Do not smoke; environmental toxins damage the liver more in individuals who smoke than in those who do not.
- Avoid using alcohol or taking drugs that can stress the liver, including aspirin, general anesthesia, and antibiotics; steroids; oral contraceptives; and drugs for managing psychotic disorders, high blood pressure, and yeast infections.

GOUT

Traditionally, gout has been depicted as a devil chewing on a poor soul's toe. The image is appropriate, since people afflicted with a gouty toe are in such pain they generally cannot even bear the touch of bedsheets. In the absence of other diseases, such as type II diabetes, gout is primarily a male medical condition, with only 7 percent of primary cases occurring in women. A systemic disease caused by the buildup of uric acid in the joints, resulting in inflammation, swelling, and pain, it usually appears in men in their forties, but in our clinic we have seen evidence of high uric acid levels in younger patients as well.

Uric acid, normally present in human urine only in small amounts, is a compound produced by the body's metabolism of purine—a white crystalline building block of DNA both made in the body and derived from food. Gout develops when the liver produces more uric acid than the body can excrete in the urine, thus putting more uric acid into the bloodstream than the kidneys can filter, usually due to drinking insufficient water or eating foods inappropriate for metabolic type. Over time, the uric acid crystallizes in the joints, most commonly in the first joint of the big toe, in the ankle joint, the knee, or the elbow. Uric acid crystals are exceptionally sharp and easily cut joint, kidney, and prostate tissues. Uric acid also damages the heart,[2] although not through tissue destruction from the sharp uric acid crystals, but through the presence of high blood pressure due to excessive uric acid.[3]

Most medical doctors view gout as a problem stemming from the excessive consumption of alcohol and rich foods, and advise their patients to stop eating rich foods, such as red meat, cream sauces, or red wine, and anything acidic, such as tomatoes. However, a diet designed to reduce uric acid needs to be tailored to the individual's metabolic type and blood test results. Beef, indeed, would produce uric acid in individuals with type A blood, though it is highly beneficial for those with type O or B blood. Similarly, red wine in small amounts is beneficial for patients with type A blood.

Unfortunately, most pharmaceutical drugs prescribed for gout by conventional physicians have side effects including nausea, vomiting, diarrhea, headache, joint pain and red skin rash or swelling, loss of appetite, and even damage to the kidneys. Interestingly, medical studies have found no statistically significant difference between treatment with the uric acid drug oral colchicine and a placebo, other than considerably more diarrhea and vomiting in the oral colchicine group.[4] So predictable is the diarrhea that doctors also use this drug to treat "lazy gut," or chronic constipation, among patients who are refractory to standard medical therapy. Colchicine's laxative effect may in fact be responsible for the subsequent lessening of pain in patients with gout.

In contrast to the standard view of faulty kidneys, clinical nutritionists and biocompatible physicians realize that most gout patients have normal kidneys but uncontrolled dietary habits often unsuitable for their metabolism. At our clinic, we treat gout patients by first checking electrolytes—sodium, potassium, chlorine, and others—as well as calcium levels, which are involved in bone metabolism, protein absorption, fat transfer, muscular contraction, transmission of nerve impulses, blood clotting, and heart function. Following the buildup of uric acid in the blood, the body becomes acidified, and to neutralize the acid it pulls out the alkalizing electrolytes of calcium and sodium from bone, which is the foundation for osteoporosis.

Next, we do a hair test to indicate the body burden of toxic metals, symptoms of which include low HDL cholesterol levels, high uric acid, increased calcium values, and decreased kidney and liver functions. We also check to see if the problem originated in the mouth, through the sustained release of mercury and other metals from tooth amalgams. These tests are followed by identification and removal or detoxification of heavy metals.

Then we establish a suitable diet based on metabolic type. Biocompatible physicians and clinical nutritionists do not attempt to suppress the uric acid by administering dubious pharmaceutical drugs but rather allow the body to deal with it naturally by keeping it soluble so it can be expelled with proper water intake. Pantothenic acid, vitamin B5, and folic acid, together with a natural vitamin B-complex formula, can all help dissolve uric acid crystals, and black cherry juice is one of the best food sources to help the kidneys wash out the uric acid.

In addition, since about 30 percent of uric acid is eliminated from the body by the bowels, we provide colon hydrotherapy (see "Colon Hydrotherapy," p. 85). This more complete form of an enema hydrates the body from above the rectum to the first part of the large intestine, flushing out excess uric acid.

THE BIOCOMPATIBLE VIEW

Biocompatible medicine views gout patients as having normal kidneys but dietary habits unsuitable for their metabolic type, as well as not drinking sufficient water. If the liver responds by producing too much uric acid or the kidneys excrete too little, the individuals will have too much uric acid in the blood and possibly develop gout. Biocompatible physicians treat gout by way of dietary changes rather than pharmaceutical drugs. As such, they acknowledge that reducing the amount of purines consumed—which are in such foods as sardines, liver, kidney, anchovies, herring, mussels, scallops, cod, trout, veal, venison, turkey, and alcohol—may be sensible. If foods high in purine are on the list of those beneficial for a person's metabolic type, they will not cause negative reactions.

The liver's production of uric acid is also viewed as symptomatic of a body burdened with heavy metals that may be obstructing the kidneys' ability to excrete uric acid. A relationship between lead poisoning and gout was noted in the medical literature of the 1870s, and gout as a common complication of subclinical lead poisoning is even described among the Roman aristocracy.[5]

WORDS OF ADVICE

- Since gout is associated with high blood pressure, kidney disease, diabetes, arteriosclerosis, uric acid kidney stones, leukemia, multiple myeloma, and psoriasis, it is imperative to be screened for these degenerative conditions.
- Learn about and correct metabolic imbalances that cause high uric acid levels.
- Avoid stress, which raises uric acid levels.
- If you are male and have a partner, participate in sexual activity to reduce your uric acid level and prevent gout.
- Drink plenty of water, preferably ten to twelve glasses a day, to wash out the urinary system and prevent stones from developing.
- To prevent gout, drink lime juice (one liter of mineral water and the juice of one lime) two hours before meals, which stimulates the formation of calcium carbonate, neutralizing acids in the body, including uric acid.
- Find a physician who will order a hair test to identify the heavy metals in your body, then locate a biocompatible physician to help in detoxification.

H

HAIR LOSS

Hair loss, like eye color, is an inherited trait. For many years physicians believed, incorrectly, that hair loss was inherited only from the mother's father, but medical science has now confirmed that baldness genes are passed down from both sides of the family, can skip generations, and affect siblings randomly.

The genes responsible for hair loss make the hair follicles on top of the head sensitive to the hormone DHT (dihydrotestosterone) and begin shrinking when the person reaches adulthood. As the hairs produced by these follicles become increasingly finer, they fail to grow to normal length, and what first appears as thinning or a receding hairline progresses to baldness when the shrinking follicles finally stop producing hair.

Unfortunately, consumers waste millions of dollars on products and treatments claimed to be effective for hair loss, when in fact hair follicles may be controlled by genetic coding, which is irreversible. In addition, medical science is starting to associate a low androgen hormone level with hair loss, another situation not addressed by products and treatments currently on the market.

In our clinic, we view premature hair loss or lackluster hair as a symptom of underlying health problems rather than automatically the result of genetic coding. When we see a large amount of hair loss, we first rule out malnutrition, or underlying diseases like diabetes or anemia, by checking the person's blood count and iron levels. Then we consider other conditions. For example, hair loss can be symptomatic of a hypoactive, or underactive, thyroid, usually the result of toxic metals or, in women, low progesterone or androgen levels. Moreover, mercury, found in dental amalgams, is especially detrimental to hair, and to the thyroid and skin as well.

In addition, we assess the individual's diet to make sure it is in accordance with metabolic type, and potential digestion and absorption problems due to parasites or nutritional deficiencies, such as iron or biotin. Once we have eliminated foods that are detrimental—not only to hair but also to overall health, such as milk, wheat products, and highly processed foods—we recommend foods that are beneficial based on metabolic type. These may include potato skins, green and red peppers, sprouts, and cucumbers, which are high in silicon and thus strengthen hair and nails.

Blood Type	A	B	AB	O
Potato skins	Avoid	Okay	Okay	Avoid
Green and red peppers	Avoid	Good	Avoid	Okay
Sprouts-Alfalfa	Good	Okay	Good	Avoid
Radish	Okay	Avoid	Avoid	Okay
Cucumbers	Okay	Okay	Good	Avoid

Lean meats and raisins, both high in iron, help control anemia. Seaweed and seafood help boost a hypoactive thyroid.

Then we give advice about imbalances and the effects of natural supplements on hair. For example, whereas a high level of copper makes hair brittle with split ends, insufficient inositol can cause eczema, hair loss, constipation, high cholesterol, and abnormalities of the eyes. The body is able to manufacture inositol from wheat germ, brewer's yeast, bananas, liver, brown rice, oat flakes, nuts, unrefined molasses, raisins, and vegetables.

Finally, we stress that striving for thicker, beautiful hair should not be considered vain. After all, hair loss or lackluster hair indicates nutritional changes are needed to attain not only better hair but better overall health.

THE BIOCOMPATIBLE VIEW

Although the continuously dividing cells of hair follicles are some of the most metabolically active cells in the body, requiring high levels of available nutrients for optimal growth, a diminished supply of nutrients causes decreased hair growth, or hair loss. Because hair is very sensitive to nutritional, metabolic or hormonal, or environmental changes, it is often one of the first areas of the body to reflect disturbances in physiological functioning. Biocompatible medicine seeks to correct such disturbances.

WORDS OF ADVICE

• Pursue a multifaceted response, including items from your metabolic type food list, herbs to treat hair loss, and scalp massage.

• To promote healthy hair growth, take vitamins B_6 and biotin, as well as zinc, copper, and silica. Zinc and copper inhibit growth of the enzyme that causes DHT production. Fifty milligrams of silica a day is thought to encourage hair growth in young men with hair loss; the herb horsetail (*Equisetum arvense*), which contains silica, can be taken as an infusion or a tea.

• If your hair loss is caused by anemia, request a test to find its root cause and seek appropriate treatment.

• Seek the care of a biocompatible physician, who might prescribe the herbal remedies saw palmetto (*Serenoa repens*) and pygeum (*Pygeum africanum*) to stop or slow hair loss. Saw palmetto is thought to halt DHT production, and pygeum influences testosterone production. We are finding that many women who take these herbs orally, as a dietary supplement, are growing much thicker hair. Alternatively, the Chinese herb He Shou Wun (*Polygonum mutiforum*) can be taken by mouth or applied as a topical formula.

• For hair loss caused by hair pulling, known as trichotillomania, consider behavioral therapy. If the hair pulling is triggered by stress, various therapies can be used to promote relaxation, such as acupuncture, flower remedies, aromatherapy, muscle relation exercises, yoga, guided imagery, or counseling.

HEADACHES

Headaches are the most common affliction worldwide, and fortunately, most are not serious. In many Eastern medical practices, especially those specializing in traditional Chinese medicine, headaches have been treated with a much higher success rate than has been the case in the Western world.

Everywhere, treatment for headaches is highly specialized depending on the type of headache a person has, his or her individual response, and any associated health conditions. Western medicine categorizes headaches into eleven main types according to symptoms and measurable biological effects. The first four types, the most common serious headaches, are *vascular headache* caused by brain arteries changing shape; *muscle contraction headache*; *traction headache*; and *inflammation headache*. Other types are *environmental* or *behavioral headaches* caused by such factors as caffeine withdrawal, eye strain, poor posture, or hunger. *Trauma headaches* often result from an injury; *sensitivity headaches* are caused by an allergic reaction to a food, chemical, or environmental substance. There are also *sinus headaches*, *dental headaches*, and *exertion headaches*.

Even though Western doctors recognize the role played by sensitivities to food, sugar, or MSG (monosodium glutamate, a flavor enhancer used in many foods), they most often treat headaches with pharmaceuticals, synthetic chemicals intended to correct chemical imbalances but with dangerous side effects of their own. Western medicine usually sees these imbalances affecting the liver, the endocrine system, or occasionally the nervous system. Frequently, treatment involves the regulation of hormones, since many women get headaches the day before or at the start of their menstrual flow—an effect of estrogen withdrawal. But taking nonsteroidal pain medication (NSAIDS, or nonsteroidal anti-inflammatory drugs, include aspirin, ibuprofen, naproxen, diclofenac, ketoprofen, and tiaprofenic acid) is ill advised and can result in serious side effects or even death. Some of the known side effects of aspirin, for instance, are damage to the lining of the stomach, prolonged bleeding time, wheezing, breathlessness, ringing in the ears, hearing loss, chronic catarrh and runny nose, headache, confusion, nausea, vomiting, gastrointestinal upset or bleeding, ulcers, rash, hives, bruising, abnormal liver function, liver damage, and hepatitis. Taking too much aspirin can also lead to kidney damage; severe metabolic derangements; respiratory or central nervous system insults; stroke; or fatal hemorrhage in the brain, spleen, liver, intestines, or lungs. Each year, NSAIDs-related deaths in the United States amount to an estimated 7,600.[1]

By contrast, traditional Chinese medicine and biocompatible physicians view headaches as reflecting disharmony within the person. Treatment for us therefore involves rebalancing the individual, which will both cure the headache and improve the person's overall health. We also believe that headaches can be caused by the toxic heavy metals that leak from dental amalgams. In our clinic, we treat headaches by first identifying the source of the head pain, taking into account interrelationships between aspects of the body. For example, slow-moving colons produce putrefaction chemicals like cadaverine and putrescine—toxic, colorless liquids with an unpleasant smell that stimulate mucus production in the sinuses and chest and produce headaches. Headaches that derive from this source can be treated effectively with colon hydrotherapy. Headaches caused by metals leaking from dental amalgams, on the other hand, are successfully treated by removing amalgam fillings safely—using protective equipment to minimize absorption of toxic mercury gas into the body—and replacing them with durable, nontoxic composite fillings.

For people who suffer from chronic or migraine headaches often accompanied by nausea, a highly effective form of treatment is acupuncture. Studies have shown that acupuncture decreases the severity and frequency of headaches, works better than using only conventional treatments, and has no negative side effects. Acupuncture used in addition to standard care also results in improved quality of life, decreased use of medication, fewer visits to general practitioners, and fewer days out of work.[2] Migraines can also be eased by resting in a dark, quiet room, or by sleep.

We treat headaches not only with acupuncture, amalgam removal, or colon hydrotherapy but also with herbs such as feverfew, polyporus, goldenseal, and dandelion. Feverfew has been used for centuries as a recommended treatment for headaches, rheumatic aches, abdominal pain, and menstrual cramps; and studies have shown that it acts as a natural anti-inflammatory, controlling the inflammation that leads to cerebral blood vessel dilation, which contributes to migraine headaches. The fungus *Polyporus officinalis* has been used historically to treat chronic diarrhea, chronic dysentery, periodical neuralgia, and headaches caused by nervousness.

Goldenseal, *Hydrastis Canadensis*, also called orangeroot, contains several alkaloids, including drastine, berberine, and berberastine, shown to be very effective at drying and cleansing mucous membranes and thinning the blood, making the herb useful for treating headaches. Goldenseal also enhances glandular, liver, kidney, spleen, and bowel function by speeding tissue restoration, which aids digestion and fights against constipation. Any one of these organ stagnations could be at the root of headache problems. I believe goldenseal offers the greatest headache relief because of its ability to increase peristaltic movement of the intestine, which pushes food along. Being able to promote healthy bowel movements twelve hours after eating a meal is a great headache averter. Fecal bacteria decomposing food left in the body beyond twelve hours, on the other hand, starts producing putrescine, which generates histamines that cause headaches.[3] This is why colon hydrotherapy (see "Colon Hydrotherapy," p. 85) works so well at helping to prevent migraine headaches. Goldenseal should be taken under the guidance of a certified clinical nutritionist.

The fourth popular herb for treating headaches, dandelion, *Taraxacum officinale*, "tooth of the lion," referring to the sharply indented leaves of the plant, dates back to before the Middle Ages when it was used as a folk medicine in the

Middle East.[4] Early colonists brought dandelion with them to North America, where the indigenous people soon recognized its value, particularly as a liver tonic.[5] Dandelion's ability to reduce headache is attributed to its blood-, liver-, and kidney-cleansing properties.[6] Historically, dandelion has been used for thousands of years in China to treat headaches.[7] Its effectiveness is ascribed to the phytochemicals it contains, including beta-carotene, beta-sitosterol, and caffeic acid. These natural substances have been repeatedly shown to cleanse the blood and liver, among other curative actions.

THE BIOCOMPATIBLE VIEW

Headaches often reflect internal disharmony and thus treating them involves rebalancing the individual to both cure the headaches and improve their health in general. Many headaches are associated with the following metabolic disorders efficaciously treated by biocompatible medicine: hypoxia, low blood-oxygen levels brought on by acid stress; hypercapnia, high blood levels of carbon dioxide from acid stress–lowering gas exchange in the lungs; mixed hypoxia and hypercapnia, both low oxygen and high carbon dioxide; hypoglycemia, abnormally low glucose levels in the blood from spiked insulin; and other metabolic abnormalities associated with heavy metals, pesticides, insecticides, and petroleum products. In addition, headaches on the temple lateral to the eye result from a liver overburdened by detoxification.

WORDS OF ADVICE

- Find a biocompatible physician to diagnose the source of your headache so that appropriate treatment can be undertaken.
- Seek acupuncture treatments; they work wonders for headaches and help to prevent future ones.
- If possible, increase the amount of oxygen delivered to your brain. Walking and learning how to breathe better are instrumental in preventing headaches.
- To prevent migraines, avoid foods listed as detrimental for your metabolic type.

HEART ATTACKS

Heart disease and heart attacks kill more people in America and other developed countries than any other medical condition. The American Heart Association estimates that about 6 million men and 6.3 million women in the United States have a history of heart problems. Of the deaths from heart attacks each year, more than half, or over 500,000, are women, a greater number than deaths caused by breast cancer, accidents, domestic violence, and diabetes combined. According to the American Heart Association, "One in three female adults has some form of cardiovascular disease (CVD). Since 1984, the number of CVD deaths for females has exceeded those for males."[8]

Heart attacks are more deadly to women than to men because of difficulty of diagnosis, lack of quick response to heart emergencies, and complications due to concurrent medical conditions. First, heart attacks can be more difficult to diagnose in women because women tend to have fewer typical symptoms such as crushing chest pain and instead are more likely than men to experience symptoms of nausea, dizziness, and anxiety. Because of the difficulty of early diagnosis of heart attack in women, it is important for them, as well as for men, to be aware of the following symptoms so they can get timely treatment:

- Chest pain, which may include discomfort in other areas of the upper body, including the arms, back, neck, jaw, or stomach
- Breathlessness when waking up
- Clammy sweating
- Dizziness or blackouts
- Anxiety, or feelings of impending doom
- Edema, fluid retention and swelling, usually of the ankles or lower legs
- Fluttering, rapid heartbeats, palpitations
- Nausea, bloating, gastrointestinal upset, especially in women
- Feeling of heaviness, pressure-like chest pain between the breasts that may radiate to the left arm or shoulder.

Second, women take much longer to seek medical care when they are having a heart emergency, even one with intense symptoms. Although men seek medical care faster, their greater tendency to drive themselves to the hospital "whilst having a [heart attack] is obviously extremely dangerous both for patients and the general public."[9] Further, once at the hospital, women may not receive appropriate treatment. Electrocardiograms initially make it difficult to tell whether or not women are having a heart attack, and women have more complications from commonly used treatments for heart attacks.

Third, in addition to difficulty of diagnosis and delay in seeking medical attention, women are half as likely as men to survive their first heart attack and, among those who do, are more likely to have a second heart attack within one year. This is because women tend to be about ten years older than men when they have a first heart attack and are more likely to have other conditions, such as diabetes, high blood pressure, or congestive heart failure. Two studies in the *New England Journal of Medicine* show that although women under fifty are less likely than men to get heart disease, when they do it is more severe. In fact, women who have a heart attack before age fifty have twice the risk of dying as a man of the same age.[10]

According to medical studies, reasons given for the higher death rates from heart disease among younger women are that women are more likely to have weakened heart muscle and dangerously low blood pressure; conditions related to artery spasms, such as migraine headaches; diabetes and clinical depression; hormonal abnormalities that make them more susceptible to heart disease, such as problems with underactive thyroid (hypothyroid); and heart attacks caused by blood clots or spasms in the arteries.[11]

Among risk factors for heart attack, some may pertain more to one sex, while others pertain equally to both. Studies show that the risk of heart attack for men increases among those with a tendency toward migraine headaches and decreases among those who drink moderately and do not smoke. One study indicates that middle-aged men who suffer from migraine headaches are 42 percent more likely to have a heart attack than men who do not have migraines, and advises that until the link between migraines and heart attacks in men is better understood, men should reduce other known heart disease risk factors.[12] Many medical studies show that men who drink moderately—two alcoholic drinks per day—have a reduced risk of heart attack. One of these concludes: "Even in men already at low risk on the basis of body mass index, physical activity, smoking, and diet, moderate alcohol intake is associated with lower risk for myocardial infarction (MI)."[13]

Still other studies indicate that men who have stopped smoking for at least two years, even when they used to be heavy smokers, have a reduced risk of heart attack. For instance, results of one study suggest that "the risk of myocardial infarction in cigarette smokers decreases within a few years of quitting to a level similar to that in men who have never smoked."[14]

A potential risk factor for heart attack in both men and women is the type of water in their living environment. Many studies show that "soft" water—that is, water containing few or no calcium or magnesium ions—can be a contributing factor in causing heart attack. Soft water usually comes from peat or igneous rock sources, such as granite, but may also derive from sandstone sources, as sedimentary rocks are usually low in calcium and magnesium. In Aruba there is soft water for a different reason—because the drinking water is distilled from seawater using a process that removes all minerals.

Another risk factor for coronary heart disease is its association with periodontal disease. But some medical studies do not find convincing evidence of a causal association between periodontal disease and coronary heart disease risk.[15] One study states: "Evidence continues to support an association among periodontal infections, atherosclerosis and vascular disease…" It goes on to say that "recommending periodontal treatment for the prevention of atherosclerotic CVD [cardiovascular disease] is not warranted based on scientific evidence. Periodontal treatment must be recommended on the basis of the value of its benefits for the oral health of patients, recognizing that patients are not healthy without good oral health."[16]

By contrast, our clinical experience validates the association between mouth infections and heart problems, and other research concurs. For example, one study asserts: "Our findings suggest an association between periodontitis and presence of [coronary heart disease]. Periodontal pathogen burden, and particularly infection with A actinomycetemcomitans, may be of special importance."[17]

Because we recognize a causal relationship between periodontal disease and risk for coronary heart disease, we send four out of ten new patients for dental treatments ranging from cleanings to oral surgery to extract dead teeth and eradicate infections in the jaws that can leach bacteria from the mouth into the bloodstream, contributing to blockages.

Implementing this philosophy of biocompatible dentistry has led to many improvements in our patients' health, including better blood circulation. This is important because blood vessels are lined with a thin layer of flat epithelial cells that protect the vessel walls, and destruction of these cells contributes to arte-riosclerotic hardening of the arteries. Similarly, other researchers have found that "intensive periodontal treatment resulted in acute, short-term systemic inflammation and endothelial dysfunction. However, six months after therapy, the benefits in oral health were associated with improvement in endothelial function."[18]

In regard to diagnosis and treatment of periodontal disease, when reviewing a panoramic X-ray, which shows in one frame a patient's teeth, nasal area, jaw joints, and surrounding bone, I check to see if either the jugular vein or the carotid artery are hardened by calcium deposits. Several medical researchers have found that carotid stenosis, or plugged carotid arteries, is associated with periodontal disease, noting, "Dental status, oral hygiene, and particularly tooth loss are associated with the degree of and predict future progression of the disease."[19]

In our clinic, we view most of these risk factors not as potential root causes of heart attacks but as symptoms of a basic metabolic imbalance that develops along with heart problems. Further, we believe that the foundation of all dis-eases is oxidative stress (see "Oxidative Stress," p. 160), the clinical markers of which are periodontal disease, physical signs of aging, the presence of any degenerative disease, signs of chronic inflammation, and fatigue. Addressing some or all of these conditions, as well as the basics of drinking sufficient water, eating the right foods for metabolic type, getting enough exercise, and iden-tifying and removing heavy metal toxins from the body, can also help prevent heart attacks.

THE BIOCOMPATIBLE VIEW

Certain metabolic imbalances develop along with heart problems that, if not corrected, can intensify negative outcomes. For instance, nearly half of all heart attack patients exhibit chronic inflammation, putting them at higher risk for heart failure. Other high-risk factors of metabolic imbalance are gouty arthritis and periodontal gum infections—the latter, before age fifty, being a predictor of early death due to heart attack or heart failure.

WORDS OF ADVICE

• Familiarize yourself with all the symptoms of heart attack to avoid misidentifi-cation of symptoms and lack of timely treatment.
• If you experience any of the symptoms listed in this section, seek emergency medical care immediately. Denying symptoms or attributing them to gastroin-testinal upset can delay treatment that could prevent heart failure.
• Visit your dentist or oral hygienist for treatment and for a frank assessment of your oral health. If you have gum infection or pockets in your gums deeper than 3 millimeters, ask that a panoramic X-ray be taken for diagnostic purposes. Otherwise, gum disease, which is not usually painful until it reaches an advanced stage, can go undetected. Regular dental checkups are crucial to diagnose and treat this "silent disease" before it becomes advanced.

HEARTBURN (REFLUX, GERD, AND HIATAL HERNIA)

More than one-third of the population is afflicted with heartburn, and more than one-tenth experience heartburn daily.[20] Although infrequent heartburn does not usually result in serious consequences, when the condition recurs more than twice a week it is considered chronic and should be taken seriously. Heartburn, also known as gastroesophageal reflux disease (GERD) and hiatal hernia, occurs when body parts used in carrying food from the mouth to the stomach malfunction.

At the junction of the esophagus and the stomach is the sphincter, a circular band of muscle that functions like a door to prevent reflux—a back flow of liquid or food into the esophagus, the narrow tube that carries food from the mouth to the stomach—but sometimes it does not function properly. Normally, the esophagus, before joining the stomach, passes through a hole in the diaphragm, the muscle that separates the chest cavity from the abdominal cavity, called the diaphragmatic hiatus. The gastroesophageal junction, the connection of the stomach and the esophagus, is usually below the diaphragm in the abdominal cavity, but for about 15 percent of Westerners the junction and part of the stomach is located above the diaphragm, a condition called hiatal hernia. Patients with a hiatal hernia have a weak sphincter muscle at the gastroesophageal junction that allows reflux, known as gastroesophageal reflux disease (GERD), which can develop into esophageal cancer.

Symptoms of heartburn are burning in the upper abdomen and chest, the sensation that something is stuck in the throat, reflux of undigested food, belching up a sour substance, and nausea, especially in the morning. Heartburn or indigestion occurs when the stomach juices are going the wrong way, back up the esophagus. Severe chest pain after eating is usually a symptom that the stomach is twisting, causing a reduced blood flow—a dangerous situation needing prompt attention.

The number one cause of heartburn and stomach pain is overeating, and consequently, obese people get heartburn more often than others. The second most frequent cause is the consumption of fatty foods, fried foods, spicy foods, carbonated soft drinks, chocolate, milk products, peppermint, alcohol, and coffee, as well as smoking. In addition, heartburn and stomach pain, while commonly thought of as being caused by excessive stomach acid, can also be brought about by insufficient stomach acid. The principle stomach juices are hydrochloric acid (HCL) and pepsin, both of which are required for the digestion of minerals and protein; and the stomach problems of many people, especially those with type A blood, are related to a deficiency in the production of hydrochloric acid, which is known to decrease with age.

Often, medication for heartburn is contraindicated. First, over-the-counter heartburn medication assumes that the stomach has too much acid and floods the stomach with a base, usually a form of aluminum, but if in fact the stomach has too little acid, as in the majority of cases, it reacts by producing more acid. The pain gets better; however, the food moves on without being digested, causing another set of problems. Finally, the stomach "rebounds" by reducing the amount of stomach acid, resulting in a vicious circle that may ultimately lead to colon cancer and other problems.

In addition, some medications cause heartburn by relaxing the lower esophageal sphincter (LES), allowing stomach contents to reflux back into the esophagus. These include the following:

Anticholinergic drugs (for urinary tract disorders, antihistamines), such as natural belladonna alkaloids (atropine, belladonna, hyoscyamine, and scopolamine) and related products

Beta-2 agonists (bronchodilators for asthma), such as Alupent, Bronkaid Mist, Primatene Mist, Proventil, Ventolin, and Ventolin Rotacaps

Calcium channel blockers (for high blood pressure), such as Cardizem, Dilacor-XR, Norvasc, Procardia, and Vascor

Diazepam (for anxiety disorders, seizures), such as Librium, Paxipam, Valium, and Xanax

Nitrates (for angina), such Nitrogard, Nitrostat, Nitroglyn E-R, and Sorbitrate

Opioid analgesics (prescription painkillers), such as morphine, oxycodone, synthetic opioid narcotics, Aerolate Sr, Choledyl, Respbid, Slo-Bid Gyrocaps, Theobid Duracaps, and Theo-Dur

Tricyclics (psychotherapeutic agents, antidepressants), such as Anafranil, Elavil, Norpramin, and Pamelor

For heartburn, most doctors prescribe antacids, drugs that lower the stomach's acid production. People spend millions of dollars on over-the-counter and prescription medications for heartburn, but ironically, using such drugs for more than eight weeks can cause the body to produce an excess of gastrin, a hormone that tells the stomach to make more acid. Many conventional doctors also recommend surgery to tighten the junction between the stomach and esophagus.

By contrast, traditional Chinese medicine and biocompatible physicians treat GERD in different ways, depending on the individual case. For instance, I usually diagnose blood types A and AB with stagnation of the stomach, whose main symptoms are a distended, bloated stomach that feels full or painful, loss of appetite, indigestion, or diarrhea. People with type A or AB blood have the lowest incidence of GERD, although those with type A blood develop more stomach cancer. Initially, stomach problems for these groups starts as gastritis caused by low stomach acid that cannot break down destructive microbes. In blood types A and AB, which do not have adequate levels of acid, bacteria thrive in the stomach and cause inflammation leading to GERD.

On the other hand, I find that the majority of patients with GERD have type O blood and send them to test their blood for the presence of the bacterium *Helicobacter pylori; H. pylori* causes stomach ulcers and eventually stomach cancer. Instead of antibiotics, which cannot reach the bacterium that have lodged in the walls of the stomach, at our clinic we prescribe bladderwrack, a seaweed that entices the bacteria to exit the stomach. Additionally, acupuncture reduces the pain and pressure in the abdomen.

The second largest group suffering from GERD are those with type B blood. Their favorite foods—usually chicken and tomato, both of which are contraindicated for this metabolic type—encourage the overproduction of acid and thickening of blood. Both blood types O and B have a propensity to produce too much stomach acid. Usually they have hyperactive liver chi attacking the stomach, the main symptoms of which are bloating that feels full or painful, discomfort after meals, and frequent belching, all of which may be aggravated by emotional upset.

Any group can present with stomach deficiencies, including irregular stomachache with a burning sensation, which is aggravated in the afternoon or when the stomach is empty and relieved after meals, dry mouth and throat, thirst, loss of appetite, and dry bowel movements. Therefore, in addition to more specific individual recommendations, at our clinic I also advise people with heartburn and stomach pain generally to eat healthily according to blood type, drink sufficient water, and avoid resting too much after eating. Taking a nap after a heavy meal actually increases pressure in the stomach, forcing it contents to reflux and making heartburn much worse. It is better to move around after eating—and, if nothing else, wash the dishes.

For heartburn sufferers without ulcers or any serious health problem, especially those with type A blood, I also advise taking food-based Betaine-HCL supplements after meals, except for meals consisting only of fruit. If your symptoms become worse, gradually increase the dose, up to seven after each meal, until you feel warmth in your stomach, which means you have taken too many for that meal and need to reduce the dose after the next meal. Once you have found the proper dose, continue taking the supplement as your stomach regains its natural ability to produce the gastric juices needed to properly digest food, then slowly reduce supplementation. In addition, I recommend colon hydrotherapy to cleanse the colon and acupuncture treatments for the stomach.

THE BIOCOMPATIBLE VIEW

Biocompatible medicine considers heartburn symptomatic of an underlying metabolic disorder. Some people with heartburn suffer from imbalances of electrolytes—sodium, potassium, and other vital molecules. Others have acid-alkaline imbalances. For example, when the stomach wall allows calcium to move into the cells, through a series of chemical reactions hydrogen eventually combines with chloride ions to produce hydrochloric acid. People who habitually drink coffee, tea, or alcohol on an empty stomach will likewise release excessive stomach acid. A rise in blood serum chloride can indicate a stomach infection due to the presence of the bacterium *Helicobacter pylori*, diabetic lactic acid poisoning, or kidney problems. Conversely, a low blood level of chlorine indicates stomach acid deficiency, which will greatly hinder protein digestion and absorption.

WORDS OF ADVICE
• Avoid taking over-the-counter antacids for heartburn since they may cause metabolic changes.
• Do not take heartburn lightly, as it could indicate a more serious problem.
• Eat small portions; eat slowly; and chew food thoroughly to aid digestion.
• Avoid substances known to contribute to heartburn such as alcohol, caffeine, fatty

foods, fried foods, spicy foods, carbonated soft drinks, chocolate, peppermint, milk products, and nicotine.

- Avoid drugs known to contribute to heartburn, such as nitrates (heart medications like Isonate and Nitrocap), calcium channel blockers (Cardizem and Procardia), and anticholinergic drugs (Pro-banthine and Bentyl). Ask your doctor if any drugs you are taking cause heartburn.
- Avoid clothing that fits tightly around the abdomen.
- Control body weight.
- Wait three hours after eating before going to bed or lying down.
- Elevate the head of your bed six to nine inches, with bricks or a wedge under the bed, to alleviate heartburn at night.
- If you have type A blood and you do not have ulcers or other health problems, consider taking Betaine-HCL supplementation.
- Consider colon hydrotherapy to cleanse the colon.
- Get acupuncture treatments for the stomach.

HORMONES

A hormone is a chemical substance produced in the body's endocrine glands and other cells that exerts a regulatory or stimulatory effect, for example, in metabolism. The word *hormone*, which means "to set in motion through an assault," was coined by early-twentieth-century medical researchers from the Greek word *horman*, to set in motion, and *horm*, meaning assault—which seems particularly apt in regard to sex hormones, the effect of which can be like an attack. In fact, I call puberty the "season of hormone hurricane."

Doctors have a saying that goes "Only fools and endocrinologists try messing around with hormones." Just trying to understand hormones can be an overwhelming task, like attempting to understand all the deities of a religious pantheon. The endocrine glands and the hormones they secrete are involved in almost all aspects of normal body functioning. And because it is so complex, the endocrine system operates in a delicate balance. If it malfunctions, a variety of problems, both great and small, will result since hormones contribute to such a vast range of functions.

For example, DHEA, known as the "mother hormone," is the most prevalent hormone produced and secreted by the adrenal glands. It circulates in the bloodstream as DHEA-sulfate (DHEAS) and is converted as needed into other hormones, including testosterone. The level of DHEA in the body declines with age; a typical seventy-year-old woman has about 5 to 10 percent of the amount produced by a twenty-year-old woman.

Then there is melatonin, a hormone produced by the pineal gland, the secretion of which is stimulated by the dark and inhibited by light. It controls sleep cycles and is also an important antioxidant, protecting the body from free radicals that cause aging and cancer.

The secretion of cortisol, another hormone, increases in response to stress in the body, whether physical or psychological, causing muscle protein to be used for activity and blood sugar levels to be elevated so the brain will have more glucose for energy. At the same time, the other tissues of the body decrease their use of glucose as fuel. Chronic cortisol production is why stubborn belly fat is almost impossible to lose through dieting or exercise.

Female Hormones

Many aspects of women's health are affected by hormones. In our clinic, over a period of time we might have as patients a nine-year-old girl whose parents are concerned that she is showing signs of sexual maturity, a woman with swollen legs suffering from water retention, and a woman with fibroids and endometriosis that make it difficult for her to conceive. Each of these patients is experiencing an imbalance of one female hormone or another.

The major female hormone is estrogen, which is actually not a single hormone but a group of them. All fetuses start as female with an abundance of estrogen, a preset option of nature that will endure if there is no surge of testosterone to change the sex to male. Estrogens cause additional fat to be deposited under the skin, in the breast, and on the hips and buttocks; make the skin soft; help the hair grow faster and stay on the head longer; influence behavior, promoting compromise and companionship over aggression; and affect almost every tissue in the female reproductive system. As the estrogen level rises around the time of puberty, secondary sex changes are followed by menstrual flow and alterations in the cervix that allow for fertility. If sufficient estrogen is not available in the first two weeks of the menstrual cycle, eggs do not develop, which can be one reason for infertility. When menstruation stops, the estrogen level falls, signaling the body to cease preparing an environment for fertilized eggs. Estrogen depletion that comes with menopause causes the uncomfortable symptoms of hot flashes and mood swings, accelerates bone loss, and increases risk of heart disease.

Healthy functioning of the female reproductive system depends also on progesterone, a hormone involved in almost every hormonal problem in women, from premenstrual syndrome (PMS) to hormone imbalance due to perimenopause, menopause, or hysterectomy. Progesterone is produced by the ovaries to prepare the womb for the fertilized egg and later by the placenta to maintain pregnancy, as well as stimulating bone-forming cells. Because of the influx of progesterone, PMS can result in bloating, headaches, mood swings, and irritability. Too much estrogen in relation to progesterone can likewise throw the body into an imbalanced state and produce physical and emotional discomfort, causing a woman to miss menstrual periods for months in a row.

Women also have a natural supply of the hormone testosterone, about one-tenth the amount found in men, for whom it is the pilot in command of male sexuality. Overproduction of testosterone in women, caused by ovarian or adrenal tumors, can lead to masculinization, including cessation of menstrual periods and excessive growth of body hair.

Birth Control Pills and Hormone Replacement Therapy

Oral contraceptives and hormone replacement therapy (HRT) entail synthetic drugs whose long-term use can increase the risk of developing serious chronic illness, as well as depleting the body of B-complex vitamins, folic acid, vitamin C, magnesium, and zinc. Many young women who use birth control pills to control their menstrual cycles, irregular bleeding, cysts, or endometriosis experience more problems as a result. Birth control pills, or the more recent patch limiting the menstrual cycle to four periods a year, mask the ovarian function, flood the body with excess estrogen that thickens the vaginal lining, chill the G-spot and epicenter nerves due to the resulting decrease in testosterone, and inhibit the pituitary gland's secretion of oxytocin, the orgasm hormone, during sex. In addition, antibiotics may interfere with the effectiveness of combination oral contraceptive birth control pills by decreasing the steroid hormone's blood concentrations.

Consequently, birth control pills never correct the underlying dysfunction for which they are taken. Rather, to control the menstrual cycle, irregular bleeding cysts, or endometriosis, it is essential to balance the adrenal glands, as the cortisol they produce modulates the female hormones, especially progesterone. In fact, most menstrual problems are related to low progesterone in the last half of the cycle.

Likewise, many women who use HRT for menopause symptoms report complications. They complain of severe abdominal pain that cannot be explained by food intake or stomach flu; severe or sudden chest pain or shortness of breath; intense headaches with dizziness or vomiting; eye problems, such as blurred vision, flashing lights, or blindness; severe leg pain or numbness in the calf or thigh; nausea; skin changes; weight changes; or fluid retention. In addition, HRT and birth control pills contain large amounts of estrogen that increase the risk of heart attacks, breast cancers, strokes, and pulmonary embolisms.

In my professional opinion, neither HRT nor birth control pills have therapeutic benefits that outweigh their enormous risks. In our clinic, we ask patients to stop using them at the end of their current cycle. Because I am sympathetic to couples who want to avoid unplanned pregnancies and women who want to temper or eliminate their hot flashes, I recommend safe and effective ways to prevent unwanted pregnancies (condoms and the sponge, both of which act as a physical barrier between sperm and the cervix), and to reduce the unwanted symptoms of menopause I recommend herbs like black cohosh.

Male Hormones

Testosterone, the most important male sex hormone, has different functions in various phases of life. In the unborn fetus, it aids in development of the male sex glands, testes, and the external male genitals. In puberty, the hormone is responsible for virilization (masculinization). In the adult male, testosterone controls all sexual functions (libido, potency, and fertility) and preserves the typical male appearance that developed in puberty. Testosterone also maintains male physical health and performance and has a decisive influence on mood and sensation of well-being.

Testosterone is much more than a sex hormone, however. It improves oxygen uptake throughout the body, helps control blood sugar, regulates cholesterol, and maintains the immune system. The body requires testosterone to maintain youthful cardiac output and neurological function, and it is also a critical hormone in the maintenance of healthy bone density, muscle mass, and red blood cell production.

This hormone makes a dramatic appearance during puberty, when boys' bodies change very rapidly. A surge of testosterone makes boys clumsy, causing them to do things like walk into door frames. It affects cognitive function as well, often interfering with their academic performance, a disadvantage that does not last long. After the pubescent period, levels of testosterone in men's bodies begin to decline. This decrease in testosterone contributes to the most significant type of hormonal imbalance in aging men, resulting in many of the debilitating health problems associated with normal aging. A primary cause for the difficulties is that the testosterone is increasingly converted to estrogen. According to one report, estrogen levels of the average fifty-four-year-old man are higher than those of the average fifty-nine-year-old woman.[21]

As men age past age forty, other hormonal changes occur that may perceptibly inhibit sexual, physical, and cognitive functions. The outward appearance of a typical middle-aged male shows increased abdominal fat and shrinkage of muscle mass, a hallmark effect of hormonal imbalance. Further, a common psychological complication of hormone imbalance is a loss of the feeling of well-being, which can manifest as depression. Until recently, these changes were attributed to "growing old," and men were expected to accept the fact that their bodies were beginning a long degenerative process leading ultimately to death, but today there are more medical options to treat these effects.

Unfortunately, doctors are increasingly prescribing drugs to treat depression, elevated cholesterol, angina, and a host of other conditions caused by an underlying hormone imbalance. Many doctors are apparently not familiar with the hormone blood tests men can use to check their blood levels of estrogen, testosterone, thyroid, and DHEA; nor are they experienced in properly adjusting hormones to reverse the degenerative changes that begin in midlife. Whereas bodybuilders tarnished the reputation of testosterone by engaging in synthetic testosterone abuse, which can have detrimental effects, this has nothing to do with the benefits a man over age forty can enjoy by having safely restored his natural testosterone to a youthful level.

Currently, it is possible to test male hormones through a simple saliva test—the male hormone profile—which is an accurate means of evaluating testosterone activity in men and uncovering disrupted testosterone secretion rhythms caused by aging, chronic illness, infection, toxic exposure, smoking, trauma, or other factors. The comprehensive version of this profile includes the measurement of cortisol, DHEA, and melatonin to deliver a more complete picture. After such tests determine the various hormone levels, they can be adjusted to reverse degenerative changes and improve overall health.

THE BIOCOMPATIBLE VIEW

Because biocompatible medicine strives to correct factors that disrupt effective metabolism, it takes into account not only the sex hormones but also the many hormones involved in metabolism, including adiponectin, adrenalin, aldosterone, cortisol, ghrelin, glucagon, human growth hormone, IGF-1, insulin, leptin, serotonin, and thyroxin, as well as various factors that affect all hormones. One factor biocompatible physicians pay close attention to is the interrelationship existing between hormones that exert a regulatory or stimulatory effect on metabolism. Biocompatible physicians also consider the coincident nature of hormones, such as the parallel between high estrogen levels and the increased absorption of copper that then stimulates the production of more estrogen. Because of this perspective, biocompatible physicians know that it is much more effective to treat the thyroid with thyroid medication without treating a coexisting sexual hormone imbalance, for instance. Identifying and correcting metabolic imbalances introduced by toxic heavy metals is a specialty of biocompatible medicine.

WORDS OF ADVICE

- If you are a woman taking oral contraceptives and experience lower sex drive, abdominal pain, chest pain, headaches, eye or speech problems, or severe leg pains, immediately contact your doctor, because any of these symptoms can be a sign of a deeper, underlying problem.
- Be aware that use of oral contraceptives and HRT increases the risk of developing chronic illness as well as depleting the body of B-complex vitamins, folic acid, vitamin C, magnesium, and zinc.
- Maintain a healthy diet and exercise regularly to prevent endocrine system disorders.
- Monitor your diet and weight to avoid obesity, which can lead to type II diabetes, the most common endocrine disorder in the United States.
- Make sure you have enough iodine in your diet to prevent goiter or enlargement of the thyroid (uncommon in developed countries).
- Avoid prolonged physical, emotional, or environmental stress, which can disrupt hormonal functioning. When stress lasts longer than a few hours, higher energy demands are placed on the body; more hormones are secreted to meet those demands; and the body's defenses are weakened, increasing the risk of infection.

HYGIENE

Although people have been led to believe that science increased life expectancy over the last one hundred years, the increase is actually due in large part to improved living and working conditions. After all, deaths from infectious diseases have declined steadily since 1900 and antibiotics were not introduced until 1945.[22]

Many factors in daily routines can impact hygiene and health. Chief among them are choices about whether antiperspirant is used, what kind of toothpaste or soap is used, how food is cooked, what household sanitation practices to adopt, and which remedies are best for infection. For example, antiperspirant can increase the risk of developing Alzheimer's disease because the aluminum content is absorbed by the body and wreaks havoc in the brain. And although deodorants are not as bad as antiperspirants, it is best to avoid using them as well unless they are natural and aluminum free.

People have been led to believe that regular soap is not good enough and that antibacterial soap is necessary for good hygiene. Unfortunately, antibacterial soaps cause more harm than good since triclosan, an antibacterial compound in most such soap, kills not only bacteria but also human cells. As it turns out, antibacterial compounds are in nearly half of all soaps sold in the United States, which is likely contributing to the spread of antibiotic-resistant bacteria. Moreover, using toothpaste containing fluoride has the same negative factors as drinking water with fluoride (see "Fluoride," p. 62).

Choices about food preparation techniques and products have long been known to affect personal hygiene and health. While food, especially chicken, should be cooked thoroughly to kill any pathogens, overcooking food, particularly at high temperatures, can deplete it of valuable nutrients and generate harmful carcinogenic substances. The best option is to consume lightly cooked, lean red meats, provided they are of high quality from healthy animals rather than the meats infused with antibiotics and hormones sold in supermarkets. And while overcooked or fried eggs can cause health problems, eggs cooked for only two to three minutes are a good source of high-quality nutrients. Similarly, vegetables lose valuable nutrients when overcooked, but juicing is an excellent way to add nutritious, raw vegetables to the diet as long as they have been washed. In addition, aluminum can enter the body from eating processed foods and using aluminum cooking utensils.

Regarding household sanitation, medical studies have found that most germs in a home setting are on kitchen sponges, dishcloths, and sinks, whereas the least are on toilet seats. Food-borne illness in the home results largely from contaminated cutting boards, counters, or utensils not properly disinfected or sanitized before preparing foods.[23] The best way to sanitize a kitchen is to soak sponges and dishcloths in 3/4 cup of regular bleach added to 1 gallon of water (45 ml bleach per liter of water) in the sink for 5 minutes, then drain. Or use half white vinegar and half hot water. In addition, we wash our vegetables in cold vinegar and water.

Finally, when treating parasites or viral or bacterial infection, neither over-the-counter remedies nor prescribed antibiotics are likely to be the remedies of choice. Antibiotics may prolong the period during which the person can infect others and may bring on more serious symptoms by upsetting the bacterial balance in the intestines, while over-the-counter diarrhea drugs allow the bacteria to invade other body organs. The best treatment for parasites as well as viral or bacterial infection is to safely wash away the offending pathogens with colonic hydrotherapy (see "Colon Hydrotherapy," p. 85) and replace the beneficial colon bacteria with probiotics.

THE BIOCOMPATIBLE VIEW

Biocompatible medicine encourages many aspects of personal hygiene as a basis for good health, including healthful living habits, cleanliness of body and clothing, a nutritious diet based on metabolic type, a balanced regimen of exercise, the practice of safe sex, elimination of substance abuse, prevention of periodontal and other types of infection, and protection from exposure to toxic materials.

Words of advice

- Breathe deeply in fresh air.
- Drink adequate pure water and maintain a comfortable body temperature.
- Strive for internal cleanliness and elimination of toxins by getting detoxification treatments such as colon hydrotherapy.
- Eat the right food for your metabolic type to minimize inflammation and disease.
- Prepare food in a sanitary manner, and avoid using toxic household cleaning materials, insecticides, and pesticides.
- Avoid using antibacterial soaps and toothpaste with fluoride.
- Exercise at least three or four times per week, integrating cardiovascular activity that doubles the breath and pulse rate, such as jogging or aerobics, and resistance activity, such as weight training or isometrics.
- Sunbathe a minimum of twenty to thirty minutes daily, or two to three hours per week, before 10 a.m. or after 4 p.m. during the hot season.
- Avoid using antiperspirants, and use only deodorants that are aluminum free.
- See a biocompatible dentist who will avoid introducing toxic dental material and help prevent periodontal infection.
- Promote mental hygiene by taking time to relax, participating in energizing social activities, focusing on interesting hobbies, and engaging in inspirational activities that enhance creativity and are spiritually uplifting.

HYPERTENSION

Because hypertension, or high blood pressure, can cause fatal strokes, heart attacks, and heart failure, while hypotension, low blood pressure, can result in loss of consciousness, everyone should be vitally concerned about their blood pressure (BP) and potential for heart and circulatory problems. High blood pressure rarely produces symptoms, so the only way to become aware of it is to have your blood pressure measured.

Blood pressure is recorded using two numbers: a high number representing the systolic BP, or the pressure of the heart pumping blood, and a low number standing for the diastolic BP, or the pressure of blood pushing against the walls of the arteries when the heart is at rest. Normal blood pressure ranges from 100/70 to 120/80. Blood pressure higher than this can indicate a risk of developing cardiovascular disease; such risk is moderate if BP is around 140/105. Blood pressure values need to be verified when patients have cardiovascular problems, other arteriosclerotic risk factors, are taking antihypertensive pharmaceuticals, and particularly before any medical procedure. This should be done by nurses or dental assistants rather than physicians or dentists, because blood pressure readings are often higher due to "white coat hypertension"—elevation of BP attributed to patient anxiety in the presence of an authoritative physician or dentist, recorded as increases of 20/10 in up to 40 percent of patients.[24]

Conventional physicians tend to treat hypertension with pharmaceuticals that can be as dangerous as the risk associated with the condition. Several long-term clinical studies that have monitored people taking blood pressure–lowering drugs, typically diuretics and beta-blockers, concluded that individuals suffer from many side effects, including impotence and an increased risk for heart disease.[25]

By contrast, traditional Chinese medicine physicians treat high blood pressure with acupuncture that nourishes the kidneys. I also stress attaining ideal body weight as perhaps the single most important means of lowering blood pressure. In my practice, I encourage patients with high blood pressure to seek the advice of a clinical nutritionist since often it can be controlled through changes in diet and lifestyle. It is advisable to avoid the standard American/Aruban SAD diet—which is high in sugar and saturated fat, and low in fiber, essential fatty acids and omega-3 fatty acids, magnesium, and vitamin C—and to monitor your sodium-to-potassium ratio. While too much salt can help cause high blood pressure, natural sea salt rather than the highly processed table salt is not harmful if your intake of potassium, found in such sources as fresh fruit, is higher. Lifestyle factors that should be taken into account include drinking coffee or alcohol, lack of exercise, stress, and smoking.

If these changes are not enough to bring blood pressure under control, hair should be tested for metabolic elemental imbalances, such as a condition in which the body does not excrete sodium. In individuals with such a condition, the use of prescription diuretics to reduce blood pressure may actually intensify the problem by lowering potassium levels.

From a broader perspective, people with metabolic syndrome, or syndrome X, currently affecting as many as 50 million Americans,[26] are at increased risk of coronary heart disease and other conditions related to plaque buildup in artery walls, such as stroke, peripheral vascular disease, and type II diabetes. It is characterized by a group of metabolic risk factors that include abdominal obesity (excessive fat around the abdomen), atherogenic dyslipidemia (blood fat disorders—high triglycerides, low HDL cholesterol and high LDL cholesterol—that foster plaque buildup in artery walls), elevated blood pressure, insulin resistance or glucose intolerance (inability to properly use insulin or blood sugar), prothrombotic state (depositing high fibrinogen or plasminogen activator inhibitor-1 in the blood), and proinflammatory state (showing up as elevated C-reactive protein in the blood).

Conventional physicians treat metabolic syndrome with liposuction; stomach stapling; pharmaceuticals for weight loss, cholesterol and blood pressure reductions, and type II diabetes; as well as blood thinners, platelet separators, and antibiotics. By contrast, biocompatible physicians treat metabolic syndrome by detoxifying the body of heavy metals, eliminating jaw and colon infections, and advising individuals to eat foods suitable for their metabolic type.

THE BIOCOMPATIBLE VIEW

Hypertension—which can cause fatal strokes, heart attacks, and heart failure—in many cases can be brought under control by changes in diet and lifestyle. Risk factors for hypertension include drinking coffee and other caffeine-based beverages, as well as alcohol, stress, and insufficient exercise.

Words of advice

- Use natural sea salt rather than processed table salt and, when doing so, consume more foods rich in potassium.
- Avoid alcohol, stress, coffee, and other caffeine-based drinks.
- Get sufficient exercise.
- Refrain from smoking.

L

LIVER DETOXIFICATION

The liver helps protect the body by converting poisons in the blood into harmless substances that can be excreted. When an individual has a high body burden of toxins, however, the liver's job becomes more difficult and the liver itself gradually becomes dysfunctional. Symptoms of liver dysfunction include uncontrollable or unexplained emotional irritation and a green hue around the mouth. The best way to take the load off the liver is by detoxification through one or more of the following methods.

Colon hydrotherapy (see "Colon Hydrotherapy," p. 85) cleans out bowel toxicities contributing to the workload of the liver; hydrates the body; cools the "fire" of dehydration and inflammation; and flushes away excess *Candida albicans,* yeast that can make losing weight more difficult, affect the liver, and promote fermentation in the colon, which produces alcohol and converts into triglycerides that deposit fat around the organs.

Exercise detoxifies by producing lactic acid, a good chelator of heavy metals; provides energy by increasing lung gas conversion that augments the amount of available oxygen; and enhances the thyroid function, which helps control insulin resistance, the foundation of type II diabetes (see "Diabetes Type II," p. 97).

Several supplements also help detoxify the liver, the most notable of which is SAMe (see "SAMe," p. 175). SAMe (S-adenosyl methionine), a chemical produced by the body, which plays an essential role in energizing chemical processes throughout the body and conducting anti-inflammatory activity. First discovered in Italy in 1952, SAMe is made from adenosine triphosphate (ATP) and the essential amino acid known as methione. It is available both as a nutritional supplement and as a prescription medicine known as Bumbaral, Samyr, Adomet, or Admethionine. The third most concentrated chemical in the liver, SAMe has been widely used to correct liver disorders such as cirrhosis and even hepatitis. Being natural, SAMe conveys none of the serious side effects associated with other liver drug treatments.[1]

Another supplement helpful in detoxifying the liver is milk thistle. This plant has been used medicinally for many years to treat dyspeptic symptoms, loss of appetite, functional disorders of the liver and gallbladder, toxic liver disease, and hepatic cirrhosis. It has been shown to reduce outbreaks of psoriasis due to liver disease and has been successfully used as an antidote to death-cap mushroom poisoning. Milk thistle also protects the liver from damage caused by overdose of acetaminophens (pain and fever reducers), butyrophenones (major tranquilizers), phenothiazines (blood pressure reducers), halothane (general anesthetics), Dilantin (antiepileptic drug related to barbiturates), and ethanol from alcoholic beverages.

A third useful supplement is glutathione (GSH). Reduced glutathione, found in almost all living cells, is the most powerful and versatile of the body's self-generated antioxidants that neutralize and prevent the formation of free radicals. It plays an important role in immune function via white blood cell production and is one of the most potent antiviral and anticancer agents manufactured by the body. In addition, it reduces vitamins C and E back to their unoxidized state; helps the liver to detoxify formaldehyde, acetaminophen, benzpyrene (a carcinogen), and many other compounds; synthesizes nucleic acid in DNA repair; assists in the cells' effective use of oxygen; promotes cellular differentiation and slows the aging process; protects the integrity of red blood cells; and maintains normal brain function. As useful as glutathione is, to work properly it must be metabolically active and therefore in reduced rather than oxidized form. Essential cofactors for generating reduced glutathione include riboflavin, niacinamide, selenium, lipoic acid, and glutathione reductase. In our clinic, we use only reduced glutathione specifically produced for us in a private compounding lab.

THE BIOCOMPATIBLE VIEW
The liver plays a key role in metabolic processes, as well as an essential part in detoxification, filtering the blood to remove large toxins, synthesizing and secreting bile full of cholesterol and fat-soluble toxins, and breaking down unwanted chemicals. Detoxification helps the liver function properly so it can protect the body by converting poisons in the blood into harmless substances.

WORDS OF ADVICE
• Exercise to help vent frustration.
• During liver detoxification, avoid drinking alcohol and eating fried foods.

LONGEVITY
Every spring at the end of Carnival in Aruba, the momo, the symbolic carnival king, is burned at the stake, taking away the sins of the community, giving the residents a fresh beginning—and always making me aware of my own mortality. These days, however, people are generally living longer. Centenarians, who live to be at least one hundred years old, are becoming increasingly common in the United States, doubling every decade, according to one group of researchers.[2] In 1950, there were 2,300 centenarians in the United States, while in 1990 there were 37,306.[3] But even though the United States spends more money on health care than other nations, it ranks twenty-fourth in disability-adjusted life expectancy, while Japan ranks first.[4] This finding suggests that the secret to longevity in the United States is not health care, which mainly focuses on treating disease rather than protecting health and preventing disease.

There are different theories about how long the human body can last and why people of certain cultures have longer life expectancies than others. Based on a study of roundworms published in 2003, some scientists believe that people may be able to live for hundreds of years. The study found that by manipulating the worms' insulin signaling and removing their reproductive systems, the worms could live six times longer than normal, corresponding to a life span of 500 human years.[5]

Many factors seem to be involved in slowing down the aging process. Certainly, one of the most significant factors is regulation of insulin levels. I believe, however, that our maximum lifespan is about 120 years and that even manipulating insulin genes would be unlikely to improve it significantly.

Another important promoter of longevity is good nutrition. For example, whereas consuming sugar and grains increases insulin levels, akin to slamming down your foot on the aging accelerator, most vegetables and fruits, especially blueberries, contain antioxidants with anti-aging properties. Sardines, rich in ribonucleic acid, help rebuild the body by replacing cells in exact replicates. And fish oil, according to many experts, is the primary reason Japanese people live the longest.[6] When choosing a fish oil brand, it is important to ensure that the oil has been purified of mercury and other toxins.

In addition, stress relief—through relaxation, sufficient sleep, social interactions, and exercise—contributes to longevity. Stress can accelerate the aging process (see "Stress," p. 189), negatively affecting telomeres, the protective structures at the ends of chromosomes that prevent DNA strands from unraveling. Telomeres play a critical role in determining the health and life span of cells, with aging occurring as cells divide and a portion of telomeric DNA dwindles away by a few base pairs, eventually diminishing the DNA so much that the cells stop dividing. In medical studies, both a prolonged stressful situation and the perception of stress had an impact on three biological factors: oxidative stress, lower telomerase activity, and shorter telomere length—all of which are related to cell longevity and disease.[7]

Other ways to slow aging are by detoxifying the body. This occurs upon removing heavy metals; eliminating infections, especially those associated with periodontal disease; having rejuvenating cell injections (see "Rejuvenating Cell Replacement Therapy," p. 169); and maintaining an active lifestyle that stimulates physical, mental, and spiritual well-being.

THE BIOCOMPATIBLE VIEW

Biocompatible medicine views accelerated aging as a complex medical condition that is caused by metabolic problems developing from chronic inflammation. Consequently, accelerated aging, like other medical conditions, can be prevented and treated using biocompatible medicine procedures and therapies.

WORDS OF ADVICE

- Detoxify the body to lower its burden of toxins.
- Eliminate infections, including those associated with periodontal disease, and find a biocompatible dentist to remove amalgams that may be contributing to gum disease.

- Consider having rejuvenating cell injections as an age-management procedure.
- Eat foods appropriate to your metabolic type to avoid the destructive consequences of insulin resistance.
- Maintain an active lifestyle that is physically, mentally, and spiritually stimulating.
- Reduce stress in your life.

N

NERVE PROBLEMS

The body's nervous system is analogous to electrical wiring in the walls of a house that can be affected by outside forces. Just as heat and dampness pervade our adobe walls in Aruba, causing power surges during hurricane season, heat and dampness can also throw the gallbladder and liver channels out of balance, producing nerve-related symptoms: headaches, shingles, and paralysis of the face (Bell's palsy), as well as poststroke syndrome, numbness, and acute, chronic pain.

Headaches

Headaches (see "Headaches," p. 131) can be treated successfully through acupuncture and prevented from recurring by "dredging the meridians," opening them up to promote blood circulation and regulating chi. Additionally, colon hydrotherapy effectively cleanses the colon and cleans the meridians to prevent future headaches. In our clinic, we see many patients suffering from headaches originating in stomach problems. Head pain that radiates down the back of the neck, immobilizing it or causing a stiff neck, needs to be checked for possible *Helicobacter pylori* infection.

Shingles

The medical name for shingles is herpes zoster—from the Greek *herpes*, "to creep," and *zoster*, "girdle"—because the rash from shingles sometimes forms a semicircle around the waist. This image gave rise to a Latin American folk belief that if the spots meet in the middle the patient is doomed. As painful and unpleasant as shingles can be, however, the condition is not fatal. The blisters from the skin rash usually heal quickly, but the nerve pain can last for months or more, unless the patient seeks out a traditional Chinese medicine physician.

Shingles develops when a person has had chickenpox with a fever that was not allowed to run its natural course for at least twenty-four hours because a fever-reducing drug, such as aspirin, was given too early. In lieu of over-the-counter medications, fevers can be controlled through the following methods: administering an enema or colonic, which lowers the temperature while hydrating the body; rubbing parts of the body with a cold cloth, while keeping the rest of the body covered to prevent chill; lying in bed under warm blankets and allowing the body to sweat out the poison while drinking adequate fluids. If despite these measures a fever persists for more than twenty-four hours or remains higher than 104°F or 40°C, seek medical attention.

When an infected individual's immune system is weakened by stress, illness, or advanced age, the varicella zoster virus that causes chickenpox and shingles can reemerge. Contact with an infected individual does not cause another person's dormant virus to reactivate, but the virus from a shingles patient may cause chickenpox in someone who has not had it before. Why the virus reactivates in some individuals and not others is unknown to most doctors.

Since shingles presents as herpes lesions, I treat this condition the way I treat herpes. Shingles responds rapidly to acupuncture treatments that focus on "removing heat" from the stomach. I also recommend treating shingles or active herpes with dietary adjustments. Since foods that have more arginine than lysine promote the formation of herpes blisters, I advise avoiding gelatin (Jell-O), chocolate, carob, coconut, oats, whole wheat or white flour products, peanuts, soybeans, wheat germ, chicken, beef, lamb, milk, cheese, beans, brewer's yeast, and mung bean sprouts. In addition, I advise supplementing the diet with 1,000 mg of the amino acid lysine. A vaccine for shingles was licensed in 2006. In clinical trials, the vaccine reduced the risks of shingles by 50 percent. It can also reduce pain in people who still get shingles after being vaccinated.

Bell's Palsy

Bell's palsy can cause paralysis of half of the face due to a problem with a facial nerve. The condition is named after Charles Bell, a nineteenth-century Scottish surgeon who studied the nerves and muscles of the face. Symptoms may come from emotional upset, immoderate diet and drinking, sexual indulgence, or environmental influences that lead to the obstruction of chi and blood circulation. Doctors are generally taught that trauma to the seventh cranial nerve causes such facial paralysis, a theory received with skepticism by patients who go to bed fine and wake up the next morning with half their face sagging.

By contrast, in cases of Bell's palsy, traditional Chinese medicine and biocompatible physicians treat different organs depending on which part of the face is paralyzed. If the forehead is the most affected, we concentrate on the heart meridian. When the right side of the face is paralyzed, we focus on the lung meridian, while a problem with the left side indicates a deficiency in the liver energy, and an affected lower lip and chin are the result of a deficit in kidney energy.

We also supplement with B-complex vitamins and reduced glutathione and use acupuncture to encourage the seventh cranial nerve of the face to respond to these treatments. Glutathione supplementation and the precursors to glutathione include the amino acids glycine, glutamate, and cysteine. Lipoic acid, one of the precursors to glutathione, also helps make vitamins C and E work better and speeds up the body's metabolism. A diet high in fresh fruits and vegetables and freshly prepared meats will usually provide enough glycine and glutamate; cysteine comes mostly from eggs, milk, and cheese that have been cooked or processed, which breaks down the dipeptides of cystine to cysteine. While still a valuable amino acid, cysteine can no longer add to glutathione levels, hence I recommend eating soft-boiled eggs that have been cooked no more than two minutes. Sources of lipoic acid include dark leafy vegetables such as spinach and collard greens, broccoli, animal foods such as lean beef, and organ meats like calf's liver.

THE BIOCOMPATIBLE VIEW

Biocompatible medicine views nerve problems as deficiencies of the liver and gallbladder. The function of the liver is to detoxify the blood and produce glutathione, which protects the nerves from oxidative damage. Toxic heavy metals, however, reduce the liver's ability to produce glutathione. Through treatment, the increasing ability of the liver to secrete glutathione into bile enhances the liver's ability to also secrete mercury and other toxins into bile. As for the gallbladder, it receives bile from the liver, which it stores until it is needed for the digestion of proteins and fats. But if the bile ducts that carry bile to and from the gallbladder are obstructed by gallstones, biocompatible physicians prescribe lecithin supplementation to thin the bile so it can better dissolve gallstones. If the liver itself is deficient in producing an adequate flow of bile as revealed in blood test analysis, supplementation with zinc and vitamin B_6 may be recommended.

WORDS OF ADVICE

- Increase glutathione levels to help maintain an advantage in the battle against free radicals and chronic inflammation and to help fight cellular damage that causes nerve deterioration.
- Take lecithin to enhance the production of good-quality bile and diminish the development of gallstones.
- Use zinc and vitamin B_6 to assure the liver is producing good-quality bile in sufficient amounts to efficiently remove detoxified material.
- Supplement with SAMe , another powerful liver and gallbladder detoxifier.

O

OBESITY

Western countries are currently experiencing an epidemic of obesity, which is defined as 20 percent more than the recommended weight for a person's height. In Aruba and the United States, eight out of ten people older than twenty-five are overweight.[1] Obesity increases a person's odds of suffering from diabetes, cardiovascular disease, and osteoarthritis, as well as a loss of productivity and an increased rate of disability—the consequences of which are costly. According to insurance companies, treating obesity-related disorders costs as much or more than treating illnesses caused by aging, smoking, and drug and alcohol abuse combined.[2]

Susceptibility to weight gain begins in childhood. Factors in children that increase the risk for adult obesity include having obese parents; lack of sound sleep; lack of exercise, often due to too many hours spent in front of TV and computers; high birth weight; rapid weight gain; quick growth in the first two years; and early body fat. In addition, parents with substance abuse problems, particularly alcoholism and cocaine abuse, often raise children plagued not only with substance abuse issues and depression but also obesity or weight-related disorders such as bulimia or anorexia.[3] Ultimately, about 70 percent of overweight adolescents become obese later in life.[4]

Overweight or obese children are at risk for a variety of health problems. One in four overweight children show early signs of type II diabetes, also known as adult-onset diabetes (impaired glucose intolerance). Many obese children have high cholesterol and high blood pressure, which are risk factors for heart disease. One of the most severe problems for obese children is sleep apnea (interrupted breathing while sleeping), which in some cases can lead to problems with learning and memory. Obese children also have a high incidence of orthopedic problems, liver disease, and asthma. Just as sadly, childhood obesity is on the rise.[5]

Despite the fact that in their quest to overcome obesity many people use expensive pharmaceutical drugs, drink "magical" liquids, and in desperation, have their stomachs stapled, the fat either never goes away or quickly returns. Certainly, high-risk stomach-stapling operations are not the answer. After a lot of fanfare about this "miracle operation" in Aruba, the eighth patient to undergo the procedure died from complications. For many, obesity reflects the reality that their "drug of choice" is carbohydrates. Processed carbohydrates and sugar, which impact the brain using the same pathway as drugs and alcohol, are likewise addicting.

As a medical anthropologist, I view obesity also as a cultural influence posing an impact on society. In most cultures, obesity symbolizes being blessed, healthy, and prosperous. For example, in Indian and Asian cultures fat deities are often associated with prosperity or universality, such as the Indian deity Ganapathi (Ganesh), the god with the elephant body that is thought to contain the whole universe. Similarly, fat Buddhas may indicate an abundance of blessings, while fertility goddess statuettes of ancient Europe and the Middle East symbolize fertility. Many Hispanic societies unconsciously equate "big" with "great" because, linguistically, *hombre grande* ("big [fat] man") is similar to *gran hombre* ("great [powerful] man").

Such positive cultural regard associated with obesity can work against health agendas. For instance, my work in the prevention and treatment of obesity among Native Americans and Pacific Islanders was complicated by their longstanding acceptance of bigness as a sign of wealth and power. Social reality, however, shows us that obesity is most often related to poverty, low economic status, and exclusion from the health system.

In addition to having to overcome culturally symbolic aspects of obesity, those seeking to lose weight are further hampered by doctors who offer false treatments. In Aruba, we have a problem with acupuncturists who come here illegally and charge a lot of money for miracle weight loss treatments that involve keeping small acupuncture needles embedded in the body until the desired weight is achieved. One fellow even claims needling and sedating the vagus nerve, which branches out from the abdomen and enters the stomach, pancreas, small intestine, large intestine, and colon, will result in weight loss. With these organs sedated and not functioning optimally for secretion and constriction of smooth muscle, people cannot digest adequately and therefore start losing weight. Although this might seem desirable, the thorax branches of the vagus nerve go to the lungs, the esophagus, and the heart, causing, in this sedated state, bronchoconstriction, peristalsis, and a slowed heart rate.

Another problem with treating weight loss is that toxicities from heavy metals, pesticides, insecticides, and petrochemicals tend to be sequestered in fat cells and released during weight reduction. This discharge produces what holistic physicians call a "healing crisis."

Given the fact that weight loss is complicated and has physical, emotional, psychological, and cultural dimensions, it is wise to seek professional help before proceeding. In truth, there is no fast and safe weight reduction program. To effect real change, a long-term multidisciplinary approach is necessary. In our clinic, to help manage weight loss we use carbohydrate addiction counseling, acupuncture, colon hydrotherapy, and clinical nutrition based on metabolic type after blood testing, while screening for toxicities. Often we need to be aggressive in helping to control the negative reactions of the vast amount of *Candida albicans* yeast dying and exiting the body. In addition, we recommend 5-hydroxytryptophan (5-HTP) and DL-phenylalanine—natural supplements that convert to serotonin, an important brain chemical involved in mood, behavior, appetite, and sleep but also influential in impulse control and therefore able to help individuals overcome their addiction to simple carbohydrates. We also recommend supplements of GTF (glucose tolerance factor) chromium, which plays an important role in regulating blood sugar levels. Each molecule of GTF, a compound that functions like a hormone and requires chromium as its central atom, works with insulin to transport glucose from the blood into the cells. When this function is not working properly, the cells resist insulin and do not absorb the glucose necessary for energy. Further, it is crucial for obese individuals with type O blood to eliminate simple carbohydrates from their diet. Finally, we help individuals, even those with limited mobility, develop an exercise program that suits them.

THE BIOCOMPATIBLE VIEW

Biocompatible medicine considers periodontal disease and obesity the major predictors of early degenerative disease and mortality. Most morbidly obese adults who cannot detach themselves from their unconscious association with obesity and personal power and who cannot admit their addiction to simple carbohydrates have no chance for a healthy life.

WORDS OF ADVICE

• Understand that obesity is a complex medical problem that does not respond well to a "magic bullet" solution.
• Confront any unconscious association you might have that equates fatness with personal power.
• Seek addiction treatments to curb your simple carbohydrate addiction.

OSTEOPOROSIS

Osteoporosis, a disease that occurs especially in postmenopausal women, causes loss of bone density so that bones break easily and heal slowly, as well as leading to curvature of the spine after the vertebrae collapse. Loss of bone density can also occur in people subjected to prolonged periods of bed rest and astronauts who fly lengthy missions under the weightless conditions of space, because weight-bearing bones of the body, such as those in the spine and legs, are then relieved of their burden, resulting in a condition known as skeletal unloading, which inhibits bone formation and reduces bone calcium. When skeletal unloading persists for several weeks, bones start to deteriorate: the number of bone cells decreases, movement into the bone of such minerals as calcium and phosphorous slows, and the production of bone-cell precursors (called osteoprogenitor cells) diminishes, all leading to brittle bones prone to fracture. And while the bones of children may eventually be able to recover from such changes, adult bones generally do not, as reflected in studies of Skylab and Salyut-6 long-term space missions, which found that astronauts on board the craft not only lost bone density during their missions but also, five years later, had failed to recover their prelaunch bone density levels.[6] Nor can drugs reverse the situation since strong bones and muscles are a response to weight-bearing stress on the skeleton.

Initially, osteoporosis may cause no symptoms. Later, it can bring about dull pain in the bones or muscles, particularly in the low back or neck, progressing to sharp, sometimes sudden pains aggravated by activity that puts weight on the area.

THE BIOCOMPATIBLE VIEW

Conventional medicine defines the endoskeleton as the internal structure composed of bone and cartilage that protects and supports the soft organs, tissues, and other parts of a vertebrate organism and considers the leading cause of osteoporosis to be a decrease in hormone production, particularly estrogen in women and androgen in men. By contrast, biocompatible physicians, trained to look at the energetic interrelationship of body parts, see the skeleton as the internal structure composed of bone and cartilage that protects, supports, and adapts to the activity of soft organs, and view osteoporosis and low hormones as being concurrent with bone loss resulting from metabolic compensation for acid stress in the body. While traditional osteoporosis researchers recommend supplementation with calcium, vitamin D and its precursors—including 7-dehydrocholesterol, which reacts with ultraviolet light to produce vitamin D—and hormones, biocompatible physicians believe these treatments do not work. In our view, people build bone density not by ingesting calcium, vitamin D, or hormones but by increasing the demand placed on bones by muscular and physical activity. Bone growth can be further stimulated by walking barefoot or in hard shoes that "shock" the bones.

WORDS OF ADVICE

- Supplement with magnesium and phosphorous rather than calcium, which can make the bones more brittle.
- Remove heavy metals from the body, eliminate infection, and correct acid stress.
- To aid bone formation, exercise with no shoes or hard shoes that "shock" the bones, or do weight-bearing exercises, such as weightlifting.
- To increase your absorption of bone-building minerals, as well as protein that enhances flexibility of the bones, eat soups made with boiled bones, vegetables, and parsley.
- Consume at least 100 mcg of vitamin K a day to help bones get the minerals necessary for operating properly and reducing your risk of hip fracture. Since parsley is loaded with vitamin K, with over 180 mcg in just half a cup, keep this herb on hand to add to your cooking.

OXIDATIVE STRESS

One of the paradoxes of life on this planet is that the molecule sustaining aerobic life, oxygen, not only drives energy metabolism and respiration but also breaks down into a form that produces oxidative stress—the seed of many diseases, including aging, arthritis, cancer, diabetes, and all other degenerative illnesses. The term "oxidative stress" describes a constant state of oxidative damage in cells, tissues, or organs, caused by burned-up oxygen, which occurs when the generation of oxygen-free radicals in the body exceeds the natural ability to neutralize and eliminate them. This damage can affect either a specific molecule or an entire organism. Reactive oxygen, such as free radicals and peroxides, exists naturally in all aerobic organisms that live only in the presence of oxygen.

Six steps lead to oxidative stress. Lack of physical exercise and eating the wrong food for one's metabolic type makes the body more acidic (see "pH Balance,"

p. 163) as the amount of oxygen delivered to the cells decreases. Then the body starts developing anaerobic metabolism as an alternate energy-producing method requiring less oxygen but producing many free radicals. To balance the excess acid, the body draws calcium out of the bones, which produces too much free calcium in the blood. All this calcium leads to chronic inflammation, a condition in which the body constantly has to fight infection or cancer. When unresolved, the body's struggle breaks down the connective tissue that holds it together. Finally, the body's ability to neutralize free radical oxidative stress is greatly reduced, accelerating aging.

This imbalance can result from a lack of antioxidant capacity caused by disturbances in production or distribution of antioxidants, by behavioral stressors, or by an overabundance of environmental pollutants. People get oxygen-free radicals from exposure to cigarette smoke, emissions from automobiles and industries, excess alcohol, asbestos, ionizing radiation, and bacterial, fungal, or viral infections. If not regulated properly, excess free radicals can damage a cell's fats, protein, or DNA, inhibiting normal functioning. Because of this, oxidative stress advances diseases as well as the aging process.

The medical condition that best demonstrates destruction of the body by free radicals is type II diabetes. Patients who do not strictly control their diabetes through diet, natural supplements, and medicines when needed can develop arteriosclerosis (hardening of the arteries), diabetes-induced heart disease, inability to hold urine, sexual impotence and inability to achieve orgasm, problems with nerves, diabetic coma, and blindness. Major features of type II diabetes include both insulin resistance and decreased secretion of insulin by the pancreas. Insulin resistance, in which the body's insulin is bound up, mostly by gluten found in wheat products, usually precedes the onset of type II diabetes by many years (see "Diabetes Type II," p. 97). My clinical observation is that more than half of nondiabetic individuals have insulin resistance in the same range as that of patients with type II diabetes. Even so, many family doctors do not ask for insulin values on their blood test requests.

As for the decreased secretion of insulin by the pancreas, it follows a period of escalating hyperglycemia, marked by excessive sugar in the blood, during which pancreatic cells compensate for the insulin resistance by secreting more and more insulin until at last the pancreas fails to secrete sufficient insulin and diabetes ensues. Changes in lifestyle, especially the movement toward consumption of high-caloric diets and lack of exercise, have increased the global prevalence of both diabetes and obesity. In fact, between 60 and 90 percent of type II diabetes cases now appear to be related to obesity, establishing a firm association between obesity and the insulin resistance that precedes the development of hyperglycemia.[7]

Given the critical role oxidative stress plays in type II diabetes, other degenerative diseases, and the aging process, it is very important for individuals to determine their level of oxidative stress due to environmental exposure to oxidants, inadequate antioxidant ingestion, or other disorders and learn how to increase antioxidant activity in the body to help regulate oxidative reactions. Blood tests available through biocompatible physicians can indicate the severity of a patient's oxidative stress and help evaluate the risk of infection. Generally, reducing oxidative stress should be a part of any health regimen—especially treatment programs for patients with type II diabetes and those exhibiting symptoms of insulin resistance, which include numbness of feet or hands, high blood pressure, high cholesterol (especially triglycerides), rapid aging, low energy, reduced muscle mass, water retention, increased facial or body hair, weight gain around the waist, sugar craving, and heart palpitations.

A crucial factor in increasing the intake of antioxidants is diet. Vegetables and fruits, especially blueberries, are loaded with antioxidants. Alpha-lipoic acid, a powerful antioxidant when consumed as a dietary supplement, is both water and fat soluble, allowing it to function effectively in cell membranes. In fact, studies have shown that alpha-lipoic acid regenerates tissue levels of vitamins E and C and significantly elevates blood levels of the antioxidant glutathione, produced by healthy livers.[8] Alpha-lipoic acid and the antioxidant vitamins chelate, or bind, metal ions in a way that prevents them from generating free radicals. There is also evidence that high doses of alpha-lipoic acid can improve insulin sensitivity in individuals with type II diabetes.

In addition to diet and supplementation, maintaining an exercise program high in aerobic activity helps regulate the acid-base balance of the body. It also makes the body more alkaline, as does avoiding simple carbohydrates.

THE BIOCOMPATIBLE VIEW

Oxidative stress, which forms the foundation of biocompatible medicine, describes the ongoing damage occurring in cells, tissues, or organs caused by burned-up oxygen, which takes place when the generation of oxygen free radicals exceeds the body's natural ability to eliminate them. Reactive oxygen, in the form of these free radicals and peroxides, is thus produced by our metabolism of oxygen and is part of the price we pay to be alive. Most free radicals, however, are reactions to the liver's detoxification of elements that come from outside the body, including cigarette smoke, environmental pollutants such as emission from automobiles and industries, consumption of alcohol in excess, asbestos, exposure to ionizing radiation, and bacterial, fungal, or viral infections.

WORDS OF ADVICE

• Watch for symptoms of oxidative stress, such as periodontal infection, bleeding gums, physical signs of aging, chronic inflammation, chronic fatigue, a tendency toward chronic infection, cracks on lips, dry skin, or anemia.
• Determine your level of oxidative stress through blood tests interpreted by a board-certified clinical nutritionist or a physician trained in biocompatible medicine, and learn how to increase antioxidant activity in your body.
• Consume foods high in antioxidants, such as fruits and vegetables, especially blueberries, to minimize oxidative stress.
• Maintain an exercise regimen high in aerobic activity to help regulate your acid-base balance and make your body more alkaline.
• To make your body increasingly more alkaline, avoid simple carbohydrates.

P

pH BALANCE

The degree of acidity or alkalinity of a substance, expressed as pH, is a measurement of the concentration of hydrogen (H) ions; the more hydrogen ions there are, the more acidic a substance is. Most people know more about the acidity or alkalinity of their garden soil than about that of the human body. Just as plants need specific amounts of nutrients like nitrogen, phosphorous, and potassium, human beings need proteins, carbohydrates, and vitamins to grow and fight off disease. If our bodies are too acidic, we suffer from oxidative stress and then develop chronic inflammation. In modern Western society, the bodies of almost all people with degenerative diseases are overly acidic,[1] which leads to oxidative stress (see "Oxidative Stress," p. 160). One reason for this outcome is that just as automobile exhaust produces toxic fumes, the human body produces waste material from oxygen; these oxidant products then cause the release of free radicals, which results in cellular degeneration, or aging. The most common antioxidants are vitamins A, C, and E, which are not produced by the body and must be obtained from the diet. The antioxidants glutathione, lipoic acid, and CoQ10 are formed naturally by the body, but their levels decline with age.

Vinegar and lemon juice are acidic substances, while laundry detergents and ammonia are basic, or alkaline. A substance that is neither acidic nor basic is neutral, such as water, with a pH of 7.0. Mixing acids and bases can cancel out their extreme effects, much like mixing hot and cold water can even out water temperatures. When the right ratio exists between acid and alkaline levels in the body, the glands and organs function properly and general health is maintained. However, the acid and alkaline values in the body are not permanently fixed; they change according to what is going on in the body.

The body works well only in a narrow range of acid-base balance,[2] and having a pH either above or below 7.4 can be harmful. A pH above 7.0 is overly alkaline and called alkaloid, while the range below 7.0 is overly acidic, verging on acidosis. The pH level of an individual can be tested from saliva and interpreted according to the following standard:

Ideal	7.41
Acceptable	6.0–7.5
High-risk acidosis	5.0–6.0

When pH drops to less than 4.5, the individual is suffering from life-threatening acid stress.[3]

Blood that is overly alkaline, due to high levels of potassium, for example, can produce profound negative effects, such as bradycardia, or slow resting heart rate, possibly leading to episodes of fainting.[4] In general, however, high alkalinity is extremely rare.

Overly acidic blood, which is much more common, can manifest other, equally serious symptoms. Fluid from the lymph glands that carries nutrition to the cells and removes acid waste products dries and slows down, promoting lymph node swelling, increasing acid storage in the tissues, and forming adhesions throughout the tissues that can interfere with both lymph fluid and blood flow (see "Skin," p. 184).[5] Also, the acidic waste products rob the blood of proper oxygenation, cause deterioration to the heart, and alter the heartbeat.[6]

Despite the fact that most people's bodies are too acidic, there are times when it may be detrimental to alkalinize since increased acidity is the immune system's means for fighting infection and certain organs of the body exist well in an acidic environment. For instance, when the vagina loses its acidity because of alkali-producing bacteria, infection occurs.[7] Similarly, the cerumen, or earwax, found in the outer ear produces an acidic environment that safeguards the ear against the growth of microorganisms. Increasing the alkalinity of the outer ear—which can occur in the presence of debris, when the ear is syringed with water, or when the ear canal is washed with soap—may enhance the risk of developing swimmer's ear or other infections.[8] In addition, people who are threatening to commit suicide are better able to cope when their internal environment is more acidic; the high alkalinity associated with decreases in cholesterol ratios has been shown to dangerously modify serotonin levels.[9] And individuals with tuberculosis are better equipped to survive when they are acidic since relative acidity in the lungs encourages the production of nitric oxide, which kills the offending bacteria.

The pH balance can change under a variety of conditions. For one thing, it is affected by emotions. In traditional Chinese medicine, anger, nervous tension, sadness, worry, fear, and overwork are each associated with a particular organ. For example, a person who is angry or frustrated starts producing more stomach acid and bile. "Anger bile," a surge of bile from the gallbladder in response to anger or frustration can produce gastrointestinal problems, which can lead to digestive difficulties, including belching, bloating, intestinal gas, regurgitation, hiccups, lack of appetite, nausea, vomiting, diarrhea, constipation, and colic in children. Irritability and inappropriate anger can affect the liver and lead to menstrual pain, headache, redness of the face and eyes, dizziness, and dry mouth. This is why in the People's Republic of China angry individuals are sometimes told, "Put away your liver." The load on the liver, whose functions include processing acid toxins from the blood and producing alkaline enzymes for the body, is much heavier when acid waste products are constantly floating in the blood, such as from food improperly digested due to digestive difficulties resulting from anger. When the liver becomes too congested with such waste, disease or death may ensue (see "Liver Detoxification," p. 149).[10]

In my clinical experience, I have also seen a shift to acid stress take place when people eat outside of their metabolic food list, suffer from infections, or react to poisons like toxic heavy metals, mercury, insecticides, pesticides, or petroleum-derived chemicals. Professionally, I believe the unremitting shift to acidic stress eventually creates an imbalance between the production of reactive oxygen and the body's ability to readily detoxify the reactive intermediates or easily repair the resulting damage.

In general, all forms of life strive to maintain within their cells a reduced oxygen free-radical environment. This means the body, at least for a while, is "designed to win," as "Sam" Queen says, the battle against the detrimental effects of free radicals produced by its antioxidant response.[11] But with persistent acid stress and a losing battle against oxidation, the body ultimately reaches a point where it has accumulated too much acid and does not have enough alkalinizing bicarbonate elements like sodium, calcium, or potassium to effectively neutralize the acid, after which the individual develops metabolic acidosis, often seen in patients suffering from a critical illness.[12]

For example, cancer begins in an acidic environment of chronic inflammation[13] but seeks an alkaline, oxygen-rich environment as it starts growing.[14] When bicarbonate and G-6-PD (an enzyme acting as the "glue" that provides the structural integrity of the skin and the red blood cells) are high, glutamine supplementation, which is sometimes recommended, can bring about the Warburg effect, an outcome described more than fifty years ago, in which tumor cells absorb more glucose and use it as a fuel source to multiply faster, thereby promoting the spread of cancer rather than fighting it.[15] During chemotherapy, the body often exhibits a marked rise in alkaline pH as chemotherapeutic agents destroy healthy cells, which then release their phosphate.[16]

Acidosis can also occur in the kidneys, organs responsible for regulating the acid-base balance in the body. In an adult, about 1 liter of blood per minute passes through the kidneys, which keep the blood alkaline by extracting acid. But kidneys overstressed by too much acidity produce kidney stones, which are composed of waste acid cells and mineral salts that have become hardened—a painful condition that may be avoided by reducing the amount of acid-forming products entering the body. So narrow is the range of acid-base balance in a healthy body that when the body is too alkaline, the urine is too alkaline, allowing calcium kidney stones to form, and conversely, when the body is too acidic, the acidity promotes bacteria that are responsible for creating uric kidney stones.

Probably the most difficult type of acidosis to regulate is diabetic ketoacidosis, which develops when ketone bodies, produced mainly in the liver, accumulate in the blood. As levels of ketone bodies rise, the blood becomes acidic, resulting in ketoacidosis. This condition also occurs in alcoholics after binge drinking, though they, unlike diabetics, tend not to have high levels of glucose in the blood or urine. Even so, alcoholic acidosis is frequently as severe as diabetic ketoacidosis.

Ultimately, the most common contributor to persistent acid stress is the modern Western diet, and the main culprits are processed and fried foods.

Symptoms indicating that the body is becoming too acidic from the foods we digest are recurring infections, gums that bleed when flossed, and excessive tartar on the teeth.

Charts from the 1930s designated all foods as being neutral, acid forming, or alkalizing. The underlying thinking was that the foods we digest metabolize, or burn, down to an ash residue which, depending on the mineral content of the food, can be either neutral, acidic, or alkaline. For example, potassium, calcium, magnesium, sodium, zinc, and iron form basic, or alkaline, ash, while sulphur, phosphorus, chlorine, and iodine leave acid ash. According to the charts, animal foods—meat, eggs, and dairy—processed and refined foods, yeast products, fermented foods, grains, artificial sweeteners, fruit, and sugars are acidifying, as are alcohol, coffee, chocolate, black tea, and sodas. Vegetables, on the other hand, are alkalizing, including a few that are technically fruits such as avocado, tomato, and bell peppers. Some nonsweet citrus fruits are classified as basic, along with sprouted seeds, nuts, and grains. Unsprouted grains, however, are acidifying, though a few (millet, buckwheat, and spelt) are only mildly so. Raw foods are more alkalizing, while cooked foods are acidifying.

The assumption was that acidifying foods were bad and alkalizing foods were good, a one-size-fits-all directive that spawned such nutritional disasters as the outdated U.S. government's Food Guide Pyramid and dietary recommendations based largely on grains, regardless of negative pH consequences. Biocompatible medicine, on the other hand, acknowledges that while the typical Western diet of processed and fried foods produces the acidity that lies at the foundation of many of today's medical problems,[17] generalized dietary rules for everyone do not work and in fact acidifying foods can turn out to have very positive effects on people of certain blood types. Most notably, while beef is acidifying for those with type A blood, it is neutral for those with type B blood and alkalizing for those with type O blood. This is why in our clinic we recommend that patients choose foods that are compatible with their metabolic type and health situation.

We also suggest ways to raise pH levels if the body is acidic or to keep it from becoming too acidic. First, we recommend raising your arms and breathing in deeply, then lowering your arms while exhaling. This exercise enhances an exchange in the lungs and increases bicarbonate, which lowers the acidity of the body. It should be done in the morning upon waking and in the evening before sleep. Second, we suggest reassessing your diet and, along with choosing foods compatible with your metabolic type and health situation, alkalinizing your blood by consuming those that contain citric acid (oranges, lemons, limes), lactic acid (yogurt), malic acid (apples, apple cider), and acetic acid (vinegar). Also, supplement with glutamine and get adequate phosphate (found in sunlight, nuts, spinach, eggs, beans, fish, brown rice, and pumpkin seeds). Third, engage in moderate exercise, which alkalinizes the body; but avoid excessive exercise, which can make the body acidic due to lactic acid buildup. Fourth, cleanse the colon of acid wastes through colon hydrotherapy, which prevents toxins from collecting in the colon walls and being reabsorbed into the bloodstream.

THE BIOCOMPATIBLE VIEW

The body works well only in a narrow range of acid-base balance, or pH. If the body becomes too acidic, it cannot properly use proteins, carbohydrates, or vitamins to grow and can ultimately exhibit signs of oxidative stress, from which chronic inflammation and degenerative disease develop.

WORDS OF ADVICE

- To maintain optimal pH balance, eat according to metabolic type and take antioxidant supplements.
- Exercise moderately and regularly to help your body regain control of your optimal pH level.
- To lower acidity by increasing bicarbonate, practice raising your arms, inhaling deeply, and exhaling while lowering your arms.
- If your body is too acidic, consume foods that contain citric acid (oranges, lemons, limes), lactic acid (yogurt), malic acid (apples, apple cider), and acetic acid (vinegar).
- If you are too acidic, supplement your diet with glutamine and get adequate phosphate, found in sunlight, nuts, spinach, eggs, beans, fish, brown rice, and pumpkin seeds.

R

REJUVENATING CELL REPLACEMENT THERAPY

For the first twenty-eight years of a person's life each atom and cell is replaced every seven years. After age twenty-eight, the number of undifferentiated blood stem cells containing new material for building the body diminishes. This is because blood stem cells cannot divide more than one hundred times, resulting in adult stem cells with limited ability to replicate. Consequently, the body deteriorates, leading to a variety of potential medical problems—all reflecting the lack of new building material. Only a few foods, such as sardines and brewer's yeast, contain available RNA and DNA material that the body can use to rebuild itself. Current stem cell research, however, offers the possibility of acquiring new building material from primal cells that retain the ability to differentiate into other cell types and thus potentially rejuvenate cells in older people or reverse degenerative physical conditions.

It is generally thought that the study of stem cells began in the 1960s, following research by Canadian scientists Ernest A. McCulloch and James E. Till. But the true history of using undifferentiated cells to rejuvenate cells of the body started much earlier, as explained by author E. Michael Molnar, MD:

> *Paracelsus, a sixteenth-century physician, stated the basic theory behind cell therapy best: "Heart heals the heart, lung heals lung, spleen heals spleen; like cures like." Paracelsus and many other early physicians believed that the best way to treat illness was to use living tissue to rebuild and revitalize ailing or aging tissue. Modern orthodox medicine lost sight of this method, so it now uses chemicals to interrupt or override living processes. While chemicals and drugs work only until the body's metabolic processes break them down, cell therapy has a long-term effect, because it stimulates the body's own healing and revitalizing powers.*
>
> *Doctors who practice cell therapy believe that cell therapy functions like an organ transplant and actually teaches the old cells to "act younger." This biological "lesson" is not quickly forgotten by the cells.*
>
> *In Europe, the effectiveness of cell therapy is widely accepted. In West Germany [sic], for example, more than 5,000 German physicians regularly administer cell therapy injections. A great proportion of those injections are funded by the West German social security system. Several million patients the world over have received cell therapy injections since the mid-1950s.*

Swiss physician Paul Niehans discovered the beneficial effects of live cell therapy quite by accident. In 1931, a colleague who had accidentally removed a patient's parathyroid glands during the course of thyroid surgery summoned Niehans. So vital are these glands to life that there was little chance that the woman could survive the day without them. A successful transplant was the only chance the surgeon had of saving her. So Niehans, who had a reputation for therapeutically transplanting organs and glands, was called in.

On his way to the hospital, Niehans stopped off at the abattoir, where the animals he used in his revitalization experiments were slaughtered. He obtained fresh parathyroid glands from a steer and proceeded to the hospital, fully intending to perform a parathyroid transplant.

However, when Niehans arrived, one look at the patient—who was violently convulsing—told him that there was simply not enough time to perform the operation. The woman would not survive long enough.

However, Niehans had an idea. He used a surgical knife to slice the steer's parathyroid glands into finer and finer pieces, taking care not to mash the individual cells. He then mixed the pieces in a saline solution and loaded it into a large hypodermic needle. To the shock and dismay of his colleagues, Niehans injected the mixture into the fatally ill woman.

Immediately, her convulsions ceased. Her condition improved—and continued improving. To everyone's surprise, including Niehans', she recovered. Niehans wrote, many years later, "I thought the effect would be short-lived, just like the effect of an injection of hormones, and that I should have to repeat the injection. But to my great surprise, the injection of fresh cells not only failed to provoke a reaction but the effect lasted, and longer than any synthetic hormone, any implant or any surgical graft."

Longer indeed. The woman went on to live another thirty years, well into her nineties.

Thus was born cell therapy. At his Clinique La Prairie in Montreaux, Switzerland, Dr. Niehans went on to administer live cell injections to thousands and thousands of patients, including many of the crowned heads, United States presidents, Pope Pius XII, and several Hollywood stars.

Dr. Niehans stated the ultimate aim of cell therapy in this way: "What I am striving after is not only to give more years to life but especially to give more life to years." Niehans' aim was to "make all the organs struck by old age capable once more of functioning properly and, at the same time, bring fresh strength to the whole body by revitalization of the sex glands."[1]

Undifferentiated cells have the unique power to turn into any type of cell found in a mammalian body. Cells from the tissue of one animal are thus able to give rise to cell types of a completely different tissue in another animal, a phenomenon known as plasticity or transdifferentiation. French scientists have used embryonic stem cells from one animal species to repair heart damage in another species. Implanting embryonic stem cells from mice resulted in healthier heart tissue in nine sheep with damaged cardiac muscle, according to a report in the

The Lancet by researchers at the National Center for Scientific Research in Montpelier and the Hospital European Georges Pompidou in Paris. No such response was seen in nine sheep with similar damage that did not get the transplants.[2]

Likewise, as Niehans discovered, cellular material from another mammal can be combined with human hormones to rebuild the body of a person over age twenty-eight whose existing differentiated cells are no longer dividing to generate pairs of daughter cells of the same type. In such instances, the cellular material, composed of relatively undifferentiated stem cells, is delivered by way of a rejuvenating injection.

From 1998 until 2008, when he passed away, I had the honor of working with Dr. C. Tom Smith, medical director of the International Clinic of Biological Regeneration (ICBR), a leading international cell therapy center that has been in continuous operation since 1981. ICBR rejuvenating cell replacement therapy was simultaneously available in Nassau, London, and in Matamoros, Mexico. Over the years of observing changes that had taken place in recipients of rejuvenating injections, I saw some dramatic results: improved skin tone and complexion, increased vitality, the return of youthful optimism and energy, and various other reversals involving the infirmities of aging. In effect, this form of cell therapy helps people become biologically younger while growing chronologically older.

Rejuvenating cell replacement therapy as practiced by biocompatible physicians, unlike these "live cell" therapies, results in cells having no trace of proteins capable of causing immune reactions. Cell material in this case is composed of organ ultrafiltrates—organ-specific preparations made up of submicroscopic cellular particles of embryonic sheep cells that are only about three nanometers in diameter. In fact, since the largest particles of the preparation are much, much smaller than any protein molecule, the German Ministry of Health classifies this material as being "protein free," suggesting there is no danger of initiating a foreign protein reaction.

Rejuvenating cell replacement therapy as practiced by biocompatible physicians also differs from other rejuvenating applications. Several European and Mexican clinics routinely inject material from the whole cell—which takes several weeks—to prevent the possibility of an allergic reaction. But only the nucleus of the cell, which contains a matrix of RNA (ribonucleic acid), has rejuvenating capacity. It is generally understood that applications containing only the RNA matrix, and free of proteins and possible viruses, are the safest and most effective cell injections.

Specifically, biocompatible rejuvenating cell replacement therapy is designed to help reverse the following degenerative conditions:

- General loss of vitality
- Physical and mental exhaustion
- Convalescence after illness
- Premature aging
- Deterioration of the brain, heart, kidneys, lungs, liver, or digestive organs
- Lack of drive and declining mental efficiency

- Weakness of the immune system
- Arthritis and other degenerative diseases of the connective tissue
- Hypo-function of the endocrine glands
- Disturbances of menopause
- Parkinsonism
- Chronic pain, migraine, headaches, neuralgia, back pain, or sciatica
- Atherosclerosis of the brain, heart, or peripheral circulation

Although rejuvenating cell replacement therapy is said to be effective for anyone suffering from one or more these conditions, I have found that some patients benefit more than others. Patients with the greatest gains are those who have undergone identification and removal of toxins, reduced their rate of infections, begun eating according to their metabolic type, and shifted to a healthier lifestyle. Improved outcomes are also linked with exercise following the injections, since increased physical activity helps the new material rebuild tissue.

Stem cell research, also called regenerative medical research, has the potential to change the face of human disease by contributing to tissue repair and organ growth. The cell therapy developed by Dr. Niehans, however, is no longer qualified for patenting by pharmaceutical companies. Thus the search is on to patent the use of human embryo stem cells.

THE BIOCOMPATIBLE VIEW

After age twenty-eight, a person's supply of undifferentiated stem cells diminishes, affecting their body's ability to repair lost functions on its own. Ongoing deterioration often leads to serious conditions, many of which can be reversed or prevented through rejuvenating cell therapy. Use of embryonic stem cells is therefore viewed as a viable means of complementing the overall biocompatible protocol.

WORDS OF ADVICE

- If you are over age twenty-eight, consume foods high in available RNA or RNA equivalent, like sardines (1.5 percent nucleic acid), liver (approximately 0.5 percent nucleic acid), muscle meat (0.5 percent nucleic acid), and such vegetables as spinach, leeks, broccoli, Chinese cabbage, cauliflower, and oyster, flat, button (whitecaps), or cep (porcini) mushrooms.
- If your health still feels compromised due to degenerative conditions associated with aging or serious illness, seek the care of a biocompatible physician, who might prescribe rejuvenating cell replacement injections.

RINGING IN THE EARS (TINNITUS)

In the United States, over 50 million people experience tinnitus, the medical term for the perception of sound in one or both ears or in the head, when no external sound is present. Approximately 12 million of them suffer from tinnitus severely enough to seek medical attention, while about 2 million are so debilitated they cannot function normally.[3] Tinnitus is often referred to as "ringing in the ears" because the word comes from a Latin term meaning "to tinkle or to ring like a bell." This symptom can be intermittent or constant; involve single or multiple tones; sound like hissing, roaring, whistling, chirping, or clicking; and range in volume from subtle to loud.

Cultures throughout the world think of tinnitus as receptivity to a special vibration or sound current. In regions of the People's Republic of China, tinnitus is welcomed as a sign of wisdom. In parts of Turkey, it portends good luck. To some yogic sects in India it signifies an intimate message from the voice of the Divine. Certain Christian denominations view it as an attunement to the word of God. On the other hand, practitioners of biocompatible medicine regard tinnitus, like other pronounced symptoms, as a message from the unconscious trying to tell us something about our state of health.

Western medicine has not yet identified the physiological cause of tinnitus, but the following circumstances are said to trigger or worsen it:

Noise-induced hearing loss—Exposure to loud noises, such as carnival parades or rock concerts, can damage hair cells, called cilia, in the inner ear, which cannot be renewed or replaced. About 30 percent of male and only 3 percent of female tinnitus patients have some level of noise-induced hearing loss.[4]

Wax buildup in the ear canal—Wax produced in the ears can compromise hearing. Excess earwax should be removed with a hollow candle that warms the wax and draws it out of the ear, rather than with a cotton swab, which may push the wax to the back of the ear canal.

Medications—Some medications that produce tinnitus are toxic to the ear, while others produce tinnitus as a side effect without damaging the inner ear. Effects, which can depend on dosage, may be temporary or permanent.

Ear or sinus infection—Many people experience tinnitus along with an ear or sinus infection. Generally, it diminishes or disappears once the infection is healed.

Jaw misalignment—Misaligned jaw joints or muscles can induce tinnitus and also affect cranial muscles, nerves, and shock absorbers in the jaw joint. Dentists who specialize in temporomandibular jaw alignment can assist with treatment.

Cardiovascular disease—Approximately 3 percent of tinnitus patients experience pulsatile tinnitus, a rhythmic pulsing, often in time to the heartbeat, which can indicate a cardiovascular condition, such as a heart murmur, hypertension, or hardening of the arteries.[5]

Tumors—A benign and slow-growing tumor on the auditory, vestibular, or facial nerves can cause tinnitus, along with deafness, facial paralysis, and loss of balance.

Physical trauma—Trauma to the head or neck can induce tinnitus, as well as headaches, vertigo, and memory loss.

Emotional problems—Emotions such as sadness and grief can weaken the lungs and heart and may lead to tinnitus.

As a doctor of traditional Chinese medicine, when I detect tinnitus I check the kidney meridian, which opens into the ears, and the gallbladder channel, which flows through the ear and can be involved in ear problems; I also ask about emotional issues, since they can produce "liver fire" that rises upward to disturb the ears, and general body problems. In addition to treatments for any problems found, I recommend acupuncture and lifestyle assessment to put patients back on the track to health. Diagnosing any imbalance in the body's energy and adjusting lifestyle to support health are critical first steps to quieting the noise in the ears.

THE BIOCOMPATIBLE VIEW

Biocompatible medicine views individuals as energy beings, and traditional Chinese medicine regards tinnitus as symptomatic of a yang energy deficiency in the kidney. Alleviating tinnitus requires restoring the yang energy through increased oxidation to the ear.

WORDS OF ADVICE

- Tinnitus is not a disease but a symptom. Because it can be caused by an underlying metabolic condition or drug reaction, seek a medical evaluation, starting with an ear, nose, and throat specialist and proceeding, if necessary, to a certified clinical nutritionist to determine the underlying cause.
- Consider taking supplements of ginkgo biloba and rosemary, which treat circulatory disorders that can contribute to tinnitus.
- Consider taking a supplement or tincture of oats, organically grown fresh aerial parts of *Avena sativa*, effective in reducing high cholesterol levels that can contribute to circulatory problems causing tinnitus.
- Avoid loud noises, which can cause trauma leading to ringing in the ears.
- Remove excess earwax with a hollow candle.
- For chronic tinnitus, take a B-complex vitamin that contains cobalamin and vitamin B_{12}.

S

SAMe

S-adenosylmethionine, or SAMe, which has been used to treat numerous medical conditions, including arthritis, depression, liver problems, and pain and inflammation, is a molecule continually produced by the body from methionine, an amino acid found in protein-rich foods, and adenosine triphosphate (ATP), an energy-producing compound in all the body's cells. The liver uses this process to make SAMe—as much as 8 grams per day when the liver is healthy. SAMe produces methylation in the body, a chemical transformation that occurs a billion times a second, regulating fetal development, brain function, the expression of genes, the preservation of fatty membranes that insulate cells, and the action of various hormones and neurotransmitters, including serotonin, melatonin, dopamine, and adrenaline.[1] Liver disease, osteoarthritis, or overuse of prescription drugs or over-the-counter medications, however, can diminish the body's SAMe production.[2]

The human body makes SAMe and then recycles it. Once a SAMe molecule loses its methyl group, however, it breaks down to form homocysteine, which is extremely toxic if it builds up within cells. Fortunately, with the help of vitamins B_6, B_{12}, as well as folic acid, the body converts homocysteine into glutathione, a valuable antioxidant, or "remethylates" it back into methionine.

The dangers of elevated concentrations of homocysteine in the blood are numerous. For one, they increase the risk for heart disease by damaging the lining of blood vessels and promoting blood clotting, which can halt the blood flow in small arteries. If the plugged artery is in the heart, a heart attack ensues; if it's in the brain, a stroke; in the legs, thrombosis. A blood clot, especially in deep veins of the leg, is a particular danger after surgery as it can either block blood flow at the point of clot formation or break free and block it elsewhere. High homocysteine levels also affect the collagen, or fibrous protein constituent, of bones, resulting in an increased incidence of broken bones in older people. In addition, high levels of homocysteine raises the risk of spina bifida and other defects that form in utero, and it has been implicated in depression.

It is possible to determine homocysteine levels through either a blood test for homocysteine or, if that's unavailable, a blood test to determine the amount of high-sensitivity C-reactive protein, levels of which rise in response to inflammation, especially inflammation related to bacterial infections. As homocysteine levels in body go up, so do the high-sensitivity C-reactive protein levels.

SAMe and homocysteine are essentially two versions of the same molecule—one benign and the other dangerous. Due to the rapid pace of methylation, people need sufficient B vitamins in their cells so that homocysteine levels stay low enough to avoid triggering health problems. The body, on its own, can generate only a small amount of SAMe; however, these levels increase following supplementation with B-complex vitamins.

In addition to its other positive effects, SAMe enhances the impact of mood-boosting messengers, such as serotonin and dopamine, either by regulating their breakdown or by speeding production of the receptor molecules they latch on to.[3] These molecules float in the outer membranes of brain cells like swimmers treading water in a pool, but if the membranes get thick and glutinous, due to age or other assaults, the receptors lose their ability to move and change in response to chemical signals. By methylating fats called phospholipids, SAMe keeps the membranes fluid and the receptors mobile.[4]

SAMe also assists in the treatment of various medical problems. In dozens of European medical trails involving thousands of patients, it has performed as well as traditional treatments for arthritis and depression, and research suggests it can also ease difficult liver conditions. In addition, researchers have found SAMe as effective as pharmaceutical treatments for pain and inflammation.[5]

SAMe apparently causes no adverse effects, even at high doses, and doctors have prescribed it successfully for two decades in the fourteen countries where it has been approved as a drug.[6] Unlike NSAIDs, SAMe shows no sign of damaging the digestive tract and, instead of speeding the breakdown of cartilage, may actually help restore it.

THE BIOCOMPATIBLE VIEW

The conversion of homocysteine to SAMe and glutathione is regularly checked by biocompatible physicians since a high blood level of homocysteine has many negative health outcomes. To support these conversions, biocompatible physicians recommend dietary supplementation with vitamins B_6 and B_{12}, folic acid, pyridoxal-5-phosphate, and trimethylglycine. Due to its relationship with SAMe, trimethylglycine may be useful as part of an oral therapy regimen for depression.

WORDS OF ADVICE

- Supplement your diet daily with B-complex vitamins, folic acid, pyridoxal-5-phosphate, and trimethylglycine to maintain the strong positive conversion of homocysteine into SAMe and glutathione.
- Protect the health of your liver since only healthy livers can produce adequate amounts of SAMe (see "Liver Detoxification," p. 149).
- Make sure you are screened for high-sensitivity C-reactive protein levels every time you have a blood test.
- If you suffer from depression, under the supervision of a certified clinical nutritionist explore substituting your present medication with SAMe, 5-hydroxytryptophan and trimethylglycine.

SEASONAL AFFECTIVE DISORDER (SAD)

Seasonal affective disorder (SAD) is a form of depression that often occurs in winter throughout the Northern and Southern Hemispheres due to lack of light and sunshine. It is rare in people living within 30 degrees of the equator, where daylight hours are long. In individuals affected by this disorder, the symptoms usually recur each winter, starting between September and November and continuing until March or April; although SAD may begin at any age, the typical age of onset is between eighteen and thirty. In addition to symptoms of depression, most sufferers show signs of a weakened immune system during the winter and thus increased vulnerability to infections and other illnesses, while in spring and autumn they may have extreme mood changes and short periods of hypomania (overactivity). For some people, SAD produces symptoms severe enough to cause considerable stress and to disrupt their lives.

A diagnosis of SAD can be made after three or more consecutive winters of symptoms, which include the following: desire to oversleep and difficulty staying awake; disturbed sleep and early morning waking; feelings of fatigue and inability to carry out normal routine; craving for carbohydrates and sweet foods, usually resulting in weight gain; feelings of misery, guilt, and reduced self-esteem, sometimes despair, apathy, and loss of feelings; irritability and the desire to avoid social contact; tension and inability to tolerate stress; and decreased interest in sex and physical contact. SAD symptoms usually disappear automatically in spring or when affected individuals travel to sunnier climates.

If a change of location is not possible, SAD can be treated in several ways. First, individuals can buy full-spectrum lightbulbs, which are similar to daylight in two ways: the light is perceived to have the bluish-white color and brightness values of daylight, as well as strong color-rendering capabilities. Daylight is a form of radiant energy that travels in waves, each of a certain length. In the visible part of the light spectrum, short waves produce a light that appears blue to the human eye, while longer waves produce a light that appears red. Daylight, because it includes all wavelengths visible to the human eye, is considered full spectrum.

When SAD leads to depression, it can be treated with standard antidepressant drugs, or if these are ineffective, relief may be found in 5-HTP (hydroxytryptophan), the precursor to serotonin, which plays an important role in regulating mood, sleep, sexuality, appetite, and vomiting. The benefits of 5-HTP, which, unlike other antidepressants, affects only the brain, are very similar to those of L-tryptophan, such as aiding sleep, alleviating age-related depression, and minimizing effects of alcohol withdrawal. But 5-HTP must not be taken with other serotonin-enhancing drugs, such as L-tryptophan or Prozac, without the supervision of a physician since the combination may cause severe side effects, including mania, anxiety, and dermatitis. In addition, depression caused by SAD can be treated with acupuncture.

The effects of SAD can be prevented or minimized through continuing physical activity during the fall and winter months. Participating in outdoor activities such as skating, skiing, or snowshoeing, or even indoor stretches and exercises such as swimming, yoga, or tai chi, are excellent ways to maintain a healthy mind and body. In addition, ensure that you get proper rest, nourishment, and emotional support.

THE BIOCOMPATIBLE VIEW

Biocompatible medicine, like traditional Chinese medicine, teaches that six external climatic forces—heat, cold, wind, dampness, dryness, and summer heat—can invade the human organism and create disharmony in body, mind, and spirit. Through acupuncture and other modalities, biocompatible medicine can help people who suffer from SAD achieve a more balanced state.

WORDS OF ADVICE

• Keep physically active during the fall and winter months to minimize symptoms of SAD.
• Get proper nourishment and rest.
• Allow yourself the necessary emotional support from family and friends to maintain a positive outlook on life.
• Install full-spectrum lightbulbs.
• Have acupuncture treatments to maintain physical and emotional balance.

SEXUAL RELATIONSHIPS

Sex, one of humanity's primary instincts, is a good indicator of health, and satisfying sexual relationships are known to confer not only physical but also psychological and social benefits. In fact, when consulting with a new patient, ideally with their significant other present, I review all parts of a traditional Chinese medicine examination to gain a fairly good understanding of the person's energetics. Toward the end of the examination, I almost always ask, "So how is your sex life?" By then I generally know if the person has enough chi, or vital life energy, to engage in sex or if they have been squandering their energy through extramarital trysts, and I want to see how honest they are willing to be with their new primary care provider.

I believe, along with my Chinese colleagues, that a moderate amount of healthy sex supports a good flow of chi and too much sex—specifically, ejaculation for men and childbearing for women—depletes the chi, blood, and kidneys. Moderate sexual activity has also been shown to release endorphins and other feel-good hormones, inspiring endocrinologists to research its impact on the central nervous system, especially its positive effects on stress.[7]

The Biology of Passion

From the perspective of biocompatible medicine, sexual intercourse consists of interactions of energy between partners. And because every cell in the human body radiates and reacts to energy, it is possible to measure the physiological changes that occur even with sexual desire. Consequently it is known that all bodily cells radiate charge as the energy fields of the partners fuse; that positive and negative charges flow back and forth between the partners until the current

equalizes; and that the orgasms of men and women resemble each other physiologically, with the same kind of excitation before climax, rhythmic convulsions
of the involuntary muscles at climax, and ebbing of excitation after climax.

Research shows a major change of body chemistry at climax, with physical,
psychological, and social implications. Primarily, acetylcholine/parasympathetic
nervous functions are enhanced, stimulating the production of sex hormones
and the chemical neurotransmitters dopamine and serotonin. Acetylcholine
supports brain, liver, cardiovascular, and reproductive health, while helping
the body absorb fat-soluble nutrients. Dopamine affects brain processes that
control movement, emotional response, and the ability to experience pleasure
and pain. Regulation of dopamine plays a crucial role in mental and physical
health. Serotonin deficiency is implicated in various disorders, including anxiety,
depression, obsessive-compulsive disorder, schizophrenia, stroke, obesity, pain,
hypertension, vascular problems, migraine, and nausea.

Frequent orgasm increases the level of the hormone oxytocin, which is linked
to personality, passion, social skills, and emotional quotient (EQ), all of which
affect career, marriage, and social life. Most notably, oxytocin, generated by the
pituitary gland and known to peak during orgasm, promotes feelings of gratification and the ongoing ability to surrender to one's own life force, free of fear and
self-conscious monitoring by the ego. Oxytocin, which is also produced in women
during childbirth and while nursing, elevates a sense of bonding, tenderness, and
gratitude toward the partner, as well as other emotional responses. For instance,
among premenopausal women in a healthy relationship the released oxytocin
helps to suppress physiological stress,[8] but when sexual excitation does not end in
a climax it can transform into anxiety.[9]

Prostaglandin, a hormone found in low concentrations throughout the body
and in semen, may be absorbed in the female genital tract, exacerbating diseases
of the female reproductive organs, including uterine cancer.[10] This could explain
why some women are allergic to their partner's sperm and why condom use is
encouraged even in stable relationships among partners not seeking birth control
measures.

Sexual Desire

Sexual desire peaks at different ages in men and women—in men at around age
eighteen and in women between thirty-five and forty. When both partners are
between the ages of twenty-five and thirty-five, they have fairly equal sex drives.
Not surprisingly, the majority of divorces in the West take place when couples
are in the thirty-five to forty age range.

Another sexual-related difference between men and women is that men are
naturally programmed to have sex more often than women. Consequently, the
proverbial notion that "all men think about is sex" has a biological foundation.

Combined, these differences put pressure on long-term monogamous relationships. Traditionally, such differences have led to various behaviors that cause
stress between partners. Young men, with their increased libido, tend to be promiscuous, while young women can feel "used" if their sexual appetite has not yet

peaked; middle-aged husbands may have affairs or leave their marriage, while wives consent to having sex with their husbands either to please them or because they feel it is their "duty"; husbands become "hen-pecked," while wives determine the rules of sexual behavior. Such behaviors can lead to serious consequences, such as divorce or separation, often in a context of misunderstanding of the emotional and physiological causes. For example, many times middle-aged men whose machismo is suffering will divorce and mate with younger women, but these women tend to have lower sexual urges than the men's former wives. By understanding these physiological differences and opening solid lines of communication, it may be possible to prevent substantial emotional trauma.

To facilitate such communication, it would be wise to break any remaining taboos limiting communication about sexual issues and to avoid judgments and stereotyping. In addition, trained natural physicians, through bodywork and counseling, can help each partner become personally responsible for his or her own sexual satisfaction, removing the burden from the partnership. Achieving sexual integrity involves a delicate balance that fosters a loving relationship.

Benefits of Sex

Satisfactory sexual expression is essential to many human relationships and provides a sense of physical, psychological, and social well-being. Having regular and enthusiastic sex confers physical advantages for both men and women, provided they are practicing safe sex, as sex with multiple partners can raise the risk of sexually transmitted diseases, such as AIDS, as well as increase the risk of cancer by up to 40 percent because of such diseases. For those who want all the benefits of sex but have no partner, masturbation is a safe alternative.

Having sex even a few times a week is associated with the following benefits:

Improved sense of smell. After sex, production of the hormone prolactin surges, which causes stem cells in the brain to develop new neurons in the brain's olfactory bulb, its smell center.

Reduced risk of heart attack and stroke. Studies debunking the presumed connection between sex and death show that in fact sexual activity seems to have a protective effect on men's health.[11]

Weight loss, overall fitness. Vigorous sex burns approximately 200 calories, about the same as running fifteen minutes on a treadmill or playing a spirited game of squash. The pulse rate in an aroused person rises from about 70 beats per minute to 150, comparable to that of an athlete, while muscle contractions during intercourse work the pelvis, thighs, buttocks, arms, neck, and thorax. Sex also boosts production of testosterone, which leads to stronger bones and muscles. *Men's Health* magazine has gone so far as to call the bed the single greatest piece of exercise equipment ever invented.

Pain relief. Immediately before orgasm, levels of the hormone oxytocin surge to five times their normal level, which releases endorphins that alleviate the pain of everything from arthritis to headaches. In women, sex also prompts production of estrogen, which can reduce the pain of PMS.

Less frequent colds and flu. According to a Wilkes University study, individuals who have sex once or twice a week show a 30 percent higher level of the antibody immunoglobulin A, which is known to boost the immune system.[12]

Better bladder control. The same muscles used in Kegel exercises for bladder control are worked during sex.

Better teeth. Seminal plasma contains zinc, calcium, and other minerals shown to retard tooth decay.

Improved prostate health. Some urologists believe a relationship exists between infrequency of ejaculation and cancer of the prostate. A study published in the *British Journal of Urology International* asserts that men in their twenties can reduce by 30 percent their chance of getting prostate cancer by ejaculating more than five times a week.[13] This may be because during the production of seminal fluid, the prostate and the seminal vesicles take such substances from the blood as zinc, citric acid, and potassium, and then concentrate them up to six hundred times before flushing them during ejaculation, a process that likewise occurs with any carcinogens present in the blood.

Less vaginal atrophy for postmenopausal women. Postmenopausal women who abstain from sex may experience vaginal atrophy, which can interfere with the muscles, nerves, and tissues that perform urinary and rectal control. Such women can also experience dysparenia, pain associated with intercourse; lower back pain and leg pain, resulting in a bent-over walking posture; and incontinence. According to Dr. Claire Bailey of the University of Bristol, a woman has little or no risk of overdosing on sex. In fact, she advises, repeated sexual activity can not only protect against vaginal atrophy but also firm the stomach and buttocks and improve the woman's posture.[14]

Ongoing sexual activity. A regular and stable pattern of sexual activity early in adult life leads to sustained sexual activity in later years.[15] Sexual activity in old age also depends on good physical health and the availability of a partner.

Sexual Problems

Without satisfactory sexual expression, individuals may experience a lack of physical, psychological, or social well-being. The origins of sexual problems run the gamut from physiological to emotional.

Loss of libido

Many epidemiological and clinical studies show impaired sexual function associated with depression and schizophrenia, due to lack of libido in both treated and untreated populations. Loss of libido is also associated with underlying medical problems such as cardiovascular problems (particularly hypertension), peripheral vascular disease, diabetes mellitus, renal failure, cancer, arthrosis, and neurological problems.

Impotence

Both men and women can be impotent, unable to achieve meaningful sexual coupling. In our clinic, we routinely observe patients with repressed sexual urges having physical, mental, or emotional symptoms, including distorted sexual behavior. In men, impotence usually shows up as either penis anesthesia (lack of feeling in the penis during sex and inability to discharge semen), premature ejaculation (the discharging of semen before penetration), or delayed ejaculation (inability to ejaculate after more than fifteen minutes). Often the underlying problem in men who ejaculate early or "withhold" their semen is seething anger, usually not directed at their partner. Also, men abusing cocaine or other drugs may have difficulty ejaculating.

Female impotence is generally based less on performance and more on emotional issues. Some women who are prone to sexual passivity, a learned behavior rooted in early experiences with strict parents or religious beliefs, may place the onus of their unsatisfactory coupling on their partner. Or they may tell their partner that sex is of no interest to them but their partner may use their body for sexual purposes. Most often such emotional and physical detachment from sex occurs in women who have been sexually violated. Withholding their climax is a way of remaining emotionally distant from their partner for fear of retriggering the earlier trauma.

In both sexes, lack of sex education, blockages associated with exhaustion or low self-esteem, or previous sexual violations can all lead to frustrated sexual responses that, in turn, may erupt in rage. Men suffering from penis anesthesia may resort to sadistic-compulsive symptoms such as rape, battering, or the constant need to hire prostitutes. Women blocked by early childhood prohibitions may angrily blame their partner for their own inability to achieve climax. Such behaviors illustrate the mind/body split of individuals who are unable to integrate their sexual self with their loving self. In these instances, counseling will most likely be needed to resolve the underlying issues and attain healthy and enjoyable sexual responses.

Erectile dysfunction

An easy way to assess a man's physical, psychological, and social health is to determine how often he wants and can have sex. For a more in-depth investigation of his health, a sperm analysis will reveal his status. A man in his mid-fifties who is interested in sex three times a week is physically doing very well. But if a man in his mid-fifties responds to an inquiry about his sex life with, "Sex? Never been better! I swallow my little pill and then I can have sex for three hours," he may be suffering from erectile dysfunction, the inability to achieve or maintain an erection long enough to engage in sexual intercourse. Normally, when a man is sexually excited, his penis fills with more blood than usual and becomes erect; when a man has erectile dysfunction, his penis does not fill with enough blood to get erect or may not stay erect long enough to complete sexual activity.

About 30 million men in the United States have erection problems and about half of men between the ages of forty and seventy are impotent to some degree. Although most men with erection problems realize their need for help, they often do not visit their physician seeking treatment for the erectile dysfunction.[16] A man who has trouble getting or sustaining an erection should seek medical assistance for this problem, however, because he most likely has an underlying medical condition such as high blood pressure, high cholesterol, diabetes, heart disease, depression, unmanaged stress or injuries, or he is suffering the consequences of smoking, drug or alcohol abuse, or the use of blood-pressure lowering drugs, heart condition drugs, cancer drugs, or certain antidepressants or diuretics.

Treatment for erectile dysfunction often hinges on pharmaceutical drugs, which can occasionally fail to decrease a man's erection after sexual activity, causing blood to continually flow into the penis rather than oxygenate the blood. As a result, the penis tissue can become damaged from oxygen starvation. An erection lasting more than four hours requires immediate medical attention, since otherwise the penis can sustain permanent damage. In lieu of taking prescription medication, a more prudent way to deal with erectile dysfunction is by correcting the physical problems that caused it.

Conflicts over sexual preference

Perhaps the greatest cause of marital friction is the attempt to maintain a socially acceptable marriage without reflecting one's underlying preference for a same-sex partner. Even though love relationships that are not heterosexual are socially taboo in nearly all traditional societies, bisexual and homosexual feelings are in fact a part of life. Worldwide, statistics reveal that 25 percent of all individuals are exclusively heterosexual, 25 percent are exclusively homosexual, and 50 percent are bisexual[17]—figures born out in my clinical practice.

Clinically, I have witnessed as well that dissatisfied bisexuals can cause many conflicts in relationships. Moreover, the fact there is a high percentage of bisexuals could be an unexplored contributing factor to social problems.

Self-awareness and self-esteem issues

Self-awareness helps people recognize when they are too stressed to have satisfying sex and is therefore a prerequisite for effective communication with sex partners. People lacking self-awareness often fail to understand themselves; as a result, they remain caught up in their own internal struggles and cannot effectively respond to their partner.

Low self-esteem has a similar impact on sexual relations. The reasons people suffer from low self-esteem include perceived lack of self-worth, uncontrollable jealousy, a relationship breakup, high levels of anxiety or stress, inability to think positively, and mild depression. Professionals trained in treating such problems holistically can help couples suffering with self-esteem or self-awareness issues develop satisfying love relationships.

THE BIOCOMPATIBLE VIEW

Biocompatible medicine stresses the importance of having a healthy sexual attitude, sufficient self-respect to avoid getting involved in harmful sexual relationships, and an ability to communicate openly about sex. It also regards healthy sexual relationships in adulthood as essential to physical, psychological, and social well-being.

WORDS OF ADVICE

- If you have low self-esteem and experience sexual problems, consider counseling with a trained professional.
- Learn to communicate with your sexual partner to enhance sexual experiences.
- If you develop disinterest in having consensual sex with your marital or relationship partner, seek assistance as this can be symptomatic of a physical, emotional, or spiritual imbalance.
- If you have sexual problems, get a medical assessment to determine any underlying physical conditions and consider sex therapy. Although sex is not all there is to a happy marriage or relationship, for most people it is an important aspect.
- If you are a parent, make sure your children, especially teens, receive proper information about healthy sex, sexual relationships, reproduction and birth control, sexually transmitted diseases, and sexual abuse. Withholding such information from children and teens puts them at risk for sexual diseases, abuse, and other needless difficulties.

SKIN

As the body's largest organ, skin reflects the state of an individual's health—and therefore general health needs to be maintained for skin to remain blemish free. Although companies that make skin care products would like people to believe that a beautiful complexion can be obtained by using such items, truly radiant, moist, and blemish-free skin is the result of having clean blood that continuously supplies beneficial nutrients to every cell in the body.

Unfortunately, keeping toxins out of the blood and organs is difficult in modern societies because the environment is full of chemicals and refined foods often lack essential nutrients for good health. Toxicity can accumulate beneath the skin from poor diet; lack of exercise; improper pH levels in soaps, skin creams, and antiperspirants; or synthetic fibers worn next to the skin. Consequently, to maintain healthy skin, it is necessary both to detoxify the body and to consume the finest nutrients. Fortunately, the body is constantly in a cleansing mode and will discharge toxins as long as it is supplied with sufficient energy. An adult can eliminate two to four pounds of toxic waste daily through the skin. Perspiration is composed of 99 percent water and 1 percent mineral salts, complex fatty substances, and waste acids being eliminated by the body.

To maintain beautiful, healthy skin, it is imperative to keep the pertinent organs nourished and detoxified. The six organs responsible for beautiful skin are the liver, kidneys, adrenals, thyroid, large intestines, and small intestines. An overworked liver or kidneys can compromise healthy skin. The liver and kidneys constantly filter wastes, which are extracted by the large intestine. In today's environment, these organs are likely to be overworked due to toxicity and bad nutrition; therefore, it is advantageous to learn from a clinical nutritionist how to protect them from harm and properly nourish them to keep skin healthy (see "Liver Detoxification," p. 149).

A weak thyroid can make skin nonresponsive to cosmetic intervention. Most underactive or hypothyroid problems are the result of toxic metals or low progesterone levels in women. Mercury, which is found in dental amalgams, is especially detrimental to thyroid and skin. Finding a biocompatible dentist is therefore one of the first steps in establishing a foundation of healthy and beautiful skin.

Other aids to obtaining healthy and beautiful skin are drinking sufficient amounts of water, eating according to metabolic type, and taking the necessary natural supplements. Skin beauty can also be enhanced by certain procedures performed by a dermatologist or other specialized practitioner. One such treatment is a full-body lymph drainage massage, in which the practitioner uses a range of gently rhythmic pumping techniques to move the skin in the direction of the lymph flow, stimulating the lymphatic vessels that carry substances vital to the defense of the body, and removing waste products. If the lymphatic system, which plays an important role in regulating the immune system, becomes blocked, lymphatic fluid builds up, causing the system to become toxic. Lymphatic drainage clears blockages, eliminates metabolic wastes and toxins, transports nutrients to cells, and increases metabolic efficiency, reducing excess fluid, assisting weight reduction, and relieving stress and tension. It is a very successful beauty treatment for the face, improving the appearance of the skin, helping to rejuvenate collagen fibers, and slowing the aging process.

Another treatment to cleanse the lymph system of toxins and improve surface circulation to keep pores open is dry skin brushing toward the heart, which encourages discharge of metabolic wastes that leads to improved ability to combat bacteria and support healthier, more radiant skin. This technique, which can be self-administered, results in tighter skin, better digestion, less cellulite, improved circulation, increased cell renewal, a clean lymphatic system, removal of dead skin layers, a strengthened immune system, and improved exchange between cells and gland stimulation. The technique, requiring the use of a natural-bristle brush with a long handle to facilitate reaching difficult areas, is as follows:

- Before bathing, brush dry skin at least once a day (twice is better). Although helpful for removing toxins from cancer patients, do not brush over an obvious skin tumor.
- Brush the soles of the feet first, from the toes to the heel.
- Brush legs, moving upward from the toes.
- Brush buttocks and lower back to each side, then up the spine to the base of the neck.
- Gently pull the brush from the back of the neck to the front; then slide the brush along the jaw from the earlobe to the underside of the chin.
- Brush down the neck to the center of the breasts.
- Brush from the fingers up to the armpits.
- Brush the armpits and upper chest toward the middle of the chest and down.
- Lightly brush the breasts from the nipple down to the base. Brush from the top of the breasts down the center, and from the sides and bottom to the solar plexus.
- On the right and left sides of the groin, rotate the brush gently counterclockwise, then clockwise, seven times each. Finish the groin area by brushing upward to the abdomen.

- Brush up the abdomen and stomach toward the solar plexus.
- If possible, take a warm bath or shower followed by a cool rinse to invigorate blood circulation and stimulate surface warmth.
- Finish with a vigorous towel rub.

Contrary to popular belief, exposing skin to the sun—but not to the point of being sunburned—is beneficial, since it is the safest way to obtain vitamin D, a powerful antioxidant that can help prevent premature aging of the skin and degenerative diseases such as skin cancer. On the other hand, sunburn, characterized by red, swollen, or blistered skin and caused by too much exposure to ultraviolet light from the sun, sunlamps, or even some workplace light sources such as welding arcs, may lead to premature skin aging and skin cancer. The risk for sunburn is higher among people with fair skin, blue eyes, and red or blond hair, and is also greatly increased by the use of sulfa drugs, some antibiotics, some water pills, and even over-the-counter antihistamines. Unfortunately, use of sunscreen is not necessarily a good means of protection from sunburn since it contains a toxic chemical that can cause systemic problems and increase the risk of disease. If you have to be exposed to the sun between 11 a.m. and 2 p.m., wear a hat, long-sleeved shirt, and long pants to block the sun's rays.

Another beneficial treatment for skin is acupuncture, a therapy based on the principle that optimal health is achieved when the body's systems are in balance. Acupuncture provides other benefits as well. For example, women who choose facial acupuncture can expect reduced depression and less anxiety, improved digestion, better sleep cycles, and fewer hot flashes and night sweats, while those who opt for abdominal acupuncture are likely to benefit from increased sex drive and fertility.

Treatments for acne, a skin condition that has become prevalent in cultures with a high consumption of refined carbohydrates and sugar, vary. Interestingly, in one study involving non-Westernized islanders of Papua, New Guinea, and hunter-gatherers of Paraguay, no cases of acne were found in either group. Comparing this outcome with the relatively high rates of acne in modernized Western societies, the researchers concluded that the discrepancy "cannot be solely attributed to genetic differences among populations but likely results from differing environmental factors."[18] We have noted similar findings in our clinic, indicating the significant role of environmental factors, such as diet and vitamin deficiencies, in acne.

Conventional treatments for acne—antibiotics and topical creams—unfortunately can be problematic because the drugs may kill the good bacteria along with the bad. Consequently, the best treatment for acne is appropriate diet for metabolic type, avoiding foods with sugar, taking appropriate supplements, and reducing toxins in the body. In terms of supplements, vitamin A has a long history of use in treating acne and, as the ingredient in Retin-A, appears to smooth out wrinkles and improve skin texture by restoring the skin's ability to produce collagen. Vitamin E improves the efficiency of vitamin A and helps keep skin tissues healthy; I recommend liquid vitamin E applied directly to the skin. In addition, vitamin C, an antioxidant that fights inflammation within the body, protects against free-radical damage and participates in the production of collagen, which supports the skin, keeping it from sagging. Brewer's yeast, a source of B vitamins, also protects the skin.

A combination of cleansing, replenishing, and protecting the body, along with good lifestyle habits, can promote radiant, blemish-free skin. Good lifestyle habits include drinking sufficient water daily to hydrate the skin; detoxifying the colon and removing heavy metals to counteract inflammatory reactions in the body that show up on the skin as acne, white yeast spots, hives, or psoriasis; eating foods appropriate for metabolic type; avoiding drinks and foods with sugar, as well as limiting grains and milk products; supplementing with zinc and collagen hydrogenase; getting acupuncture treatments; following an appropriate exercise program, which benefits the skin by cleansing toxins and increasing circulation; and using natural skin cleansing and skin protection products.

THE BIOCOMPATIBLE VIEW
Biocompatible medicine associates the skin with the lungs and large intestines. Consequently, biocompatible physicians believe that problems in these organs manifest on the skin surface and can be treated by treating the skin.

WORDS OF ADVICE
• If you have blemishes, acne, itching or dry skin, do not merely cover it up with cosmetics but have it checked medically to determine the underlying pathology.
• Avoid smoking, drinking, or abusing drugs.
• Sunbathe at least fifteen minutes a day in the tropics and thirty minutes in northern latitudes before 10:00 a.m. and after 3:00 p.m.
• Take supplements of vitamin A, vitamin E, and vitamin C, as well as brewer's yeast.
• Drink sufficient water, 1 to 3 liters per day, to hydrate the skin.
• Detoxify the body through colon hydrotherapy.
• Eat according to metabolic type; avoid drinks and foods with sugar; and limit grains and milk products.
• Supplement with zinc (25 to 30 mg daily) and collagen hydrogenase.
• Exercise regularly to release toxins and increase circulation.
• Use natural skin cleansing and skin protection products.
• Get acupuncture treatments.

SLEEP
Sleep is a basic human need, as important for good health as diet and exercise. When people sleep, their bodies rest while their brains remain active, contributing to productivity and healing. Currently, 10 to 25 percent of individuals have chronic insomnia or other sleep problems, and approximately $98 million a year is spent in the United States alone on over-the-counter sleep aids.

Most people need eight hours of sleep nightly, but research shows that in developed countries the typical night's sleep has decreased since the beginning of the century, from nine hours to seven and a half hours. On average, a woman aged thirty to sixty sleeps only six hours and forty-one minutes per night during the workweek. Conditions unique to women, such as the menstrual cycle, pregnancy, and menopause—all of which involve changing levels of hormones like estrogen and progesterone—can affect how well a woman sleeps.

Getting sufficient sleep is vital. I believe that seven hours is an absolute minimum, and most people would benefit from nine hours. Those who give up sleep to make more time for work and leisure, or who have sleep disorders, are accelerating the aging process and putting themselves at greater risk of stress-related problems, poor performance on the job and in school, sickness, and weight gain. Chronic sleep loss hinders metabolism and hormone production in a way similar to aging and the early stages of diabetes, and may speed the onset or increase the severity of conditions such as type II diabetes, high blood pressure, obesity, and memory loss. Medical researchers have shown that just one week of sleep deprivation can alter hormone levels and the ability to metabolize carbohydrates.[19]

During sleep deprivation, men's blood sugar levels can take 40 percent longer than usual to drop and the ability to secrete and respond to the hormone insulin, which helps regulate blood sugar, can drop by 30 percent, reflecting the effects of insulin resistance. In addition, sleep-deprived men have elevated nighttime concentrations of the hormone cortisol, which also helps regulate blood sugar and lower the level of thyroid-stimulating hormone, a condition often seen in older people that may be involved in age-related insulin resistance and memory loss.

Sleep disorders can be caused by a variety of physical, psychological, or environmental problems, including eating, drinking alcohol, or exercising too close to bedtime; consuming caffeine; being in an environment unconducive to sleep; anxiety; or fundamental physical problems. In children, many sleep problems are related to irregular sleep habits or anxiety about becoming separated from parents.

Treating chronic sleep loss usually requires a visit to a holistic physician to determine the cause of the problem, then adherence to a treatment plan. General suggestions for optimizing sleep can include anything from establishing a new bedtime routine or environment to avoiding food, caffeine, nicotine, alcohol, or exercise just before bedtime. Supplements such as 5-HTP or SAMe may be recommended to aid sleep, or melatonin for resetting the sleep cycle.

THE BIOCOMPATIBLE VIEW

Biocompatible medicine encourages adequate sleep since it rejuvenates and energizes the body and brain, positively affecting all physical and metal processes. Lack of sleep has dramatic negative effects on physical and mental performance and lowers the body's ability to repair itself.

WORDS OF ADVICE

• Maintain a regular schedule for bedtime and waking, even on weekends.
• Create an environment conducive to sleep—dark, quiet, comfortable, and cool.
• Establish a relaxing bedtime routine, such as taking a hot bath, reading a book, or listening to music.
• Use the bedroom only for sleep and sex, making sure to remove work materials, computers, and the TV.

- After a bad night's sleep, get up and go about your day to avoid disturbing your internal clock.
- If you wake at night, relax in bed to see if you can go back to sleep, then if that doesn't work get up and engage in a quiet activity until you are sleepy again.
- Before bedtime, write down any concerns you may have about what you will do the next day.
- Eat a healthy diet and finish eating at least two to three hours before bedtime.
- Avoid eating chocolate or drinking coffee, tea, and soft drinks that contain caffeine before bedtime, as the body needs four to five hours to reduce by half the amount of caffeine in the blood.
- Avoid nicotine (cigarettes and tobacco products) and alcohol close to bedtime.
- Exercise regularly during the day but stop at least a few hours before bedtime.
- Take 5-HTP or SAMe with a little fruit juice thirty minutes before a meal to aid sleep; take melatonin to reset your sleep cycle if it has been altered due to travel or a work shift change. Avoid taking sleeping pills, however, as they are habit forming and do not produce the deep restorative sleep needed to regain health.
- Have acupuncture treatments to balance the body and encourage restful sleep.
- If sleep disruption persists, see a holistic physician to determine if it is being caused by an underlying physiological problem.

STRESS

Stress is the condition resulting from the body's reaction to one or more stressors. An individual under stress goes through numerous physiological changes: the body releases adrenaline along with glucose from the liver; the body begins to sweat, causing the blood sugar to rise and blood pressure to increase; and the heart beats fasters and pumps blood harder, the arteries narrow, and digestion slows. As a result, the individual may experience poor sleep, bad temper, repeated sickness, a propensity for accidents, frustration, and an increase in alcohol intake that can have additional negative consequences, both socially and physiologically.

Under the effects of constant stress, the thymus gland, spleen, and lymph nodes shrink; the immune system loses its ability to fight off infection; excess stomach acid is produced; blood pressure becomes continuously high; the brain releases the stimulating chemical norepinephrine; and levels of sex hormones almost always decline. The emotional center of the brain, now starved for norepinephrine, can cause a person to experience biological depression or anxiety; metabolically, this can lead to anhedonia, the inability to feel emotional pleasure. Chronic stress can also result in heart disease, cancer, or diabetes.

Despite the negative consequences of stress, a manageable amount of stress over a short period can be healthy since the brain's release of norepinephrine initially has a beneficial effect. It promotes a positive mood and helps learning by moving short-term memory into long-term storage.

Interestingly, the decisive factor guiding the impact of stress is not so much what happens to people but their response to events. People who go through horrendous situations and view them as challenging adventures may not suffer the negative consequences of stress. By contrast, regarding such circumstances as a matter of survival may stimulate the body to release cortisol, which I call the "suicide chemical," also known as hydrocortisone. Cortisol is produced to help handle stressors, but its secretion is detrimental in three ways: it starves the brain of glucose, wreaks havoc with brain chemicals, and ultimately kills brain cells. Learning to take control by perceiving a stressful situation as a challenge rather than a threat is probably the most critical element in defeating the negative consequences of stress.

Most people who experience chronic stress cannot identify the root of the problem. They blame it on emotional stressors—lack of money, marital problems, job hassles, and the constant demands of children. Consequently, they may go to a psychiatrist to discuss what they believe is bothering them or to receive a prescription for antidepressant drugs with dangerous side effects. By contrast, rather than attempting to eliminate stress from people's lives, biocompatible physicians seek to increase people's ability to cope with stress by advising them to maintain an appropriate diet for metabolic type, especially people with type A blood—since inappropriate diets are seen as principal stressors. In our clinic, we also do blood tests and hair analysis to check for any physical reasons for stress and to identify existing environmental toxins (insecticides, pesticides, petrochemicals, or heavy metals) that may be further stressing the body. Once toxins are identified, a certified clinical nutritionist, chelation therapist, or homeopath can help with various types of detoxification. In addition, a holistic physician can provide concrete recommendations for stress relief through one or more of the many available therapies, such as the following:

Bodywork
Acupuncture. Used alone or in conjunction with other therapy modalities, acupuncture helps reduce a racing heartbeat, anxiety, and elevated blood pressure.
Chiropractic adjustments.
Massage, especially shiatsu and rolfing. A comprehensive method of hands-on, connective tissue manipulation and movement education can release stress patterns.

Complementary therapies
Clinical nutrition counseling.
Homeopathic treatments.
Bach flower remedies.

Psychological/spiritual techniques
Energy healing of the spirit.
Chakra therapy.
Hypnotherapy.
Meditation and other relaxation therapies.

In addition, rather than taking antidepressants with dangerous side effects as a treatment for stress, natural products can help, such as 5-HTP, SAMe, and St. John's Wort, provided individuals are not on antidepressants. Even a cup of chamomile tea at bedtime might be all a person needs to calm down enough to sleep.

Relaxation is a great boon in coping with stress. When the body is relaxed, stress symptoms can reverse, leading to an experience of control instead of the helplessness that often accompanies stress. Means for inducing relaxation include engaging in hobbies or sex, which releases chemicals that provide a sense of well-being (endorphins, adrenaline, serotonin, and dopamine) and helps maintain or restore supportive relationships. In our clinic, we have found that a primary form of stress reduction, especially among thirty-five- to forty-five-year-old women, is increased sexual stimulation.

Finally, regular exercise relaxes tense muscles and builds resistance to the negative consequences of stress by improving the circulation, releasing mood-elevating chemicals, and strengthening the immune system. Studies show that people who exercise regularly are less likely to suffer from stress-related illness.[20]

THE BIOCOMPATIBLE VIEW
Biocompatible medicine regards stress as a natural part of being alive, and some stress as having a positive effect on health. Instead of attempting to eliminate stress, biocompatible medicine strives to increase people's ability to cope with what they consider negative stressors so these will not impair their health. Stress can be managed by maintaining a diet appropriate for metabolic type; detoxification; various therapies; and making lifestyle changes, including learning relaxation techniques.

WORDS OF ADVICE
• Learn ways to relax, such as by participating in a hobby, sexual activity, listening to music, or reading.
• Reduce the clutter in your life.
• Deal head-on with anything that has been bothering you, since resolving problems will eliminate them.
• Get sufficient sleep to "reboot" for more challenges.
• Eat according to metabolic type.
• Try some therapy modalities to increase your ability to cope with stress.
• Exercise regularly.

SUGAR
Too much sugar in the diet can be detrimental to health since products rich in sugar metabolize too fast in the bloodstream, resulting in harmful spikes in blood sugar, rapid depletion of energy, and damaging stress symptoms. Although the World Health Organization (WHO) guidelines for nutrition advise that a healthy diet should consist of no more than 10 percent sugar, the sugar industry in the United States has officially stated that "a quarter of our food and drink intake can safely consist of sugar" and demanded that Congress end its $406 million funding unless WHO scrapped its guidelines on healthy eating.[21]

The sugar industry tried to substantiate its position by declaring its experts "found that a higher intake of sugar did not negatively affect micronutrient intake and that high consumption of sugars was not associated with a poorer quality diet. In a study of 143 children, ages eleven and twelve years, a seven-day weighed and recorded food inventory revealed that as the proportion of energy from sugars increased, there was no decline in dietary fiber or micronutrient intake, with the exception of niacin, which exceeded recommended levels."[22]

In fact, informed nutritionists know that refined white sugar provides only "empty" calories and is metabolized through the depletion of enzymes that contain thiamin, vitamin B_1, niacin, and other B vitamins, thereby increasing the requirement for these vitamins in populations subjected to diets rich in sugar, including Americans and Arubans.

In addition, it is known that refined white sugar kills the friendly bacteria in the colon that help produce B-complex vitamins, which play a major role in converting vegetable protein to L-glutamic acid, the only amino acid metabolized in the brain and vital for brain and parasympathetic nervous system function. In our clinic, we routinely recommend the use of L-glutamic acid in the treatment of fatigue, Parkinson's disease, schizophrenia, mental retardation, muscular dystrophy, alcoholism, and cocaine addiction, all of which have been linked to the high consumption of refined white sugar. Metabolizing refined white sugar also forces the body to deplete its stores of essential minerals such as calcium, potassium, magnesium, and zinc, making sugar also a key contributor to osteoporosis.

There are more immediate symptoms of sugar intolerance as well. These include hyperactivity in children, a strong craving for sweets, falling asleep after meals, allergies, gas and bloating, distended stomach after meals, joint pains, headaches, chronic fatigue, constipation, diarrhea, weight gain, skin problems, and high blood pressure.

From a neurological perspective, refined white sugar can be considered a dangerous drug. In fact, for many individuals this simple carbohydrate is the first addictive substance they ingest. Using the same neurological pathways as cocaine, it stimulates the release of serotonin in the hypothalamus, which then metabolizes into dopamine, inducing a "high" that often manifests as hyperactivity in children. With repeated exposures, refined white sugar programs children's brains for other addictive substances.

Breaking the sugar habit can be almost as difficult as overcoming drug addiction. One approach is to lower refined white sugar consumption by eating sweet alternatives such as fruit, the sweet herb stevia, and natural sugars like maple syrup, blackstrap molasses, or honey in small amounts; artificial sweeteners, however, are not recommended as they are carcinogens. Also, an increased consumption of water and protein can lower cravings for sugar. In fact, a desire for sweets is a symptom of dehydration and an indication that not enough protein and too many carbohydrates have been eaten.

In our clinic we use acupuncture treatments, chiropractic adjustments, and the supplements 5-HTP and DL-phenylalanine to help control carbohydrate addiction. Another helpful supplement is chromium glucose tolerance factor (GTF), a trace mineral that works with insulin to transport glucose from the blood into the cells; however, cells resistant to insulin will not absorb the glucose needed for energy. Finally, studies have shown that individuals who increase their aerobic activity by 38 minutes per day, walking about 2.2 miles or 4,400 steps, even without losing weight will experience a noteworthy reduction in blood sugar, as well as total cholesterol, triglycerides, and blood pressure.[23]

THE BIOCOMPATIBLE VIEW

Biocompatible medicine, which focuses on the body's metabolism, maintains that products containing refined white sugar metabolize too fast in the bloodstream, resulting in unhealthy spikes in blood sugar, rapid depletion of energy, and damaging stress symptoms. Reducing such items in the diet makes it possible to better control weight, increase energy levels, and reduce the risk of heart disease.

WORDS OF ADVICE

• Reduce the consumption of foods containing refined white sugar by eating sweet alternatives, such as fruit, stevia, blackstrap molasses, maple syrup, or honey.
• Drink sufficient water and eat enough protein to reduce the craving for sweets.
• Exercise to decrease your blood sugar level.
• Take supplements to regulate your blood sugar level.

T

THYROID

The thyroid, the largest endocrine gland in the human body, secretes the iodine-rich hormones thyroxin and triiodothyronine, which regulate metabolic rate. If the thyroid gland is not functioning optimally, it can produce a myriad of symptoms, described as follows.

Symptoms of an underactive or low-functioning thyroid, also known as hypothyroidism:

- Fatigue
- Feeling run down and sluggish
- Depression
- Difficulty concentrating; brain fog
- Unexplained or excessive weight gain
- Dry, coarse, or itchy skin
- Dry, coarse, or thinning hair
- Feeling cold, especially in the extremities
- Constipation
- Muscle cramps
- Increased menstrual flow; more frequent periods
- Infertility; miscarriage[1]

Symptoms of an overactive or high-functioning thyroid, also known as hyperthyroidism:

- Nervousness
- Irritability
- Increased perspiration
- Thinning skin
- Fine, brittle hair
- Muscular weakness, especially in the upper arms and thighs
- Shaky hands
- Panic disorder
- Insomnia

- Racing heart
- Frequent bowel movements
- Weight loss despite a good appetite
- Lighter menstrual flow; less frequent periods[2]

Thyroid and sex hormones stimulate each other, which is why many women with low progesterone are initially misdiagnosed as thyroid deficient. In our clinic, when not enough progesterone is produced in the cycle to balance the effects of estrogen, we see estrogen dominance. Symptoms include swollen breasts, bloating, food cravings, mood swings, cyclical migraine headaches, lack of sexual desire, short cycles, heavy bleeding cycles, and growing fibroids. Estrogen dominance is often experienced by perimenopausal women and premenopausal women with subclinical hypothyroidism or T3 (thyroid hormone triiodothyronine) deficiency, or women who have had one ovary removed, tubal ligation, or exposure to chemical endocrine disruptors. In premenopausal women, estrogen dominance is a common cause of PMS. Irregular periods, often leading to needless hysterectomies, and breast disease are common results of hypothyroidism.

Too little thyroid production may also cause increased prolactin levels[3] and persistent estrogen stimulation.[4] Levels of prolactin, the hormone that stimulates breastmilk production, rise naturally during pregnancy and breastfeeding. But high prolactin levels at other times, most often resulting from malfunction of the controlling pituitary gland, causes menstrual irregularity—especially light and less frequent periods, or cessation of menstruation—and production of milk from the breasts. The opposing actions of thyroid and estrogen can be envisioned as estrogen causing calories to be stored as fat and thyroid hormone causing fat calories to be turned into energy. Thus even in the presence of normal serum levels of thyroid hormone, excess estrogen may inhibit thyroid action in the cells, interfering with the binding of thyroid to its receptor, disrupting thyroid functioning, and producing the hypothyroid symptoms of fatigue, weight gain, and low body temperature.

Up to 10 percent of Westerners, including as many as 20 percent of women over age sixty, have a thyroid problem[5]—one that has most likely not been properly diagnosed. One reason thyroid problems have not been correctly assessed is that thyroid levels constantly fluctuate and all individuals have their own ideal level, which can vary at different ages. Therefore, thyroid diagnoses based on standard blood tests are often inaccurate because they do not reflect the normal level for a particular person according to prior baseline data.

Acutely aware of this situation, "Sam" Queen, of the Institute for Health Realities, alerts his students to the danger of treating "test results" instead of people's symptoms. For example, a test may indicate that a thirty-year-old's thyroid level is in the normal range, say 5.5, but if the individual had been tested at age nine and found to have a higher hormone level the latest findings would indicate an underactive, rather than a normal, thyroid function. Ideally, baseline testing would occur in the late teens or early twenties, when the thyroid is at peak levels, to establish a norm against which later tests can be compared.

A second reason thyroid tests are often inaccurate is that they show only the hormone level sent on the day of testing, which can depend largely on what the individual has eaten, since the food consumed each day has an immediate impact on how much hormone the thyroid secretes. For example, a sushi meal eaten the night before a thyroid blood test will skew the results. This is because the portion of the meal consisting of seaweed, which contains about "a thousand times as much iodine as any other food,"[6] will prompt the thyroid gland to increase the amount of hormone it secretes. This also explains why the Japanese population is virtually free of thyroid problems.

A third reason for the inaccuracy of thyroid tests is that they do not indicate if the thyroid hormone is actually entering the cells. For instance, an individual's thyroid can be manufacturing plenty of hormone, but his cells may have become resistant to it and unable to utilize it, a condition known as Wilson's syndrome.

Since it is not possible to determine accurate hormone levels from standard thyroid tests, to diagnose thyroid problems I recommend blood spot hormone testing, which measures the "free" thyroid hormone level, as opposed to the protein-bound, inactive level picked up by standard blood tests. The comprehensive thyroid profile resulting from this test provides the most accurate gauge of thyroid function that currently exists.

I also recommend saliva tests, which can be done at home, to measure the free, "bioavailable" fraction of steroid hormones that have moved out of the bloodstream and into the tissue. Saliva tests afford the most reliable calculation of tissue uptake with respect to topical hormone supplementation; are painless, non-invasive, and needle free (stress caused by a conventional blood draw can alter test results); are private, convenient, and allow for optimal collection time; are stable at room temperature for up to three weeks, allowing for worldwide shipment to labs; are less expensive than conventional blood testing; and allow for routine monitoring of hormone levels and adjustment of hormone supplementation as needed.

An additional test used to evaluate metabolic impacts on the thyroid is the hair element analysis. Hair is an excretory tissue, and therefore hair tests identify toxicities the body is discharging.

Universally, the thyroid problem most often diagnosed is hypothyroidism. The traditional treatment for this condition is thyroid hormone replacement, a prescription drug composed of T4 (thyroid hormone thyroxine), T3 (thyroid hormone triiodothyronine), or a combination product containing synthetic T4 and synthetic T3. By contrast, treatment for low-functioning thyroid in our clinic involves removing the toxic heavy metals, especially cadmium and mercury, then correcting the zinc-copper ratio to about 5:1 for women and 10:1 or higher for men. If an individual has too much dietary intake of zinc, estrogen will accelerate the thyroidal functioning (hyperthyroidism); and if a person has too much copper, estrogen will cause the body to slow down thyroidal functioning (hypothyroidism). In general, the thyroid can be nourished best through a diet that includes the good fats (coconut oil, pumpkin seed oil, raw butter, cod liver oil, and egg yolks) and mineral-rich foods (dark green leafy vegetables, sea salt, and ocean veggies like seaweed, if these are suitable for the person's blood type).

If, after removing the toxic heavy metals and adjusting the zinc-copper ratio, the thyroid still functions slowly, we recommend Armour Thyroid, a naturally derived thyroid replacement containing both T3 and T4. Since all parts of the body are interconnected, medicating the thyroid is not in an individual's best interests; however, when properly monitored, thyroid medication composed of this natural glandular material has been found to be nearly risk free.[7]

In our clinic, the minority of thyroid patients with blood test results indicating hyperthyroidism, the cause is usually low blood protein levels or a need for protease that helps break down protein. The most common reason for hyperthyroidism in reproductive-aged women is elevated levels of thyroid receptor antibodies, a condition known as Graves' disease.

THE BIOCOMPATIBLE VIEW

The approach of biocompatible medicine to both low- and high-functioning thyroid is to correct the metabolic process by removing heavy metals and returning the zinc-copper ratio to a healthy balance. When a patient first presents with a thyroid imbalance, the biocompatible physician will verify the results through a blood test then order a hair element analysis report to determine cadmium levels and ensure that zinc is active. In the presence of a zinc deficiency, thyroid-stimulating hormone thyroxine (T4) tends to decrease, so it is important to also verify that the zinc will not be compromised by high levels of either cadmium or copper.

Copper deficiency, on the other hand, enhances the effects of an underactive thyroid that develops when the thyroid gland fails to produce or secrete as much T4 as the body needs. By contrast, an excess of copper can lead to Wilson's disease, involving enlargement of the thyroid gland via one or more nodular goiters. To excrete the excess copper, the body needs to use valuable zinc stores.

WORDS OF ADVICE

• If you have PMS, about two weeks before your menstrual period start using a natural progesterone cream to help reduce the likelihood of thyroid problems.
• To help balance the thyroid gland, take 500 to 1,000 mg of tyrosine for three to six months.
• Take either flaxseed or fish oil (3,000 to 6,000 mg a day of a combination of flaxseed and fish oil) and eat nuts, fish, and seeds to get fatty acids, which help produce and balance hormones and reduce thyroid problems.
• If you have hypothyroidism, do aerobic exercise, to stimulate your thyroid function. Building muscle can help raise your metabolism and accelerate weight loss.

U

ULCERS

Every year, ulcers affect about 4 million Americans, more than 40,000 of whom end up having surgery because of persistent symptoms.[1] Ulcers are characterized by pain in the stomach made worse by eating (gastric ulcers) or pain relieved by eating only to return two to three hours later (duodenal ulcers); excessive weight gain or loss; gnawing or burning pain in the abdomen between the breastbone and navel, usually occurring between meals and in the early hours of the morning; nausea, with blood in vomit or stool; indigestion; and bloating.

At one time, ulcers were thought to be caused by stress, spicy foods, or too much stomach acid. But a persistent Australian physician named Barry J. Marshall, whose theory that bacteria called *Helicobacter pylori* (*H. pylori*) caused peptic ulcers was ignored for years, ultimately substantiated his theory by using himself as a guinea pig. Drinking the bacteria, he proved that exposure to it temporarily caused the inflammation and gastric irritation we call an ulcer or gastritis, and consequently his ideas were accepted by Western medicine. *H. pylori* have since been implicated in gastritis, peptic ulcer disease, gastric cancer, cancers of the stomach's lymphatic system (called gastric lymphoma), and most recently, heart disease.[2] Also, it has been found that *H. pylori* favor type O blood. These bacteria are like molecular Velcro for the O antigen, while the A and B blood type antigens do not give *H. pylori* much to stick to, causing people with type O blood to have more ulcers.[3] Other commonly recognized causes of ulcers include not eating well, vitamin and mineral deficiencies, smoking, inability to control anger, and some pharmaceutical drugs (selective COX-2 drugs are safer for the gastrointestinal tract than older NSAIDS used in arthritis).[4]

Unfortunately, ulcers often go undiagnosed by conventional doctors, many of whom do not test for *H. pylori* and instead perform repeated endoscopies and biopsies, and prescribe bismuth and courses of antibiotics. But most patients whose ulcers are treated with bismuth and antibiotics become infected again with *H. pylori* within a year.[5] Also, some doctors mistakenly diagnose ulcer patients with GERD (gastroesophageal reflux disease) when the cause could be *H. pylori* infection, in which case the GERD medication is the worst possible remedy. Most prescriptions for stomach treatments are contraindicated for *H. pylori*, especially those that contain bismuth, even over-the-counter bismuth subsalicylate preparations such as Pepto-Bismol.

Many doctors believe that bismuth and several antibiotics used to prevent the bacteria from developing resistance to any one of them, can kill *H. pylori*; however, the bacteria, buried deep in the stomach mucus, are not easily eliminated through these means. Also, bismuth, which is a toxic metal, can produce gray staining of the teeth and mouth and cause constipation, diarrhea, and blackening of the stool; a state of extreme excitement or emotion; delusions, hallucinations, incoherence, and distorted perceptions of reality; inability to coordinate the movements of muscles; muscular spasm; and seizures. Antibiotics, for their part, may cause a bad taste in the mouth, dizziness, tingling in the arms and hands, stomach upset, diarrhea, and occasionally, death.

By contrast, in our clinic we view *H. pylori* infection as a sexually transmitted disease and insist that the patient's sexual partner be screened also since the exchange of saliva through kissing is enough to transmit the infection. For treatment of ulcers, we first recommend eating foods appropriate to blood type. Eating poorly and deficiencies in zinc, vitamin A, glutamine, and vitamin E dramatically increase the incidence of ulcers in the duodenum; and smoking after a meal, which decreases bicarbonate and slows down the stomach function, impairs digestion.

Second, acupuncture works wonders in easing the pain and stiff neck and shoulders associated with ulcers. It can reduce the excess "stomach fire" as well, and thus prevent bleeding gums, irritability, stomach ulcers, and other conditions.

Third, friendly probiotic bacteria should be an important part of the healing strategy because they act as natural antagonists to *H. pylori* and should always be used to prevent antibiotic-induced disturbances of the friendly bacteria.

Fourth, specific lectin-blocking sugars found in foods and natural herbs, such as D-fucose, a simple sugar found in bladderwrack, kelp, and broccoli, can be eaten to make the cells of the stomach wall much more slippery so *H. pylori* will be unable to adhere to them. People who weigh in excess of 150 pounds (68 kilos) should take two capsules of bladderwrack 30 to 60 minutes before meals, while people who weigh less should take one capsule and refrain from snacking between meals.

Fifth, the herbs goldenseal (*Hydrastis canadensis*), which should only be taken for short periods of time, and coptis (*Coptis chinensis*), which should be taken under the direction of a clinical nutritionist, can be used as dietary supplements to inhibit the growth of *H. pylori*. Further, licorice, which is also antagonistic to *H. pylori*, can be taken provided that its glycyrrhizin—which, when taken in high amounts, can cause fluid retention, increased blood pressure, and loss of potassium—has been removed; deglycyrrhizinated licorice (DGL), found in health food stores, can help repair the walls of the stomach and intestines.

THE BIOCOMPATIBLE VIEW

Biocompatible medicine views ulcers primarily as a symptom of other diseases, especially those caused by colonization of *H. pylori* in the stomach wall. Instead of waging war against the *H. pylori*, biocompatible physicians eradicate the bacterium slowly by prescribing bladderwack kelp to be taken on an empty stomach to move its contents over a three-month treatment period.

- Eat three small meals and three snacks evenly spaced throughout the day, avoiding both periods of hunger and overeating.
- Eat slowly and chew foods well.
- Be relaxed at mealtime.
- Sit up while eating and for one hour afterward to prevent against trapping air in your stomach.
- Avoid eating within three hours before bedtime, which can cause gastric acid secretion during the night.
- Cut down on caffeine-containing foods and beverages, citrus and tomato products, and chocolate if these foods cause discomfort.
- Include a good source of protein (milk, meat, eggs, cheese) at each meal and snack.
- Take antacids, according to the prescribed dose, one hour after meals and three hours prior to bedtime, to keep the acidity of the stomach at the most stable and lowest level.
- Do not consume milk products as antacid therapy because, although milk has an initial neutralizing effect on gastric acid, it is also a potent stimulator.
- If you have a stomach ulcer caused by *H. pylori*, take two capsules of bladderwrack 30 minutes to 1 hour before eating.
- Take deglycyrrhizinated licorice (DGL) to stimulate the natural protective factors in the digestive tract, which helps relieve stomach discomfort.
- Use bifidobacterium lactis as a dietary supplement to improve the intestinal microbial balance leading to enhanced immune response.
- Take a leisurely stroll after meals to help stimulate digestion.

URINARY TRACT INFECTION

Urinary tract infection (UTI), an inflammatory condition that affects millions of people around the world annually,[6] can be life threatening if it involves the kidneys. The urinary tract is comprised of the two kidneys; the ureters, tubes that connect the kidneys to the bladder; the bladder, which is like a dammed reservoir; and the urethra, the channel that carries urine from the bladder out of the body. In traditional Chinese medicine, this system, called the lower burner, is responsible for separating "clean" from "dirty" body fluids and facilitates the excretion of urine from the body.

Based on chemist Louis Pasteur's work in the nineteenth century, many doctors claim that bacteria, viruses, and fungi cause UTI, classified as either urethritis, infection of the urethra; cystitis, infection of the bladder; or pyelonephritis, infection of the kidneys. Urethritis occurs when microorganisms, usually *Escherichia coli* (*E. coli*), pathogens in the colon that help synthesize vitamin B_{12} from the remnants of digested meat, enter the urethra, causing the inflammation. Cystitis develops when microorganisms are transferred from the bowel through the urethra into the bladder. Pyelonephritis, much more serious, results from infection in the blood spilling over into the kidneys.

Upon developing a UTI, a person experiences pain on urination, either in the urethra or the bladder, frequent urination, mental confusion, and sometimes blood in the urine or pain in the mid-back, over the kidneys, and fever higher than 102°F persisting for more than two days. Most often when patients present with these symptoms, conventional doctors will prescribe antibiotics to kill bacteria, or other symptom-relieving drugs to fight viruses or fungi. Women, in particular, are given antibiotics because doctors believe that since the urethra is shorter in women bacteria can enter their urinary system more easily. Indeed, up to 50 percent of women will have at least one UTI in their lifetime; the risk of infection increases with age, use of a catheter, and diabetes. Among both men and women diagnosed with UTI, approximately 80 percent will undergo recurrence.[7]

Departing from the views rooted in Pasteur's findings, biocompatible medicine distinguishes the etiology and treatment of lower UTI (urethritis and cystitis) from that of the more systemic upper UTI (pyelonephritis). Lower UTI is regarded as either a postdefecation hygiene problem or a pH imbalance. In terms of the latter, it recognizes that a cause of UTI in women is the decline in hormone levels after menopause or hysterectomy. Before this decline, hormones in a woman's sexual organs provide an acidic pH that protects the body from many pathogens that can cause urinary tract infections. But after the decline, when women have unprotected sex, they can develop a urinary tract infection because sperm, being more alkaline, disturb the delicate acidic balance of the vagina, making a woman more prone to infection. For this reason, I recommend that such women use condoms during sex. Similarly, I advise women with urinary tract inflammation to avoid wearing pantyhose or tight underwear, especially if made of nylon, which stops the flow of lymph, restricts airflow, and traps moisture against the vagina, causing a fungal infection of the skin called eczema marginatum or crotch rot. In men, for whom eczema marginatum is three times more common, it is called jock itch.[8] Bras, especially those with underwires, can also stop the flow of lymph. In these cases, the culprit is thrush, a yeastlike bacteria called *Candida albicans*, which infects the urinary tract and spreads rapidly under warm, moist conditions (see "Yeast Overgrowth," p. 205).

Also in contrast to the methods of conventional doctors, physicians trained in traditional Chinese medicine do not use antibiotics to treat UTI. Following guidelines delineated 2,300 years ago in *The Yellow Emperor's Classic of Medicine*, in the majority of cases acupuncture treatments, healthy diet, homeopathic remedies, and herbs, along with commonsense lifestyle suggestions, can generally resolve UTIs quickly and without side effects such as the yeast infections resulting from antibiotics.

In our clinic, we group symptoms into patterns, each of which has its own treatment protocol. For example, "damp heat" symptoms can be grouped into three patterns: "damp heat pouring down," "toxic heat accumulation," and "kidney deficiency." To treat toxic heat accumulation—a consequence of consuming hot spicy foods, meals high in fats and sweets, or alcohol, taking certain medications, or improper personal hygiene—I use acupuncture to ease the back and abdominal pain and to allow the damp heat to run off. To treat kidney deficiency, due to chronic illness, aging, pregnancy, menopause, or emotional stress, I employ acupuncture and herbs.

In addition, I advise patients with a UTI to drink as much water as possible; cut out sweets and simple carbohydrates; avoid caffeine and nicotine, which irritate the bladder; and take plenty of vitamin C, which, by increasing the acidity of urine, helps decrease the number of harmful bacteria that may be present in the urinary tract. The best remedy we have found is an all-natural sugar compound, D-mannose, that occurs in peaches, apples, and berries, especially cranberries; D-mannose literally "washes away" urinary bacterial infections.[9] We recommend drinking 100 percent pure cranberry juice since processed juice has too much sugar in it to be helpful.

Additionally, many women report that performing Kegel exercises has helped alleviate problems with urinary tract infection. To do these exercises, first locate the pubococcygeus muscles, or PC muscles, by repeatedly stopping urine in midstream and starting again. Then practice squeezing these muscles while not urinating. If your stomach or buttocks move, you are not using the right muscles. Hold the squeeze for three seconds then relax for three seconds. Repeat the exercise ten to fifteen minutes per session. Do at least three Kegel exercise sessions per day.

THE BIOCOMPATIBLE VIEW

Biocompatible physicians believe it is important to identify whether an infection is a lower or upper UTI so it can be properly treated. In the majority of cases, UTIs can be effectively treated with acupuncture, healthy diet, homeopathic remedies, and herbs.

Biocompatible physicians also encourage their patients to prevent recurrences of UTI. More and more women patients in Aruba, for example, elect to remove their pubic hair or keep it closely trimmed. In the absence of a bladder infection, urine is sterile but a rich medium for bacterial growth, as is urine-saturated pubic hair, especially in the tropics. Removing or closely cropping pubic hair helps keep the skin around and between the rectum and vagina clean after washing with soap and water.

Women also realize that natural cotton panties are healthier than those made of other fabrics, and most women will at least opt for panties with a cotton crotch. Cotton lets moisture escape, while other fabrics can trap moisture, creating a potential breeding ground for bacteria. Some women with recurring UTIs find that wearing cotton "G-strings" that barely cover the vaginal lips and changing them several times a day reduces the incidence of reinfection.

Showering instead of bathing helps prevent bacteria from entering the urethra and causing a UTI. And washing the genital area both before and after sexual intercourse protects against transferring bacteria to the urethra or vaginal area.

WORDS OF ADVICE

• Keep the genital area clean, and after using the toilet remember to wipe from front to back to reduce the likelihood of introducing bacteria from the rectal area to the urethra.

• Urinate immediately after sex to help eliminate any bacteria that may have been introduced during intercourse and reduce the risk of developing cystitis.

- Use a condom during sexual activity, both for purposes of safe sex and to protect against the alkalinity of bacteria in sperm, especially after menopause or a hysterectomy.
- If you have recurrent or chronic UTIs, see a doctor about the possible implication of allergies.
- Avoid allergic foods, and stick to your metabolic food list.
- Increase your intake of fluids to between 64 to 128 ounces a day to encourage frequent urination that flushes bacteria from the bladder. Drink natural cranberry juice to prevent bacteria from attaching to the wall of the bladder.
- To help prevent or treat UTIs caused by *E. coli*, take D-mannose supplements (1 teaspoon, 5 ml, dissolved in water or juice every two to three hours while awake). If you are pregnant, use this supplement with caution.
- Take the enzymes bromelain (1 capsule) and trypsin (1 capsule) before each meal to serve as an anti-inflammatory agent and to enhance the effect of antibiotics in treating UTI.
- Take vitamin C supplements (250 to 500 mg two times per day) to make your urine acidic and thus inhibit bacterial growth.
- Take beta-carotene supplements (25,000 to 50,000 IU per day) and zinc supplements (30 to 50 mg per day) to support your immune system and keep mucous membranes healthy.
- Do Kegel exercises regularly to help strengthen the muscles that control the flow of urine and reduce problems with urinary tract infections.

YEAST OVERGROWTH

The overgrowth of yeast, a family of minuscule single-cell fungi that normally live on membranes of the intestines, digestive tract, and vagina, has become a major problem by breaking through into the bloodstream or deeper tissue of many people. This out-of-control behavior of yeast is caused by the widespread use of broad-spectrum antibiotics in animals, food, and people, as well as the modern high-fat, low-fiber, high-sugar diet and prolonged use of cortisone and cortisone-like drugs and also immunosuppressant drugs. When a person's immune system is strong, yeast organisms are not able to break through in this way, but when it is weak they can have wide-ranging effects, especially on the immune system itself.

Perhaps the greatest factor contributing to yeast overgrowth in women is the use of birth control pills because they cause hormonal imbalances by releasing into the body a continual stream of estrogen. In today's world, where common lifestyle choices include antibiotics and a highly refined bread-and-sugar diet, coupled with high stress levels—all of which depress immunity—birth control pills profoundly impact an already depressed immune system and lead to the overgrowth of the most widespread form of yeast, *Candida albicans*, which exists naturally in the descending colon, where it produces B-complex vitamins from the outer coverings of ingested whole grains.

Another risk factor contributing to yeast overgrowth is exposure to a hospital setting, which usually is a breeding ground for the transmission of other *Candida* species, such as *Candida tropicalis, Candida glabrata, Candida parapsilosis, Candida krusei,* or *Candida lusitaniae.* Collectively referred to as "nosocomial candidiasis," this secondary medical problem associated with being treated in a hospital is unrelated to an affected patient's presenting condition.[1] Considered iatrogenic, meaning "brought forth by a healer," such effects almost exclusively signify ill health or a complication arising from medical treatment.

Yeast overgrowth that shows up in the form of *Candida albicans* is also known as candidiasis or moniliasis. When *Candida albicans* affects the tongue or mouth, the condition is called oral thrush; when it affects skin folds, it is called intertriginous rash; in the corners of the mouth, perlèche; in the vagina, vulvovaginitis; on the head of the penis and sometimes the scrotum of diabetic or uncircumcised men, penile candidiasis; in nail beds, candidal paronychia; and so forth.

Symptoms of yeast overgrowth range from migraines to infertility, endometriosis, psoriasis, PMS, depression, fibromyalgia, digestive disorders, and many other symptoms so seemingly unrelated that it is difficult for most doctors to comprehend that there could be a single underlying cause. For example, on one occasion a father, mother, and two children came to my clinic for a consultation. Both parents acknowledged they were suffering from fatigue, joint pains, muscle stiffness, cold hands and feet sometimes developing into numbness and tingling, and loss of libido. The husband had chronic heartburn that had been diagnosed at times as gastritis and other times as colitis. The wife was being treated by a gynecologist for chronic vaginitis. The fifteen-year-old daughter, who had previously been doing very well in school, was now forgetting facts and losing her ability to concentrate. Her twelve-year-old brother suffered from breathing problems and took asthma medication. My nose helped diagnose the problem when I realized they smelled like fresh bread or beer—like yeast, in this case *Candida albicans*.

William G. Crook, MD, author of *The Yeast Connection*, asked people the following questions to help them determine if they had a yeast problem:

- Have you taken repeated or prolonged courses of antibacterial drugs?
- Have you been bothered by recurrent vaginal, prostate, or urinary infections?
- Do you feel "sick all over," yet the cause hasn't been found?
- Are you bothered by hormone disturbances, including PMS, menstrual irregularities, sexual dysfunction, sugar craving, low body temperature, or fatigue?
- Are you unusually sensitive to tobacco smoke, perfumes, colognes, and other chemical odors?
- Are you bothered by memory or concentration problems? Do you sometimes feel "spaced out"?
- Have you taken prolonged courses of prednisone or other steroids; or have you taken "the pill" for more than three years?
- Do some foods disagree with you or trigger your symptoms?
- Do you suffer with constipation, diarrhea, bloating, or abdominal pain?
- Does your skin itch, tingle, or burn; or is it unusually dry; or are you bothered by rashes?[2]

Treatment for yeast overgrowth requires a multilevel approach employing the following procedures:

- Elimination of antibiotics, birth control pills, and other hormone-altering substances.
- Use of natural antifungal agents such as olive leaf for people with type A or AB blood or ulcers and grapefruit seed extract for people with type O or B blood to help destroy *Candida albicans*, including daily probiotics (acidophilus or lactobacilli) regardless of blood type.

- Modification of the blood-type-specific diet to eliminate all sources of fermented foods, yeast, fungus, and sugars, such as those found in alcohol, dried fruit, vinegar, fermented soy sauce, cheese, mushrooms, pickled foods, breads with yeast, lactose-containing dairy products except for unsalted butter, and to limit fruit juice to only 100 percent natural with no added sugars.
- Washing yeast organisms from sinuses and throat using seawater or a saline (saltwater) solution in a small pot designed for this purpose, usually available in pharmacies and health food stores.
- Cleaning out excess wax from the ears with ear candles, which can be purchased at health food stores. *Candida albicans* in the ears causes pressure, pain, and hearing problems.
- Avoiding tobacco smoke, perfume, hair spray, or gasoline fumes, which can aggravate symptoms.
- Soaking affected fingers or toes in peroxide, or in 3 to 5 drops of grapefruit seed extract or lemon juice, mixed in 1 cup of water.
- Using a condom or abstaining from sexual intercourse to prevent the spread of vaginal yeast infections to a partner, as well as testing for other sexually transmitted infections.
- Using vitamin E in capsule form (1,000 mg per day) as a suppository to reduce inflammation and provide antioxidants to help protect the sexual organs.
- Bathing in the sea or using a sitz bath to cleanse inflamed areas.

THE BIOCOMPATIBLE VIEW

Biocompatible medicine views yeast overgrowth in the body as a failing immune system. Most yeast problems are the result of *Candida albicans*, which exist naturally in the descending colon. Problems occur when a compromised immune system fails to control *Candida albicans*, which then increases the body's acidity and contributes to the overall acid stress leading to chronic inflammation. The only real solution, according to biocompatible medicine, is to restore efficiency to the immune system through eating according to metabolic type and correcting factors leading to the inflammation.

WORDS OF ADVICE

- Watch for the following symptoms, which may indicate the presence of yeast overgrowth, particularly *Candida albicans*: gas, indigestion, heartburn; bowel irregularities; food cravings, especially for carbohydrates or sweets; mood swings; headaches; menstrual problems; respiratory problems; dry, itchy skin or hives; fingernail or toenail fungus; vertigo or balance problems; joint or muscle pain; bad breath despite good oral hygiene; allergies; malabsorption; vaginal yeast infections; acne; cravings for chocolate, peanuts, pistachios, or alcohol; adrenal problems or low-functioning thyroid; hemorrhoids; insomnia; chronic fatigue; feeling cold and shaky; weight imbalances; poor memory or inability to concentrate; puffy, dry, or burning eyes; urinary tract problems (infections, prostatitis, incontinence); premature aging; chemical sensitivity (especially to colognes or fabric dyes); blood sugar imbalances; thrush or receding gums; or numbness, especially in the hands.

- Avoid the following factors, all of which can promote yeast overgrowth: frequent or long-term use of antibiotics, such as tetracycline for acne; frequent use of broad-spectrum antibiotics for recurrent infections, such as in the ears, bladder, vagina, or throat; infections, which lower the immune system, creating an imbalance in innate flora; poor diet (not eating according to your metabolic type and consuming junk and sugary foods); wheat and milk products (for individuals with type O blood); stress or trauma; painkillers; exposure to toxic heavy metals and environmental pollutants; use of cortisone-type drugs or stimulants and depressants (caffeine, nicotine, alcohol); eating disorders (starvation, vomiting, taking laxatives); vaccinations and immunizations; and humid climates.
- Eliminate or minimize the use of antibiotics, steroids, immune-suppressing drugs, and oral contraceptives (after consulting with your healthcare provider or physician).
- Try colon hydrotherapy to remove excess amounts of yeast organisms.
- Avoid wearing nylon underwear, panty hose, tight jeans, close-fitting exercise clothing, or wet bathing suits, since moisture retention encourages yeast overgrowth.
- Stick to a diet that will not promote the overgrowth of yeast—one low in carbohydrates and containing no yeast products or sugar in any form. Eliminate fruit and fruit juices, sugar and other sweeteners, including honey; cheese and other dairy products; soy sauce; mushrooms; bread and baked goods with yeast (substitute yeast-free bread made with gluten-free grains such as millet and quinoa); refined foods and foods to which you are allergic; coffee, soda, and alcoholic beverages; and fermented foods. Eat plenty of vegetables and lean protein, including the following beneficial foods: most vegetables, especially broccoli, kale, garlic, turnip greens, onions, and cabbage; eggs; fish and chicken (if you have type O or A blood) and beef (if you have type O or B blood). Limit your consumption of potatoes, beets, carrots, and corn, and drink plenty of mineral or spring water.
- Take acidophilus and bifidus supplements to help restore the normal balance of flora in the colon and vagina.
- Use olive leaf to help control the growth of yeast if you have type A or AB blood.
- Use grapefruit seed extract to help control the growth of yeast if you have type O or B blood.
- Supplement with ground flaxseeds, which are rich in omega-3 fatty acids, antioxidants, and phytochemicals called lignans.
- Take zinc citrate supplements (twice a day for thirty days) to support the immune system and destroy *Trichomonas*, the single-celled organism responsible for vaginitis.
- Take vitamin E supplements (1,000 IU) as vaginal suppositories every night to help your body develop resistance to *Trichomonas*, maintain a healthy hormonal balance, and alleviate vaginal dryness if you are menopausal.
- Exercise and do deep breathing to help improve immune function, stimulate lymph flow, and cleanse the body of *Candida albicans* and accumulated toxins.

The Biocompatible Treatment Protocol

In Western medicine, prevention is synonymous with getting yearly physicals, vaccinations, mammograms, and other diagnostic tests, whereas prevention in traditional Chinese medicine means looking at energetic rather than physiological imbalances and taking steps to regain balance. *The Yellow Emperor's Classic of Medicine,* a Chinese medical text written in the second century BC, reveals: "The sages of ancient times emphasized not the treatment of disease, but rather the prevention of its occurrence. To administer medicine to disease that has already developed and to suppress revolts that have already begun is comparable to the behavior of one who begins to dig a well after he has become thirsty. Would these actions not be too late?... A doctor who treats a disease after it has happened is a mediocre doctor; a doctor who treats a disease *before it happens* is a superior doctor."[1]

Holistic physicians, who are not obstructed by socialized medicine or insurance company protocols, are free to revise treatment and prevention plans so they elicit more positive outcomes. At our clinic, biocompatible procedures continuously evolve. When I realize there is a missing piece in our approach, the Healing Spirit sends the information and authority to guide me.

Over the years, we have developed a treatment protocol composed of three steps to help restore the health of our patients:

Identify and eliminate toxins that produce chronic inflammation, which accelerates aging and negatively affects health.

Provide healing constituents, the right foods and supplements based on metabolic type to start rebuilding functions of the body.

Find balance in all aspects of life.

Step One: Identify and Eliminate Toxins

The first step in our protocol is to identify the source of chronic inflammation that is producing the ill health. Through blood tests we can detect the chemical and environmental toxins (see "Environmental Toxins," p. 115) that are causing harm to the body and then detoxify the body, all the while reducing further exposure to these pollutants. To find a person's level of exposure to lead, mercury, and other potentially toxic elements, we utilize hair elemental profile testing. In conjunction with blood tests and patient symptoms, we use this test for early detection of toxins because changes often appear in hair prior to overt body symptoms. In addition, we rely on comprehensive blood tests, hair analysis reports, digital infrared thermal photographs (thermograms), dental panoramic X-rays, and dental reports to create a clear picture of an individual's overall medical status, looking in depth at causes of their problems and arriving at restorative solutions. One of my mentors, "Sam" Queen, often reminds me that our bodies are "made by design to win," meaning that the Healing Spirit within us all is always trying to return us to a state of health.

Detoxification of the body lies at the foundation of biocompatible medicine. To eliminate waste, the body uses five primary organs: the liver, kidneys, colon, lungs, and skin.

Liver: This organ regulates most chemical levels in the blood and excretes bile, which helps carry away waste products from the liver. All blood leaving the stomach and intestines passes through the liver, which breaks down the nutrients and drugs into forms that are easier for the rest of the body to use. More than five hundred vital functions have been identified with the liver—among them the fact that the liver is the only organ in the body that can regenerate itself and can lose three-quarters of its cells before it stops functioning. Maintaining a healthy liver depends on a regularly functioning colon. In fact, constipation causes toxins that have been eliminated in bile to be reabsorbed in the small intestine during protein and fat digestion.

Kidneys: The kidneys remove wastes and excess water collected by and carried in the blood as it flows through the body. About 190 liters (335 pints) of blood enter the kidneys every day via the renal arteries. Millions of tiny filters called glomeruli, inside the kidneys, separate wastes and water from the blood. Most of these unwanted substances come from what we eat and drink, and include, for example, urea from protein catabolism and uric acid from energy production (see "ATP," p. 107). The kidneys automatically remove the right amount of salt and other minerals from the blood to leave just the quantities the body needs. The cleansed blood then returns to the heart and recirculates through the body, while the excess wastes and fluid leave the kidneys in the form of urine.

Colon: The function of the colon is to receive water from the lungs and collect toxic waste from every part of the body. We believe that most health problems have the common denominator of chronic inflammation stemming from the colon, a natural breeding ground for both healthy and unhealthy bacteria. Procedures for cleaning the colon have been in place since biblical times. Colon irrigation, as we know it today, performs a cleansing, antiseptic, solvent action on the intestines whereby putrefied material—including impacted old content, excess mucous, pus and infected tissue, and even parasites—is removed from the colon and toxins are diluted and flushed out, increasing the elimination potential of the kidneys and skin (see "Colon Hydrotherapy," p. 85).

Lungs: Most people normally use only about 10 percent of their lung capacity and, unless engaging in heavy exercise, rarely breathe deeply enough to optimize the lungs' ability to use oxygen and to remove toxins. By contrast, while doing abdominal deep breathing as taught in scuba diving, singing, yoga, and other disciplines, an extensive exchange of lung gases takes place. Carbon dioxide is removed from the body, allowing breathing to slow down and increasing the lungs' capacity to exchange toxic carbon dioxide for oxygen. A good exercise to do first thing in the morning to help the lungs function effectively is to take five deep breaths. Resting both arms at the sides of the body and then lifting them overhead while breathing in, has the added benefit of helping to move stagnant lymph fluid.

Skin: The skin not only flushes out toxins through sweating but also acts as a first line of immune defense. Because humanity has lost its natural means of stimulating the skin, such as having it rubbed by clothing made of animal hides, it is beneficial to scrub the skin with rough loofahs in order to clean it and stimulate the body's filtering system, known as lymph. Dry skin brushing is another good technique for stimulating lymph (see "Skin," p. 184). Flowing just under the skin and ready to attack foreign bodies, lymph is a transparent fluid that contains white blood cells, mostly lymphocytes, and a few red blood cells. Lymph that has stagnated in the lymph nodes grows thick, and over time, engorged lymph nodes may become cysts that turn cancerous.

Removing toxic materials through an organ of elimination involves the use of various substances. In my clinical experience of removing heavy metals from patients' bodies, I have observed that lead, silver, tin, and nickel either chelated or detoxified in response to EDTA injections (see "EDTA Chelation," p. 103), while mercury, arsenic, and cadmium are sequestered by EDTA and cholesterol in the liver then excreted through the bile. Any aluminum attached to the EDTA needs silica supplementation to successfully egress the body. All the while, many of these toxins are exiting through the skin as well. Removal of pesticides and insecticides that are locked in fat cells, on the other hand, requires oil-based detoxicants and baths. Successful outcomes almost always depend on patient participation in the decision-making process.

Avoiding toxins in the environment means steering clear of cleaning detergents, pesticides, and industrial chemicals that are linked to hormonal, reproductive, neurological, or immune disorders. [3] The use of nontoxic products, both in personal care and cleaning, at home and at work, is essential.

Step Two: Provide Healing Constituents

The second step in our treatment protocol is to encourage our patients to eat the right foods and supplements for their metabolic type so they can start rebuilding their bodily functions using natural medicine. For individuals with type A blood, we strengthen digestion and immunity. For those with type O blood, who have very aggressive immune responses, we support healthy elimination and reinforce adrenal activity. For people with type B blood, we protect against immune system disorders, such as lupus and chronic fatigue syndrome. For people with type AB blood, we fortify the sensitive digestive tract that otherwise may remain vulnerable to viruses. Additionally, we build brain power and develop weight loss strategies for older patients.

In this regard, the biocompatible protocol again calls for natural medicine. Here the healing constituents are food, water, and supplements.

Food: In the first century BC, Hippocrates, the "father of medicine," said, "Let food be thy medicine," but today we would have to insist that the food be whole, nonaltered, and unprocessed. It is also important to take into account the fact that the same food items do not have the same effect on all people. Metabolic type, as established by blood type, is an essential element to consider in choosing the right foods. For individuals with type A or AB blood, a low-fat, high-complex-carbohydrate diet works well. People with type O or B blood feel much healthier with a high-protein diet that includes many vegetables and very few starches (see "Blood Type Diet," p. 65).

Adele Davis, who trained in dietetics and nutrition at the University of California at Berkeley and earned an MS degree in biochemistry from the University of Southern California in 1938, was the first nutritionist to state, in her popular book *Let's Eat Right to Keep Fit*, "You are what you eat." The next generation of nutritionists went further, claiming that people are not only what they eat but also what they absorb. Today's clinical nutritionists realize that people are what their bodies can process, as well.

The food we eat and how we process it either sustains our health or undermines it. Indeed, the paradox of modern life is that while convenience foods have freed us from cooking, we have as a result become enslaved by ill health. In developed countries, millions of people are dying annually of heart disease, cancer, kidney disease, cirrhosis of the liver, or diabetes. More have arthritis, asthma, bronchitis, hypoglycemia, venereal disease, dental problems, or mental illness. And while life expectancy in the United States has effectively doubled over the past two hundred years,[4] with similar improvements observed in other developed nations and, although less pronounced, in the Global South,[5] notable reductions are predicted due to substantial increases in obesity, insulin resistance, and as a result, diabetes mellitus.[6]

Even though it has been shown repeatedly that the most nutritious foods are whole, unaltered, and unprocessed, food today is genetically altered, waxed shiny for supermarkets, frozen, and canned; and snack food, junk food, fast food, instant dinners, and microwave specials are popular despite their nutritional deficiencies. In foods "spoil-proofed" or precooked for convenience, complex carbohydrates have been modified into simple carbohydrates that lack nutrients. White sugar, white flour, table salt, soft drinks, coffee, alcohol, and other amenities are responsible for 80 percent of our medical problems.[5]

Among the most nutritious foods, on the other hand, are whole grains. In addition to the ever-popular brown rice, there is a wonderful sorghum called maishi rabo; amaranth, the ancient grain of the Aztecs, which is high in fiber and protein; and whole wheat berries, which can be either sprouted or cooked as a cereal. For people who cannot tolerate wheat products, quinoa and millet are gluten free and easy to digest.

Water: Many people do not realize the importance of water and instead consume drinks that rob the body of water. Drinking lots of clean water is essential for the assimilation of nutrients, digestion, and elimination, and for transporting nutrients through the arteries to the brain and all bodily tissues, as well as numerous biochemical processes. Water intake helps prevent chronic inflammation; enhances and moistens lung surfaces for gas exchange; aids in regulation of body temperature; and supports communication between cells, organs, and all parts of the body.

A body deficient in water is dehydrated (see "Dehydration," p. 93). Symptoms of water deficiency include stiff bones and joints, hardening of body canals, sluggish colon, hearing difficulties, faulty eyesight, irritated nerves, a wrinkled face, and the brain ailments and temperament changes common to elderly patients. In our clinic, we stress the importance of drinking sufficient water and have seen dramatic improvements in patients' health after several months of adequate water intake, such as the disappearance of arthritic symptoms.

Supplements: Because much of today's food is nutrient deficient, many people are at risk for developing such chronic illnesses as diabetes and heart disease. A good solution is to supplement the daily diet with extra vitamins, minerals, amino acids, enzymes, fatty acids, and phytonutrients. In addition, synthetic vitamins, which are not absorbed properly in the body, may utilize more energy than they provide, the most effective supplements are those made from organically grown whole foods.

Step Three: Find Balance

The third step in our biocompatible treatment protocol is to help individuals find balance in all aspects of life—body, mind, emotions, relationship to the environment, and spirit. Energy imbalances can lead to illness on various levels, while being energetically balanced results in good health and can be achieved by getting adequate rest, making time for play and relaxation, having meaningful work and social interactions, eating nutritious food, and getting regular exercise.

Traditional Chinese medicine focuses on interrelationships between various dimensions. For example, it is understood that excessive emotions arise because of internal organ malfunctions and disorders in the circulation of chi and blood. Therefore, patients exhibiting excessive emotions are encouraged to find internal balance by regulating their daily lives: rising early, eating nutritious foods, working effectively, avoiding overindulgences in sexual activity, dressing appropriately for the weather, being kind and compassionate to others, and going to sleep at a reasonable hour.

The next phase in regaining health is to balance rest and exercise. Most people erroneously equate rest with the cessation of activity, but rest actually requires the presence of yin energy. By contrast, people going to bed very late and being too overtired to sleep have exhausted their yin energy.

Sufficient sleep is the most fundamental natural medicine, yet nearly one out of every three people in industrialized countries experiences insomnia on a regular basis. Such people, looking for a quick fix to their problems, take prescription or over-the-counter medications despite the fact that typical sleeping pills, or tranquilizers (benzodiazepines), have serious side effects and can become addictive. In addition, such individuals may develop a vicious cycle: (1) they take a sleeping pill to fall asleep; (2) the sleep it provides lacks normal episodes of rapid eye movement (REM), during which the body is rejuvenated and dreaming takes place; (3) they therefore do not wake up refreshed; (4) they ingest coffee and other stimulants to get going in the morning; and (5) wired once again, they have trouble falling asleep at night.

We often tell patients with sleep and rest problems to begin an exercise program. Exercise can improve not only sleep and rest but also general health. Exercise enhances the way the body handles dietary fat; reduces risk of heart attack; helps lower blood cholesterol and triglycerides; raises HDL (good cholesterol); helps alleviate calcium deposits in the soft tissues of joints; reduces the risk of osteoporosis; improves immune function; aids digestion and elimination; increases endurance and energy levels; promotes lean body mass and burns fat; helps the body handle stress; and benefits the musculoskeletal system, heart and blood vessels, and mental processes. Perhaps the least expensive, safest, and easiest-to-perform exercise is walking briskly four times a week for twenty minutes, gradually increasing to an hour for maximum benefit.

Among other opposites to be balanced are work and relaxation, including vacation time. It is important to take time out from work periodically—with either frequent short vacations or less frequent longer ones—to support physical, mental, and emotional health, as well as to maintain good relationships with family and friends.

Another duality to balance is spiritual activity and worldly pleasures. Pursuing one to the exclusion of the other can lead to self-centeredness or greed. To be truly healthy, it is just as important to play and enjoy life as it is to engage in reflection and spiritual concerns.

An additional aspect of finding balance is to seek harmony with the environment. Disharmony with one's surroundings affects families, communities, and ultimately nations. Traditional Chinese medicine seeks to put people in harmonious balance with their surroundings through the five-element theory—transforming bodily phases of fire, earth, metal, water, and wood to correspond with those found in nature—and the practice of feng shui, which literally means "wind, fire" and involves the application of yin and yang principles to the analysis of energy. For instance, using a special compass, a feng shui practitioner can determine the energy characteristics of a building and its influence on the occupants, then balance the energy so it will have a positive effect. In this way, people can develop greater harmony with their surroundings and thus receive health benefits.

APPENDIX B
Getting Back on Track
A Patient's Viewpoint
Armand Hessels, age 54, January 3, 2006

After I started working as a physical education teacher in 1975, my nickname became Zuf-zuf[1] because I was always on the run. I would fill any spare time with work for my job at school; meetings connected with several businesses I had in and outside of Aruba; sports, social, union, and political events; and activities with my wife and two children.

In 1992, I experienced a particularly stressful time in my life: I divorced, remarried, moved to Holland, got a new job, and started writing a book. In 1995, I returned to Aruba. Then in 1998, I started having health problems while renovating an old house, feeling constantly exhausted. In an attempt to "recharge my batteries," I went on a Caribbean cruise, but when I returned I was as exhausted as before and became progressively worse, to the point where I couldn't perform the slightest physical activity without losing my breath.

In November 1999, my cardiologist sent me to Houston for tests after discovering an aneurysm of about 2.4 inches in my aorta ascendens. Analysis in Houston confirmed the discovery, and a radical decrease in my physical activities was recommended.

Over the subsequent years, I gradually increased my activity level, with swimming, biking, and occasionally playing tennis; however, such sports always gave me a headache and made me feel dizzy, negative effects that caused me to resist physical activities. During everyday life, my body felt tired and broken, as if I had carried big bags of cement all day, or been beaten by several people with baseball bats—symptoms that, according to my cardiologist, were not typical of an aneurysm.

By the end of 2004, my health had deteriorated significantly. One day at work in November 2004, I felt severe pressure on my chest and broke out in a cold sweat, sensations I experienced several times over the next few days. My physician ordered me to rest for two to three months because of severe burnout, but after a few weeks I felt guilty about not working, as I did not really feel ill.

Back at school in January 2005, I began participating in many different activities but within days felt worse than before my rest, experiencing exhaustion and severe pain in my joints, especially in my feet upon waking up in the morning. My exhaustion even prevented me from falling asleep, which had never before been a problem, and I had to walk briskly on the beach at night in order to eventually fall asleep. I began taking Celebrex daily to suppress my muscle and joint pains. Then I went to see a psychiatrist to find out what all my anxiety was about and how to fight it. The psychiatrist prescribed antidepressants.

Next, a colleague advised me to see Dr. Viana, a natural healer, and feeling desperate I decided to try my luck. As we sat under a tree during our first meeting, Dr. Viana checked me out, including my eyes and teeth. He then recommended that I have the amalgam fillings in my teeth and all four wisdom teeth removed. I thought the man was crazy but managed to say I would think about it. Then he gave me an acupuncture treatment for my anxiety, which had been my greatest concern. To my surprise, from the moment the needles were inserted, I no longer focused on obsessions but went completely blank, which was a great feeling, and afterwards I was more relaxed.

In the three weeks that followed, eager to relive that experience I returned three times a week, eventually coming less often. Two or three months later, I no longer needed treatments. Yet I still balked at doing anything about my teeth.

As time passed, however, I encountered people who had experienced a similar persistent tiredness and, after following Dr. Viana's advice to have their amalgam fillings removed, had noted great improvement in their sense of well-being. Their stories convinced me to submit to the procedure.

In one shot, I had a severely inflamed tooth plus the wisdom teeth pulled on one side of my mouth and all the amalgam fillings replaced, then followed the dentist's advice to have an acupuncture treatment from Dr. Viana to prevent too much swelling of my jaw, which succeeded although I still needed pills prescribed by the dentist for inflammation and pain. After three weeks, I had the other two wisdom teeth removed. Following this, in keeping with Dr. Viana's protocol, I had colon hydrotherapy and an extended suppository treatment to remove toxic metals from different organs.

After these procedures, to my astonishment I no longer felt sharp pains in my joints, which, according to the dentist, had been caused by inflammation in my tooth and jaw. Moreover, I was much less tired and able to participate in more rigorous physical activities without experiencing headaches, dizziness, or other problems. I was even able to stop taking the Celebrex and to get off the antidepressants. The only problem that still remains is my back, which, according to X-rays, is worn out.

As a result of my progress, I believe that Dr. Viana's theories and protocol are very effective. This means a lot coming from someone who began his healing journey as a cynical man.

NOTES

Introduction

1. G. Singh, "Recent Considerations in Nonsteroidal Anti-Inflammatory Drug Gastropathy," *American Journal of Medicine* 105 (July 1998): 31S–38S.

2. D.W. Bates et al., "Incidence of Adverse Drug Events and Potential Adverse Drug Events: Implications for Prevention," *Journal of the American Medical Association* 274, no. 5 (July 5, 1995): 29–34.

3. Institute of Medicine Report Brief, *Preventing Medication Errors* (Washington, DC: National Academies Press, 2006).

4. Ivan Illich, *Medical Nemesis: The Expropriation of Health* (London: Marian Boyars, 1975).

5. Gong-Soog Hong and Jeff Grabmeier, "Research Communications," a presentation at the annual conference of the American Council on Consumer Interests (April 9, 2005).

6. National Institute of Health Office of the Director, Office of Budget, Budget Reporting and Legislative Branch, http://nccam.nih.gov/.

7. Richard Dawkins, *A Devil's Chaplain* (New York: Houghton Mifflin Company, 2003).

A

1. D. M. Eisenberg et al., "Trends in Alternative Medicine Use in the United States, 1990–1997: Results of a Follow-Up National Survey," *Journal of the American Medical Association* 280 (1998): 1569–75.

2. Donna Kalauokalani, MD, MPH, Daniel C. Cherkin, PhD, and Karen J. Sherman, PhD, "A Comparison of Physician and Nonphysician Acupuncture Treatment for Chronic Low Back Pain," in "Childhood Abuse and Pain in Adulthood," special issue, *Clinical Journal of Pain* 21, no. 5 (September–October 2005): 406–11.

3. National Institutes of Health, news release, "NIH Panel Issues Consensus Statement on Acupuncture," November 5, 1997, http://www.nih.gov/news/pr/nov97/od-05.htm.

4. World Health Organization, review, "Acupuncture: Review and Analysis of Reports on Controlled Clinical Trials," http://whqlibdoc.who.int/publications/2002/9241545437.pdf.

5. Mark F. Blaxill, *What's Going On? The Question of Time Trends in Autism*, Public Health Reports 119, no. 6 (November–December 2004): 536–51, doi: 10.1016/j.phr.2004.09.003.

6. "Fighting Autism," *Autism: Statistics, Incidence, Prevalence,* http://www.fightingautism.org/idea/index.php.

7. American Psychiatric Association, *Diagnostic and Statistical Manual of Mental Disorders* IV (*DSM-IV*) (Washington, DC: American Psychiatric Association, 2000).

8. Robert Berkow, MD, ed., *The Merck Manual* (Rahway, NJ: Merck Sharp & Dohme Research Laboratories, 1987).

9. American Psychiatric Association, DSM-IV.

10. Berkow, *Merck Manual.*

11. American Psychiatric Association, *DSM-IV.*

12. Wikipedia, *Merck Manual,* http://en.wikipedia.org/wiki/Merck_Manual_of_Diagnosis_and_Therapy.

13. Vaccination Risk Awareness Network, "New Research Suggests Link between Vaccine Ingredients and Autism, ADHD," http://www.vran.org/vaccines/mercury/research-link-mer.htm (February 3, 2004).

14. See articles on mercury toxicity on the Web site of Boyd Haley, PhD, http://www.whale.to/v/haley.html.

15. Anju I. Usman, MD, "Journey to Recovery: Finding a Safe Path to Heavy Metal Detoxification," slide 7 (presentation at the Autism One Conference, Chicago, Illinois, May 2006). Presentation available at http:// www.autismone.org/uploads/2006/UsmanAnju_Autism_One_Handouts_06.ppt.

16. Hyperbaric Healing Institute, http://www.hhi-kc.com/.

17. Diana L. Vargas et al., "Neuroglial Activation and Neuroinflammation in the Brain of Patients with Autism," *Annals of Neurology*, published online November 15, 2004, doi: 10.1002/ana.20315.

18. Paul Whiteley et al., "A Gluten-Free Diet As an Intervention for Autism and Associated Spectrum Disorders: Preliminary Findings," *Autism* 3, no. 1 (1999): 45–65.

19. Richard A. Collins, "Biomedical Intervention and Prospects for Recovery from Autism," report from the Asian Autism Conference held in Hong Kong, *The Biomedical Scientist*, November 2006: 1–5.

20. Kenneth Blum et al., "Reward Deficiency Syndrome: A Biogenetic Model for the Diagnosis and Treatment of Impulsive, Addictive, and Compulsive Behaviors," *Journal of Psychoactive Drugs* 32, nos. 1 and 2 (2000).

21. See the Web log on compulsive craving behaviors at: http://rewarddeficiencysyndrome.blogspot.com.

22. Melvyn R. Werback, MD, *Nutritional Influences on Mental Illness* (Tarzana, CA: Third Line Press, 1991).

23. S. J. S. Flora and S. N. Dube, "Modulatory Effects of Alcohol Ingestion on the Toxicology of Heavy Metals," *Indian Journal of Pharmacology* 26, no. 4 (1994): 240–48.

24. Roger D. Masters et al., "Zeroing In on Pollution Criminality Connection," Crime Times 3, no. 4 (1997): 4; 2, no. 2 (1996): 1; 2, no. 4 (1996): 7.

25. "Toxins, Health and Behavior: The Implications of 'Toxicogenomics' for Public Policy," draft of paper for meeting of the American Political Science Association, 2002, http://www.dartmouth.edu/~rmasters/tbcba.htm.

26. Substance Abuse and Mental Health Services Administration, *Results from the 2005 National Survey on Drug Use and Health: National Findings* (Rockville, MD: Office of Applied Studies, NSDUH series H-30, DHHS publication no. SMA 06-4194, 2006), http://www.drugabusestatistics.samhsa.gov/NSDUH/2k5NSDUH/2k5results.htm.

27. James T. Stevens and Darrell D. Summer, "Herbicides," in *Handbook of Pesticide Toxicology*, vol. 3, Classes of Pesticides, edited by Wayland J. Hayes and Edward R. Laws, 1317–91 (New York: Academic Press, 1991).

28. Robert L. Siblerud et al., "Psychometric Evidence That Mercury from Silver Dental Fillings May Be an FBI Factor in Depression, Excessive Anger, Anxiety," *Psychological Reports* 74 (1994): 67–80.

29. Sherry A. Rogers, MD, *Detoxify or Die* (Sarasota, FL: Sand Key Company, 2002).

30. James L. Wilson, Adrenal Fatigue: The 21st Century Stress Syndrome (Petaluma, CA: Smart Publications, 2001).

31. Freedonia Group, "Anti-aging Products." Report is available through http://www.marketresearch.com.

32. Gilbert N. Ling, PhD, *Life at the Cell and Below-Cell Level* (Melville, NY: Pacific Press, 2001).

33. Joel Fuhrman, MD, *Disease-Proof Your Child: Feeding Kids Right* (New York: St. Martin's Press, 2005).

34. Ishmael Kasvosve et al., "Ferroportin (SLC40A1) Q248H Mutation Is Associated with Lower Circulating Plasma Tumor Necrosis Factor-a and Macrophage Migration Inhibitory Factor Concentrations in African Children," *Clinica Chimica Acta* 411, no. 17–18 (2010): 1248–1252, http://www.sciencedirect.com/science/article/pii/S0009898110003086.

35. Richard D. Smith and Joanna Coast, *Antimicrobial Resistance: A Global Response*, Bulletin of the World Health Organization 80, no. 2 (2002).

36. "Antibiotics," Merck Manuals Online Medical Library, http://www.merck.com/mmhe/sec17/ch192/ch192a.html.

37. S. Almond, "Neck Swellings in Children," *Journal of Surgery* (Oxford) 22, no. 9 (2004): 204–8.

38. "Strep Throat," Medline Plus, http://www.nlm.nih.gov/medlineplus/ency/article/000639.htm.

39. Marian Melish, MD, "Most Childhood Infections DON'T Need Antibiotics," *Kapi'olani Kids* 2, no. 1 (May 2004), Kapi`olani Medical Center for Women & Children, Honolulu, http://kapiolani.startingouthealthy.com/archive/issue204/story3.html.

40. "Class Suicidality Labeling Language for Antidepressants" (a label required on antidepressant drugs). For current information on antidepressants, see http://www.fda.gov/cder/drug/antidepressants/default.htm.

41. C. Patrono et al., "Platelet-Active Drugs: The Relationships among Dose, Effectiveness, and Side Effects," *Chest: Journal of American College of Chest Physicians* 119, no. 1, suppl. (January 2001): 39S–63S.

42. Charles W. Shilling, ed., *The Physician's Guide to Diving Medicine* (New York: Plenum Press, 1984), 94.

43. M. Lethbridge-Çejku, J. S. Schiller, and L. Bernadel, *Summary Health Statistics for U.S. Adults: National Health Interview Survey, 2002, Vital Health Statistics* series 10, no. 222 (2004).

44. Ling, "Life at the Cell and Below-Cell Level."

45. Cornelia E. Farnum and Norman J. Wilsman, "Lectin-Binding Histochemistry of Intracellular and Extracellular Glycoconjugates of the Reserve Cell Zone of Growth Plate Cartilage," *Journal of Orthopaedic Research* 6, no. 2 (February 18, 2005): 166–79.

46. W. Tang et al., "Detection of Disease-Specific Augmentation of Abnormal Immunoglobulin G in Sera of Patients with Rheumatoid Arthritis," *Glycoconjugate Journal* 15, no. 9 (September 1998): 929–34.

47. Gabor Maté, MD, *When the Body Says No: Understanding the Stress-Disease Connection* (Hoboken, NJ: John Wiley & Sons, 2003).

48. Peter D'Adamo, MD, *Eat Right for Your Type* (New York: G. P. Putnam's Sons, 2001).

49. Michael B. Keller and Steven R. Lowenstein, "Epidemiology of Asthma," *Seminars in Respiratory and Critical Care Medicine* 23 (2002): 317–30, doi: 10.1055/s-2002-34327.

50. V. Mishra, "Effect of Obesity on Asthma among Adult Indian Women," *International Journal of Obesity* 28, no. 8 (August 2004): 1048–58.

51. D. A. Stempel et al., "The Economic Impact of Children Dispensed Asthma Medications without an Asthma Diagnosis," *Journal of Pediatrics* 148, no. 6 (June 2006): 819–23D.

52. Michael J. H. Akerman, Catherine M. Calacanis, and Mary K. Madsen, "Relationship between Asthma Severity and Obesity," *Journal of Asthma* 41, no. 5 (January 2005): 521–26, http://www.informaworld.com/smpp/title%7Econtent=t713597262%7Edb=all%7Etab=issueslist%7Ebranches=41-v41.

53. Rosalind Anderson and Julius Anderson, "Acute Respiratory Effects of Diaper Emissions," *Archives of Environmental Health* 54 (September 1999): 202–9.

54. Food and Drug Administration, *FDA & You: News for Health Educators and Students*, issue 2 (Winter 2004), http://www.vaccinecheck.com/vacinfo_4-2.jsp?vac=4-2.

55. Catalin S. Buhimschi, MD, and Irina A. Buhimschi, MD, "Advantages of Vaginal Delivery: Do We Need to Advocate for Vaginal Delivery?" *Clinical Obstetrics and Gynecology* 49, no. 1 (March 2006): 167–83.

56. Marsha Wills-Karp and Joerg Koehl, "New Insights into the Role of the Complement Pathway in Allergy and Asthma," *Current Allergy and Asthma Reports* 5, no. 5 (September 2005), doi: 10.1007/s11882-005-0007-y.

57. Yousuke Takemura et al., "The Relationship between Fish Intake and the Prevalence of Asthma: The Tokorozawa Childhood Asthma and Pollinosis Study," *Preventive Medicine* 34 (February 2002): 221–25.

58. S. Suissa, "Inhaled Corticosteroids: Impact on Asthma Morbidity and Mortality," *Journal of Allergy and Clinical Immunology* 107, no. 6 (June 2001): 937–44.

59. M. Thomas et al., "Atopic Wheezing and Early Life Antibiotic Exposure: A Nested Case-Control Study," *Pediatric Allergy and Immunology* 17 (2006): 184–88.

60. Surovi Hazarika, Michael R. Van Scott, and Robert M. Lust, "Airway Inflammation Increases Infarction after Myocardial Ischemia-Reperfusion in Mice" (presented at the thirty-fifth congress of the International Union of Physiological Sciences, San Diego, California, March 31–April 5, 2005).

61. Aeesha Malik, NJ, and William Cutting, AM, "Breast Feeding: The Baby Friendly Initiative," *British Medical Journal* 316 (1998): 1548–49.

62. Chris Willette, "Introduction to Use of UV Light for the Control of Air Handler Contamination," www.freshaireuv.com.

B

1. Harris H. McIlwain and Debra Fulghum Bruce, *The Pain-Free Back: 6 Simple Steps to End Pain and Reclaim Your Active Life* (New York: Owl Books, 2004).

2. Ken Dychtwald, *Bodymind* (New York: Jeremy P. Tarcher/Putnam, 1977).

3. International Academy of Oral Medicine and Toxicology, http://iaomt.org/.

4. H. L. "Sam" Queen, *The Basic 100: A Health Model-Based Interpretation of Clinical Chemistry Parameters* (Colorado Springs: Institute for Health Realities, 1997), http://www.healthrealities.org/.

5. Ibid.

6. N. Danchin, X. Duval, and C. Leport, "Prophylaxis of Infective Endocarditis: French Recommendations 2002," *Heart* 91 (2005): 715–18.

7. A. J. Finestone and S. R. Boorujy, "Diabetes Mellitus and Periodontal Disease," *Diabetes* 16 (1967): 336–40.

8. Thaddeus Waters et al., "C-Reactive Protein and Periodontal Disease at One Month Post-Partum in Women with a Recent Pre-Term Birth: Prospective Data from the Preterm Prevention Project," *American Journal of Obstetrics and Gynecology* 195, no. 6, suppl. 1 (December 2006): S203.

9. M. O. Gonçalves et al., "Periodontal Disease As Reservoir for Multi-Resistant and Hydrolytic Enterobacterial Species," *Letters in Applied Microbiology* 44, no. 5 (2007): 488–94, doi:10.1111/j.1472-765X.2007.02111.x.

10. P. J. Ford et al., "Inflammation, Heat Shock Proteins and Periodontal Pathogens in Atherosclerosis: An Immunohistologic Study," *Oral Microbiology and Immunology* 21, no. 4 (August 2006): 206–11, doi:10.1111/j.1399-302X.2006.00276.x.

11. J. Franke et al., "Industrial Fluorosis," *Fluoride* 8, no. 2 (April 1975): 61–83.

12. R. D. Masters et al., "Association of Silicofluoride Treated Water with Elevated Blood Lead," *Neurotoxicology Journal* 21, no. 6 (December 2000): 1091–1100.

13. International Academy of Oral Medicine and Toxicology (IAOMT), "Policy Position on Ingested Fluoride and Fluoridation," undated, 24–25, http://iaomt.org/.

14. American Dental Association (ADA), "Mercury in Dental Amalgams: An Examination of the Science," a statement by the ADA to the Government Reform Committee, U.S. House of Representatives, November 14, 2002, http://www.ada.org/prof/resources/positions/statements/statements_amalgam.pdf.

15. F. L. Lorscheider, M. J. Vimy, and A. O. Summers, "Mercury Exposure from Silver Tooth Fillings: Emerging Evidence Questions a Traditional Dental Paradigm," *Federation of American Societies for Experimental Biology Journal* 9 (April 1995): 504–8.

16. Paul B. Tchounwou et al., "Review: Environmental Exposure to Mercury and Its Toxicopathologic Implications for Public Health," *Environmental Toxicology* 18, no. 3 (May 6, 2003): 149–75, doi: 10.1002/tox.10116.

17. Mercury Info, a mercury environmental health database, http://www.mercuryexposure.org/index.php?page_id=61.

18. G. E. Fagala and C. L. Wigg, "Psychiatric Manifestations of Mercury Poisoning," *Journal of the American Academy of Child Adolescent Psychiatry* 31, no. 2 (March 1992): 306–11.

19. Peter D'Adamo, MD, *Eat Right for Your Type* .

20. Richard J. Farrell, MD, and Ciarán P. Kelly, MD, "Diagnosis of Celiac Sprue," *The American Journal of Gastroenterology* 96, no. 12 (December 2001): 3237–46, doi:10.1111/j.1572-0241.2001.05320.x.

21. Bana Jabri, Donald D. Kasarda, and Peter H. R. Green, "Innate and Adaptive Immunity: The Yin and Yang of Celiac Disease," *Immunological Reviews* 206, no. 1 (August 2005): 219–31, doi:10.1111/j.0105-2896.2005.00294.x.

22. M. Hermann, R. Margreiter, and P. Hengster, "Molecular and Cellular Key Players in Human Islet Transplantation," *Journal of Cellular and Molecular Medicine* 11, no. 3 (May–June 2007): 398–415, doi:10.1111/j.1582-4934.2007.00055.x.

23. Jabri, Kasarda, and Green, "Innate and Adaptive Immunity."

24. Robert W. McGilvery, PhD, and Gerald W. Goldstein, MD, *Biochemistry: A Functional Approach*, 3rd ed. (Philadelphia: W. B. Saunders, 1983).

C

1. American Cancer Society, *Facts and Figures* 2005 (Atlanta: American Cancer Society, 2005).

2. L. Derogatis, M. Abeloff, and C. McBeth, "Cancer Patients and Their Physicians in the Perception of Psychological Symptoms," *Psychosomatics* 17 (October 1976): 197–201.

3. Peter D'Adamo, MD, *Eat Right for Your Type*.

4. Derogatis, Abeloff, and McBeth, "Cancer Patients and Their Physicians."

5. J. D. Veldhuis and A. Iranmanesh, "Physiological Regulation of the Human Growth Hormone (GH)-Insulin-Like Growth Factor Type I (IGF-I) Axis: Predominant Impact of Age, Obesity, Gonadal Function, and Sleep," *Sleep: Journal of the American Sleep Disorders Association* 19, no. 10, suppl. 10 (December 1996): S221–S224.

6. Richard Stevens, "Electric Power Use and Breast Cancer: A Hypothesis," *American Journal of Epidemiology* 125, no. 4 (April 1987): 556–61.

7. H. L. "Sam" Queen, "The Forensic Approach to Blood Chemistry: Part 1," handout, Institute for Health Realities, http://www.healthrealities.org/.

8. Johan Goudsblom, Eric L. Jones, and Stephen Mennell, *The Course of Human History: Economic Growth, Social Process, and Civilization*. (New York: M. E. Sharpe, 1996).

9. William J. Sinclair, Semmelweis, *His Life and Doctrines* (Manchester, England, 1909).

10. Annette Summers, "Sairey Gamp: Generating Fact from Fiction," Nursing Inquiry 4, no. 1 (March 1997): 14–18.

11. S. B. Nuland, "The Enigma of Semmelweis: An Interpretation," *Journal of the History of Medicine and Allied Sciences* 34 (1979): 255–72.

12. Pranee Liamputtong, PhD, et al., "Traditional Beliefs about Pregnancy and Childbirth among Women from Chiang Mai, Northern Thailand," *Midwifery* 21, no. 2 (June 2005): 139–53.

13. Vicki Van Wagner, RM, et al., "Reclaiming Birth, Health, and Community: Midwifery in the Inuit Villages of Nunavik, Canada," *Journal of Midwifery & Women's Health* 52, no. 4 (July–August 2007): 384–91.

14. Marylou Carr, CNM, MSN, Maria Luiza, and Gonzalez Riesco, Ph.D., "Rekindling of Nurse-Midwifery in Brazil: Public Policy and Childbirth Trends," *Journal of Midwifery & Women's Health* 52, no. 4 (July–August 2007): 406–11.

15. Gabriela Cob, "Impact of the Hospitalization of the Childbirth" (thesis, Primal Association, Costa Rica, 2002).

16. Deborah Walker, CNM, DNSc, FACNM, et al., "Midwifery in Action," *Journal of Midwifery & Women's Health* 52, no. 2 (March–April 2007): 180.

17. Leonie A. M. van der Hulst, MA, et al., "Dutch Women's Decision-Making in Pregnancy and Labour As Seen through the Eyes of Their Midwives," *Midwifery* 23, no. 3 (September 2007): 279–86.

18. Wendy Christiaens, MA, and Piet Bracke, PhD, "Assessment of Social Psychological Determinants of Satisfaction with Childbirth in a Cross-National Perspective," *BMC Pregnancy and Childbirth* 7 (October 2007): 26–29.

19. Margaret L. Holland, MS, and Eliza S. Holland, CNM, MSN, "Survey of Connecticut Nurse-Midwives," *Journal of Midwifery & Women's Health* 52, no. 2 (March–April 2007): 106–15.

20. Goodman, "Piercing the Veil."

21. Alan H. DeCherney and Martin L. Pernoll, *Obstetric and Gynecological Diagnosis and Treatment* (Englewood Cliffs, NJ: Appleton and Lange, Prentice Hall, 1994), 570.

22. Mona Lydon-Rochelle, MPH, PhD, CNM, et al., "Association between Method of Delivery and Maternal Rehospitalization," *Journal of the American Medical Association* 283 (2000): 2411–16.

23. V. A. Kazandjian and T. R. Lied, "Cesarean Section Rates: Effects of Participation in a Performance Measurement Project," *Journal on Quality Improvement* 24, no. 4 (1998): 187–96.

24. DeCherney and Pernoll, *Obstetric and Gynecological Diagnosis*, 560.

25. Rhona Mahony et al., "Outcome of Second Delivery after Prior Macrosomic Infant in Women with Normal Glucose Tolerance," *Obstetrics & Gynecology* 107 (2006): 857–62.

26. William M. Gilbert, MD, et al., "Vaginal versus Cesarean Delivery for Breech Presentation in California: A Population-Based Study," *Obstetrics & Gynecology* 102 (2003): 911–17.

27. Yinka Oyelese, MD, and John C. Smulian, MD, MPH, "Placenta Previa, Placenta Accreta, and Vasa Previa," *Obstetrics & Gynecology* 107 (2006): 927–41.

28. Deidre Spelliscy Gifford, MD, MPH, et al., "Lack of Progress in Labor As a Reason for Cesarean," Obstetrics & Gynecology 95 (2000): 589–95.

29. Steven L. Bloom et al., "Decision-to-Incision Times and Maternal and Infant Outcomes," *Obstetrics & Gynecology* 108 (July 2006): 6–11.

30. Mark B. Landon, MD, et al., "Risk of Uterine Rupture with a Trial of Labor in Women with Multiple and Single Prior Cesarean Delivery," *Obstetrics & Gynecology* 108 (2006): 12–20.

31. Joy Melnikow, MD, et al., "Vaginal Birth after Cesarean in California," *Obstetrics & Gynecology* 98 (2001): 421–26.

32. R. Gonen, MD, et al., "Obstetricians' Opinions regarding Patient Choice in Cesarean Delivery," *Obstetrics & Gynecology* 99 (2002): 577–80.

33. Susan P. Walker et al., "Cesarean Delivery or Vaginal Birth: A Survey of Patient and Clinician Thresholds," *Obstetrics & Gynecology* 109 (2007): 67–72.

34. Arialdi M. Miniño, MPH, et al., *Deaths: Final Data for 2004*, National Vital Statistics Reports 55, no. 19 (August 21, 2007).

35. James M. Alexander et al., "Fetal Injury Associated with Cesarean Delivery," *Obstetrics & Gynecology* 108 (2006): 885–90.

36. P. D. Sutton and T. J. Mathews, "Trends in Characteristics of Births by State: United States, 1990, 1995, and 2000–2002," *National Vital Statistics Reports* 10, no. 52 (May 2004): 1–152.

37. R. G. Faix and S. M. Donn, "Immediate Management of the Traumatized Infant," *Clinics in Perinatology* 10, no. 2 (1983): 487–505.

38. C. A. Dickman et al., "Pediatric Spinal Trauma: Vertebral Column and Spinal Cord Injuries in Children," *Pediatric Neuroscience* 15 (1989): 237–56.

39. J. Gardosi and S. Sylvester, "Alternative Positions in the Second Stage of Labor: A Randomized Controlled Trial," *British Journal of Obstetrics and Gynaecology* 11, no. 6 (1989): 1290–96.

40. T. D. Gastaldo, "Labor Posture," *Birth* 19, no. 4 (1992): 230.

41. Ibid.

42. Mary Lou Moore, PhD, RNC, LCCE, FACCE, "Adopting Birth Philosophies to Guide Successful Birth Practices and Outcomes," *Journal of Perinatal Education* 10, no. 2 (Spring 2001): 43–45.

43. S. Budd, "Moxibustion for Breech Presentation," *Complementary Therapies in Nursing and Midwifery* 6, no. 4 (2000): 176–79.

44. US Food and Drug Administration, Center for Drug Evaluation and Research, "Baycol Information," http://www.fda.gov/cder/drug/infopage/baycol/default.htm.

45. R. J. Baldessarini, "Neuropharmacology of S-adenosyl-L-methionine," *American Journal of Medicine* 83, no. 5A (November 20, 1987): 95–103.

46. H. L. "Sam" Queen, "The Forensic Approach to Blood Chemistry: Part 1" Institute for Health Realities, http://www.healthrealities.org/.

47. Erez Ben-Menachem and D. James Cooper, "Hormonal and Metabolic Response to Trauma," *Anaesthesia & Intensive Care Medicine* 12, no. 9 (2011): 409–11.

48. J. Peiris et al., "Coronavirus As a Possible Cause of Severe Acute Respiratory Syndrome," *Lancet* 361, no. 9366 (April 19, 2003): 1319–25.

49. S. Yousem, "Alveolar Lipoproteinosis in Lung Allograft Recipients," *Human Pathology* 28, no. 12 (January 1997): 1383–86.

50. Centers for Disease Control and Prevention, "Trends in Tuberculosis Incidence: United States, 2006," Morbidity and Mortality Weekly Report, http://www.cdc.gov/mmwr/preview/mmwrhtml/mm5611a2.htm.

51. William A. Wells, "Curing TB with Sunlight," *Journal of Cell Biology* 172, no. 7 (March 27, 2006): 958–58.

52. C. Weber, "Screening and Prevention of Carcinoma of the Colon and Rectum," *Therapeutische Umschau* 63, no. 5 (May 2006): 333–37.

53. Ian Magrath and Jorge Litvak, "Cancer in Developing Countries: Opportunity and Challenge," *Journal of the National Cancer Institute* 85, no. 11 (June 2, 1993): 862–74.

54. Robert J. Genco, Frank A. Scannapieco, and Harold C. Slavkin, "Oral Reports," *The Sciences* 40, no. 6 (November–December 2000): 27–30.

55. http://www.arthritis-msm-supplements.com/CORAL_CALCIUM.HTM.

56. http://www.okicent.org/coral_calcium/coral-calcium.html.

D

1. W. I. Rosenblum and R. M. Asofsky, "Effects of Dehydration on Blood Viscosity and on Distribution of Plasma Proteins in Experimental Macroglobulinaemia," Nature 30, no. 216 (December 1967): 1327–28.

2. S. Rovio et al., "Leisure-Time Physical Activity at Midlife and the Risk of Dementia and Alzheimer's Disease," *The Lancet Neurology* 4, no. 11 (November 1, 2005): 705–11.

3. V. Chandra, N. E. Bharucha, and B. S. Schoenberg, "Patterns of Mortality from Types of Dementia in the United States, 1971 and 1973–1978," *Neurology* 36, no. 2 (February 1986): 204–8.

4. Ock Kyoung Chun, Sang Jin Chung, and Won O. Song, "Estimated Dietary Flavonoid Intake and Major Food Sources of U.S. Adults," *Journal of the American Society for Nutrition* 137, no. 12 (May 2007): 1244–52.

5. Robert G. Cumming and Robin J. Klineberg, "Aluminum in Antacids and Cooking Pots and the Risk of Hip Fractures in Elderly People," *Age and Ageing* (November 1994).

6. Howard I. Maibach, ed., *Toxicology of the Skin* (Philadephia: Taylor and Francis, 2001).

7. J. Kandiah and C. Kies, "Aluminum Concentrations in Tissues of Rats: Effect of Soft Drink Packaging," Biometals 7, no. 1 (January 1994): 57–60.

8. J. A. T. Pennington, "Aluminium Content of Foods and Diets," *Food Additives and Contaminants* 5 (1988): 161–232

9. Ibid.

10. World Health Organization, *The World Health Report 1997: Conquering Suffering, Enriching Humanity.* (Geneva: World Health Organization, 1997).

11. Kerri L. Cavanaugh, MD, "Diabetes Management Issues for Patients with Chronic Kidney Disease," *Clinical Diabetes* 25 (2007): 90–97.

12. American Diabetes Association, position statement, "Diabetic Retinopathy," *Diabetes Care* 25, suppl. 1 (2002): S90–S93.

13. Ingrid Kruse, DPM, and Steven Edelman, MD, "Evaluation and Treatment of Diabetic Foot Ulcers," *Clinical Diabetes* 24 (2006): 91–93.

14. American Diabetes Association, consensus statement, "Peripheral Arterial Disease in People with Diabetes," *Clinical Diabetes* 22 (2004): 181–89.

15. Karmeen D. Kulkarni, "Food, Culture, and Diabetes in the United States," *Clinical Diabetes* 22 (2004): 190–92.

16. Jennifer Chapman, MD, et al., "Complicated Diverticulitis: Is It Time to Rethink the Rules?" *Annals of Surgery* 242, no. 4 (2005): 576–83.

E

1. Environmental Working Group (EWG), "Study: People Carry Many Environmental Pollutants," July 14, 2005, http://www.ewg.org/node/15125.

2. ——— "Body Burden: The Pollution in Newborns," July 14, 2005, http://archive.ewg.org/reports/bodyburden2/.

3. H. L. "Sam" Queen, "The Forensic Approach to Blood Chemistry: Part 1," Institute for Health Realities, http://www.healthrealities.org/.

4. Institute of Medicine, *Dietary Reference Intakes for Thiamin, Riboflavin, Niacin, Vitamin B_6, Folate, Vitamin B_{12}, Pantothenic Acid, Biotin, and Choline* (Washington, DC: National Academy Press, 1998), 390–422.

5. Ross Pelton, RPh, PhD, *Mind Food and Smart Pills* (New York: Doubleday Dell, 1989), 70–71.

6. M. J. Chang et al., "Toxic Elements in Cigarette Smoke," *Journal of Environmental Monitoring* 7 (2005): 1349.

7. D. V. Aminot-Gilchrist and H. D. I. Anderson, "Insulin-Resistance-Associated Cardiovascular Disease: Potential Benefits of Conjugated Linoleic Acid," *American Journal of Clinical Nutrition* 79, (2004): 1159S–1163S.

8. Barbara Starfield, MD, MPH, "Medical Errors a Leading Cause of Death," *Journal of the American Medical Association* 284, no. 4 (July 26, 2000): 483–85.

9. David Snashall, "ABC of Work Related Disorders: Occupational Infections," *British Medical Journal* 313 (August 1996): 551–54.

10. Stanley Weinberger, CMT, Parasites: *An Epidemic in Disguise* (Larkspur, CA: Healing within Products, 1993), 1.

11. Allan R. Gold, "Tight Limits Proposed for Popular Farm Chemical," *New York Times*, December 5, 1989, Health section.

12. Environmental Working Group (EWG), "Body Burden."

13. A. Rotchford, "What Is Practical in Glaucoma Management?" *Eye* 19 (October 2005): 1125–32.

14. S. Arora et al., "Eye Nutrient Products for Age-Related Macular Degeneration: What Do They Contain?" *Eye* 18 (May 2004): 470–73.

G

1. C-J. Tsai et al., "Dietary Carbohydrates and Glycaemic Load and the Incidence of Symptomatic Gall Stone Disease in Men," *Gut* 54 (2005): 823–28.

2. W. S. Waring, S. R. J. Maxwell, and D. J. Webb, "Uric Acid Concentrations and the Mechanisms of Cardiovascular Disease," *European Heart Journal* 23 (December 2002): 1888–89.

3. Shirmila Syamala, Jialiang Li, and Anoop Shankar, "Association between Serum Uric Acid and Prehypertension among U.S. Adults," *Journal of Hypertension* 25, no. 8 (August 2007): 1583–89.

4. M. J. Ahern et al., "Does Colchicine Work? The Results of the First Controlled Study in Acute Gout," *Australia and New Zealand Journal of Medicine* 17 (1987): 301–4.

5. J. O. Nriagu, "Saturnine Gout among Roman Aristocrats: Did Lead Poisoning Contribute to the Fall of the Empire?" *New England Journal of Medicine* 308, no. 11 (1983): 660–63.

H

1. Robin Tamblyn et al., "Unnecessary Prescribing of NSAIDs and the Management of NSAID-Related Gastropathy in Medical Practice," *Annals of Internal Medicine* 127, no. 6 (September 15, 1997): 429–438.

2. Andrew J. Vickers et al., "Acupuncture for Chronic Headache in Primary Care: Large, Pragmatic, Randomised Trial," *British Medical Journal* 328 (March 15, 2004): 744.

3. I. Steinbrecheri and R. Jarisch, "Histamin und Kopfschmerz=Histamine and Headache," *Allergologie* 28, no. 3 (2005): 85–91.

4. Dursun Esiyok, Senik Otles, Eren Akcicek, "Herbs as a Food Source in Turkey," *Asian Pacific Journal of Cancer Prevention* 5, (2004): 334–9.

5. Lily Raveh et al., "Efficacy of Antidotal Treatment Against Sarin Poisoning: The Superiority of Benactyzine and Caramiphen," *Toxicology and Applied Pharmacology* 227, no. 1 (February 15, 2008): 125–35.

6. A. Pieroni, "Medicinal Plants and Food Medicines in the Folk Traditions of the Upper Lucca Province, Italy," *Journal of Ethnopharmacology* 70 (2000): 235–73.

7. G. S. Chen et al., *The American Journal of Chinese Medicine* 7, no. 4 (1979): 384–91.

8. American Heart Association, "Women and Cardiovascular Diseases: Statistics" (2004), http://www.americanheart.org/downloadable/heart/1136818052118Females06.pdf.

9. S. O'Donnell et al., "7% of Men Drive Themselves to Hospital During a Heart Attack," *Journal of Advanced Nursing* 53 (February 2006): 268–76.

10. Nanette K. Wenger, Leon Speroff, and Barbara Packard, "Cardiovascular Health and Disease in Women," *New England Journal of Medicine* 329, no. 4 (July 22, 1993): 247–56.

11. "Studies of Acute Coronary Syndromes in Women: Lessons for Everyone," editorial, *New England Journal of Medicine* 341, no. 4 (July 22, 1999): 275–76.

12. T. Kurth et al., "Migraine and Risk of Cardiovascular Disease in Men," *Archives of Internal Medicine* 167, no. 8 (April 23, 2007): 795–801.

13. Kenneth J. Mukamal, Stephanie E. Chiuve, and Eric B. Rimm, "Alcohol Consumption and Risk for Coronary Heart Disease in Men with Healthy Lifestyles," *Archives of Internal Medicine* 166 (October 23, 2006): 2145–50.

14. L. Rosenberg et al., "The Risk of Myocardial Infarction after Quitting Smoking in Men under 55 Years of Age," *New England Journal of Medicine* 12, no. 313 (December 1985): 1511–14.

15. Philippe P. Hujoel, PhD, et al., "Periodontal Disease and Coronary Heart Disease Risk," *Journal of the American Medical Association* 284, no. 11 (September 20, 2000): 1406–10.

16. Ryan T. Demmer, PhD, and Moise Desvarieux, MD, PhD, "Periodontal Infections and Cardiovascular Disease: The Heart of the Matter," *Journal of the American Dental Association* 137, no. 2, suppl. 2 (2006): 14S–20S.

17. Axel Spahr, DDS, et al., "Periodontal Infections and Coronary Heart Disease: Role of Periodontal Bacteria and Importance of Total Pathogen Burden in the Coronary Event and Periodontal Disease (CORODONT) Study," *Archives of Internal Medicine* 166, no. 5 (March 13, 2006): 554–59.

18. Maurizio S. Tonetti, DMD, PhD, et al., "Treatment of Periodontitis and Endothelial Function," *New England Journal of Medicine* 356, no. 9 (March 1, 2007): 911–20.

19. Thomas Schillinger et al., "Dental and Periodontal Status and Risk for Progression of Carotid Atherosclerosis: The Inflammation and Carotid Artery Risk for Atherosclerosis Study Dental Substudy," *Stroke* 37 (2006): 2271.

20. Michael Siegel, DDS, MS, Jed J. Jacobson, DDS, MS, MPH, and Robert J. Braun, DDS, MS, "Diseases of the Gastrointestinal Tract," in *Burket's Oral Medicine: Diagnosis and Treatment*, 10th ed., edited by Martin S. Greenberg, DDS, and Michael Glick, DMD, (Hamilton, Ontario: B. C. Decker, 2003), 390.

21. S. M. Harman, "Testosterone in Older Men after the Institute of Medicine Report: Where Do We Go from Here?" *Climacteric* 8, no. 2 (June 2005): 124–35.

22. World Bank, report, "Life Expectancy," http://www.worldbank.org/depweb/english/modules/social/life/print.html.

23. "How to Help Avoid Foodborne Illness in the Home," http://www.pueblo.gsa.gov/cic_text/food/foodborn/foodborn.htm.

24. Patrick Owens et al., "Diagnosis of White Coat Hypertension by Ambulatory Blood Pressure Monitoring," *Hypertension* 34 (1999): 267–72.

25. Johns Hopkins Health Alerts, "Coping with Side Effects of Blood Pressure Medication," http://www.johnshopkinshealthalerts.com/reports/hypertension_stroke/378-1.html.

26. American Heart Association, "Metabolic Syndrome," http://www.americanheart.org/presenter.jhtml?identifier=4756.

L

1. Charles S. Lieber, "S-Adenosyl-L-Methionine: Its Role in the Treatment of Liver Disorders," *American Journal of Clinical Nutrition* 76, no.5 (November 2002): 1183S–1187S.

2. Constance A. Krach and Victoria A. Velkoff, *Centenarians in the United States*, U.S. Bureau of the Census, Current Population Reports, series P23-199RV (Washington, DC: U.S. Government Printing Office, July 1999), 14.

3. Ibid., 15.

4. World Health Organization, press release, "WHO Issues New Healthy Life Expectancy Rankings," released in Washington, DC, and Geneva, Switzerland, June 2000, http://www.who.int/inf-pr-2000/en/pr2000-life.html.

5. N. Arantes-Oliveira et al., "Healthy Animals with Extreme Longevity," *Science* 302 (October 24, 2003).

6. "The Benefits of Fish Oil," Papers of the Week, *Journal of Biological Chemistry* 282 (August 2007): 2225466.

7. Elissa S. Epel et al., "Accelerated Telomere Shortening in Response to Life Stress," *Proceedings of the National Academies of Sciences* 101, no. 49 (December 7, 2004): 17312–15.

O

1. David M. Nathan, MD, and Linda M. Delahanty, MS, RD, *Beating Diabetes: Lower Your Sugar, Lose Weight, and Stop Diabetes and Its Complications in Their Tracks* (New York: McGraw Hill, 2005).

2. Klea D. Bertakis and Rahman Azari, "Obesity and the Use of Health Care Services," *Obesity Research* 13 (2005): 372–9.

3. J. J. Webster et al., "The Childhood and Family Background of Women with Clinical Eating Disorders: A Comparison with Women with Major Depression and Women without Psychiatric Disorder," *Psychological Medicine* 30, no. 1 (January 2000): 53–60.

4. A. Must et al., "Long-Term Morbidity and Mortality of Overweight Adolescents: A Follow-Up of the Harvard Growth Study of 1922 to 1935," *New England Journal of Medicine* 327 (1992): 135055.

5. Carol Torgan, PhD, "Childhood Obesity on the Rise," *The NIH Word on Health*, June 2002, http://www.nih.gov/news/WordonHealth/jun2002/childhoodobesity.htm.

6. Pauline Beery Mack and Fred B.Vogt, "Roentgenographic Bone Density Changes in Astronauts During Representative Apollo Space Flight," *American Journal of Roentgenology* 113, no. 4 (December 1, 1971): 621–33.

7. S. M. Haffner et al., "Increased Insulin Resistance and Insulin Secretion in Nondiabetic African-Americans and Hispanics Compared with Non-Hispanic Whites: The Insulin Resistance Atherosclerosis Study," *Diabetes* 45 no. 6 (June 1996): 742–8.

8. Lester Packer, Eric H. Witt, and Hans Jürgen Tritschler, "Alpha-Lipoic Acid as a Biological Antioxidant," *Free Radical Biology and Medicine* 19, no. 2 (August 1995): 227–50.

P

1. H. L. "Sam" Queen, "The Forensic Approach to Blood Chemistry: Part 1," Institute for Health Realities, http://www.healthrealities.org/.

2. ——— *The Basic 100: A Health Model-Based Interpretation of Clinical Chemistry Parameters* (Colorado Springs, CO: Institute for Health Realities, 1997), http://www.healthrealities.org/.

3. Ibid.

4. K. Noble and C. Isles, "Hyperkalaemia Causing Profound Bradycardia," *Heart* 92 (2006): 1063.

5. W. G. Siems et al., "Oxidative Stress in Chronic Lymphoedema," *QJM: An International Journal of Medicine* 95, no. 12 (2002): 803–9.

6. L. Belardinelli, J. C. Shryock, and H. Fraser, "Inhibition of the Late Sodium Current As a Potential Cardioprotective Principle: Effects of the Late Sodium Current Inhibitor Ranolazine," *Heart* 92, no. 4, suppl. 4 (2006).

7. Erich Saling, Monica Schreiber, and Thomas Al-Taie, "A Simple, Efficient and Inexpensive Program for Preventing Prematurity," *Journal of Perinatal Medicine* 29, no. 3 (2001): 199–211.

8. M. B. Strauss and R. L. Dierker, "Otitis Externa Associated with Aquatic Activities (Swimmer's Ear)," *Clinical Dermatology* 5, no. 3 (1987): 103–11.

9. Jyrki Penttinen, "Hypothesis: Low Serum Cholesterol, Suicide, and Interleukin-2," *American Journal of Epidemiology* 141, no.8 (1995): 716–8.

10. S. Møller and J. H. Henriksen, "Cirrhotic Cardiomyopathy: A Pathophysiological Review of Circulatory Dysfunction in Liver Disease," *Heart* 87 (2002): 9–15.

11. H. L. "Sam" Queen, "The Forensic Approach to Blood Chemistry: Part 1," handout, Institute for Health Realities, http://www.healthrealities.org/.

12. John A. Kellum, Mingchen Song, and Jinyou Li, "Extracellular Acidosis and the Immune Response: Clinical and Physiologic Implications," *Critical Care* 8 (2004): 331–36.

13. R. J. Gillies and R. A. Gatenby, "Hypoxia and Adaptive Landscapes in the Evolution of Carcinogenesis," *Cancer and Metastasis Reviews* 26, no. 2 (June 2007): 311–17.

14. A. Di Sario et al., "Selective Inhibition of Ion Transport Mechanisms Regulating Intracellular pH Reduces Proliferation and Induces Apoptosis in Cholangiocarcinoma Cells," *Digestive and Liver Disease* 39, no. 1 (January 2007): 60–69.

15. R. Bartrons and J. Caro, "Hypoxia, Glucose Metabolism and the Warburg's Effect," *Journal of Bioenergetics and Biomembranes* 39, no. 3 (June 2007): 223–29.

16. Ralph J. DeBerardinis et al., "Brick by Brick: Metabolism and Tumor Cell Growth," *Current Opinion in Genetics & Development* 18, no. 1(February 2008): 54–61.

17. H. M. MacDonald et al., "Low Dietary Potassium Intakes and High Dietary Estimates of Net Endogenous Acid Production are Associated with Low Bone Mineral Density in Premenopausal Women and Increased Markers of Bone Resorption in Postmenopausal Women," *American Journal of Clinical Nutrition* 81, no. 4 (2005): 923–33.

R

1. E. Michael Molnar, MD, *Forever Young: The Practical Handbook of Youth Extension* (West Hartford, CT: Witkower Press, 1985), 179–91.

2. B. McLachlan et al., "Transfer of Mouse Embryonic Stem Cells to Sheep Myocardium." *The Lancet*, 367, no. 9507 (September 17, 2005): 301–2 C.

3. American Tinnitus Association, "Frequently Asked Questions" (August 12, 2007), http://www.ata.org/about_tinnitus/consumer/faq.html.

4. J.L. Stouffer and Richard S. Tyler, "Characterization of Tinnitus by Tinnitus Patients," *Journal of Speech and Hearing Disorders* 55 (August 1990): 439–53.

5. A Heller, "Classification and Epidemiology of Tinnitus," *Otolaryngologic Clinics of North America* 36, no. 2 (April 2003): 239–48.

S

1. C.W. Fetrow and J.R. Avila, "Efficacy of the Dietary Supplement S-adenosyl-L-methionine," *Annals of Pharmacotherapy* 35, no.11 (November 2001): 1414–25.

2. D. Mischoulon and M. Fava, "Role of S-adenosyl-L-methionine in the Treatment of Depression: A Review of the Evidence," *American Journal of Clinical Nutrition* 76, suppl. 5 (November 2002): 1158S–1161S.

3. A Czyrak et al, "Antidepressant Activity of S-adenosyl-L-methionine in Mice and Rats," *Journal of Basic Clinical Physiology and Pharmacology* 3 (January-March 1992).

4. S. Genedani et al., "Influence of SAMe on the Modifications of Brain Polyamine Levels in an Animal Model of Depression," *Neuroreport* 21, no. 12(18) (December 2001): 3939–42.

5. Agency for Healthcare Research and Quality, "S-Adenosyl-L-Methionine for Treatment of Depression, Osteoarthritis, and Liver Disease," *Summary, Evidence Report/Technology Assessment, no. 64. AHRQ Publication no. 02-E033*, (August 2002) http://www.ahrq.gov/clinic/epcsums/samesum.htm.

6. J.L. Goren et al., "Bioavailability and Lack of Toxicity of S-Adenosyl-L-Methionine (SAMe) in Humans," *Pharmacotherapy* 24, no.11 (November 2004): 1501–07.

7. Jon E Levine, "Editorial: Stressing the Importance of Sex," *Endocrinology* 143, no. 12 (2002): 4502–04.

8. Mattie Tops et al., "Anxiety, Cortisol, and Attachment Predict Plasma Oxytocin," Psychophysiology 44, no. 3 (March 2007): 444–49.

9. Wilhelm Reich, *The Function of the Orgasm* (New York: Farrar, Straus and Giroux, 1973), 8.

10. David J Sharkey et al., "Seminal Plasma Differentially Regulates Inflammatory Cytokine Gene Expression in Human Cervical and Vaginal Epithelial Cells," *Molecular Human Reproduction* 13, no. 7 (May 5, 2007): 491–501.

11. George Davey Smith, Stephen Frankel, and John Yarnell, "Sex and Death: Are They Related? Findings from the Caerphilly Cohort Study," *British Medical Journal* 315, no. 7123 (December 20, 1997): 1641.

12. Alan Farnham, "Is Sex Necessary?" Forbes (2002), http://www.forbes.com/2003/10/08/cz_af_1008health.html.

13. Ibid.

14. Ibid.

15. André Ludovic Phanjoo, "Sexual Dysfunction in Old Age," *Advances in Psychiatric Treatment* 6 (2000): 270–277.

16. B.J. de Boer, MD, et al., "The Prevalence of Bother, Acceptance, and Need for Help in Men with Erectile Dysfunction," *The Journal of Sexual Medicine* 2, no. 3 (April 11, 2005): 445–50.

17. Kar Nilamadhab, MD, Koola Nilamadhab, MD, and Matthew Maju, "A Pilot Survey of Sexual Functioning and Preferences in a Sample of English-Speaking Adults from a Small South Indian Town," *The Journal of Sexual Medicine* (August 2, 2007), http://www.blackwell-synergy.com/doi/abs/10.1111/j.1743-6109.2007.00543.x.

18. L. Cordain et al., "Acne Vulgaris: a Disease of Western Civilization," *Archives of Dermatology* 138, no.12 (December 2002): 1584–90.

19. K. Knutson et al., "The Metabolic Consequences of Sleep Deprivation," *Sleep Medicine Reviews* 11, no.3 (2007): 163-178.

20. Sam T. Donta et al., "Cognitive Behavioral Therapy and Aerobic Exercise for Gulf War Veterans' Illnesses: A Randomized Controlled Trial," *Journal of the American Medical Association* 289 (March 2003): 1396–1404.

21. Sarah Boseley, "Sugar Industry Threatens to Scupper WHO," *The Guardian* (April 21, 2003).

22. Anne L. Mardis, MD, MPH, "Current Knowledge of the Health Effects of Sugar Intake," *Family Economics and Nutrition Review*, http://www.ussugar.com/sugarnews/industry/health_effects.html.

23. Sam T. Donta et al., *Journal of the American Medical Association*, 1396–1404.

T

1. Christian Meier et al., "TSH-Controlled L-Thyroxine Therapy Reduces Cholesterol Levels and Clinical Symptoms in Subclinical Hypothyroidism: A Double Blind, Placebo-Controlled Trial (Basel Thyroid Study)," *The Journal of Clinical Endocrinology & Metabolism* 86, no. 10 (2001): 4860–66.

2. K Boelaert, B. Torlinska, and J. Franklyn, "Elderly Patients Presenting with Hyperthyroidism Have a Paucity of Symptoms and Signs: A Cross-Sectional Study of 3563 UK Patients," *Endocrine Abstracts* 19 (2009): OC37.

3. Geoffery P. Redmond, "Thyroid Dysfunction and Women's Reproductive Health," *Thyroid* 14, suppl. 1 (2004): 5–15.

4. Robert P. Kauffman and V. Daniel Castracane, "Premature Ovarian Failure Associated with Autoimmune Polyglandular Syndrome: Pathophysiological Mechanisms and Future Fertility," *Journal of Women's Health* 12, no.5 (2003): 513–20.

5. Gharib R. Hossein et al., "Subclinical Thyroid Dysfunction: A Joint Statement on Management from the American Association of Clinical Endocrinologists, the American Thyroid Association, and The Endocrine Society," *The Journal of Clinical Endocrinology & Metabolism* 90, no. 1 (2005): 581–85.

6. J. F. McClendon and Takeo Imai, "Iodine and Goiter: with Special Reference to the Far East," *Journal of Biological Chemistry* 102 (September 1933): 91–9.

7. A.P. Weetman, "Fortnightly Review: Hypothyroidism: Screening and Subclinical Disease," *British Medical Journal* 314, no.9 (April 1997): 1175.

U

1. D.K. Chow and J.J. Sung, "Is the Prevalence of Idiopathic Ulcers Really on the Increase?" *Nature Clinical Practice of Gastroenterology & Hepatology* 4, no. 4 (April 2007): 176–77.

2. M. F. Go, "Natural History and Epidemiology of Helicobacter Pylori Infection," *Alimentary Pharmacology & Therapeutics* 16, no. 1 (March 2002): 3–15.

3. Peter D'Adamo, MD, *Eat Right for Your Type*.

4. N. D. Yeomans et al., "Prevalence and Incidence of Gastroduodenal Ulcers during Treatment with Vascular Protective Doses of Aspirin," *Alimentary Pharmacology & Therapeutics* 22, no.9 (November 2005): 795–801.

5. B. J. Marshall et al., "Prospective Double-Blind Trial of Duodenal Ulcer Relapse after Eradication of *Campylobacter pylori*," *Lancet* 2, no. 8626–8627 (1988): 1437–1441.

6. Eric L. Buckles et al., "Role of the K2 Capsule in *Escherichia coli* Urinary Tract Infection and Serum Resistance," *The Journal of Infectious Diseases* 199, no.11 (June 2009): 1689–97.

7. Anthony J. Schaeffer, "Urinary Tract Infection," *The Journal of Urology* 163, no. 1 (January 2000): 384–90.

8. Hugo Degreef, "Clinical Forms of Dermatophytosis (Ringworm Infection)," *Mycopathologia* 166, no. 5–7 (November, 2008): 257–65.

9. Ulrich Dobrindt, and Jörg Hacker, "Targeting Virulence Traits: Potential Strategies to Combat Extraintestinal Pathogenic E. coli Infections," *Current Opinion in Microbiology* 11, no. 5 (October 2008): 409–13.

Y

1. M.A. Pfaller, "Nosocomial Candidiasis: Emerging Species, Reservoirs, and Modes of Transmission," *Clinical Infectious Disease* 22, suppl. 2 (May 1996): S89–S94.

2. William G. Crook, MD, *The Yeast Connection: Medical Breakthrough* (Jackson, TN: Professional Books, 1984), 93.

Appendix A

1 .Su Wen, *The Yellow Emperor's Classic of Medicine* (Maryland: Williams & Wilkins, 1949).

2. M. J. Tobin et al., "Breathing Patterns. 1. Normal subjects," *Chest* 84, no. 2 (August 1983): 202–205.

3. D. Lindsey Berkson, *Hormone Deception: How Everyday Foods and Products Are Disrupting Your Hormone—and How to Protect Yourself and Your Family* (New York: McGraw-Hill, 2001).

4. Caleb E. Finch, "Evolution of the Human Lifespan and Diseases of Aging: Roles of Infection, Inflammation, and Nutrition," *Proceedings of the National Academy of Sciences* (December 4, 2009): 1–7, http://ts-si.org/files/doi101073pnas0909606106.pdf.

5. Richard G. Rogers and Sharon Wofford, "Life Expectancy in Less Developed Countries: Socioeconomic Development or Public Health?" *Journal of Biosocial Science* 21 (1989): 245–52.

6. Simon Capewell et al, "Life-Years Gained Among US Adults From Modern Treatments and Changes in the Prevalence of 6 Coronary Heart Disease Risk Factors Between 1980 and 2000," *American Journal of Epidemiology* 170, no.2 (2009): 229–36.

7. William Dufty, *Sugar Blues* (Padnor, PA: Chilton Book Co., 1975).

Appendix B

1. Zuf-zuf (pronounced, in Dutch, zoef-zoef) imitates the sound of something or someone moving by very quickly.

INDEX

5–HTP (5-hydroxythyptophan)
Treatment for
Cancer, 70
Carbohydrate addiction, 192
Insomnia, 188
Obesity, 158
Seasonal affective disorder (SAD), 177
Stress, 189, 190
Abuse
Caused by
Heavy metals (alcohol), 31
Low serotonin levels, 31
Emotional maturation and, 34
Teenagers and drug, 31
Type
Antibiotic, 39–41, 84, 116, 138, 145, 147, 186, 200, 202, 205
Cocaine, 30, 85, 157,182
Drug, 30, 31
Sexual, 183, 184
Substance, 28, 30, 146, 157
Testosterone (bodybuilders), 143
Acetaminophen
Causing
Asthma, 54
Liver damage, 82
Poisoning, herbal remedy for, 82, 150
Acetylcholine (See also Choline and Lecithin), 111, 112, 179
Aches
Type
Backaches, 86
Headaches (See Headache)
Muscles, 57
Acupuncture, 25-28
Method, 23
Therapeutic effect, 26
Treatment for
Adrenal stress, 37
Anxiety attacks, 45, 216
Arteriosclerosis, 48
Back pain, 58, 59
Bell's palsy, 154
Breech baby, 78
Cancer, 69
Carbohydrate addiction, 192
Cholesterol, 81

Eyesight, 119
Hair loss, 131
Headaches, 132, 133, 153
Heartburn, 138, 139, 140
Hypertension, 147
Liver chi stagnation, 26
Seasonal affective disorder (SAD), 177, 178
Shingles (herpes zoster), 154
Skin, 186, 187
Stress, 189, 190
Tinnitus, 174
Ulcers, stomach, 200
Urinary tract infections, 202, 203
Weight loss, 100, 158
Unethical (weight reduction), 99, 158
Adenosine triphosphate (ATP)
Depletion implicated in
Arteriosclerosis, 46
Strenuous activity, 113
Essential for
Cardiac energy, 113
D-ribose production, 112
Detoxification, 115, 149
Hormone stimulation, 113
Magnesium production, 108, 114
Muscle relaxation, 113
Krebs cycle, produced in, 107, 114
SAMe precursor, 175, 149
Adrenal extracts, 37
Adult-onset diabetes (See Diabetes type II)
Alpha-lipoic acid
Antioxidant, 162
Glutathione precursor, 97
Alpha-tocopherol (See Vitamin E)
Aluminum, 24, 62, 64, 95, 96, 97, 105, 115, 137, 144–146, 211
Anemia, 39- 41, 129, 130, 162
Caused by
G6PD deficiency, 40, 41, 106
Iron deficiency, 66, 110
Toxic metals, 49
Type
Hemolytic, 51
Macrocytic, 40
Microcytic, 40
"Anger bile," 164

Angina (chest pain), 94, 138, 143
Antimony, 29, 51, 52, 105
Arsenic, 104, 105, 115, 211
Arteriosclerosis, 46-48, 91, 103, 106,
    127, 161
Arthritis, 13, 24, 36, 49-53, 125, 136, 160,
    172, 175, 176, 180, 199, 212
    Caused by
        Albumin deficiency, 51
        ATP deficiency, 113
        Colon toxicity, 86
        Dehydration, 48, 94
        Fasting, 121
        Toxic metals, 52
    Type
        Inflammatory, 66
        Metabolic, 52
        Osteoarthritis, 58, 91, 157, 175
Ascorbic acid (See Vitamin C)
Asthma, 53- 55, 63, 121, 138, 212
    Caused by
        Colon toxicity, 86
        Dehydration, 94
        Fungal toxins, 64, 116, 206
        Magnesium deficiency, 108
        Mercury toxicity, 54, 62
        Obesity, 53, 157
Athlete's foot, 19

B
B-complex vitamins, 29, 40, 83, 87, 107,
    110-112, 114, 127, 142, 144, 115, 154,
    174, 176, 192, 205
Back pain, 17, 57- 59, 172
    Caused by
        Dehydration, 59, 94, 230
        Pregnancy, 79
        Vaginal atrophy, 58, 181
Bacterial infections (See Infections,
    Bacterial)
Bad Breath, 61, 65
    Caused by
        Colon toxicity, 86
        Yeast infection, 207
Bell's palsy, 153, 154
Betaine HCL (hydrochloride), 139, 140
Biocompatible medicine, 13, 14
    Assumptions, 29, 43, 70, 84, 87, 97, 99,
        145, 162, 173, 178, 187, 191, 200,
        202, 207
    Defined, 22, 23, 27

Main premise, 18, 22, 29, 33
Metabolic corrections, 22, 31, 35-37,
    59, 82-84, 143, 151, 198
Modalities
    Acupuncture, 13, 19, 25-28, 37, 45,
        48, 58, 59, 78, 81, 85, 99, 100, 119,
        131-133, 138-140, 147, 153, 154,
        158, 174, 177, 178, 186, 187, 189,
        190, 192, 200, 202, 203, 216
    Blood tests, 13, 17, 23, 29, 30, 39, 58,
        69, 162, 209
    Chinese medicine, 13, 16, 26, 27, 31,
        49, 59, 69, 112, 178, 201, 209, 214
    Colon hydrotherapy, 13, 23, 42, 58,
        59, 69, 70, 85, 88-90, 95, 101,
        122, 127, 132, 139, 140, 146, 153,
        158, 166, 187, 208, 216
    Counseling, 23, 27, 34, 38, 69, 131,
        180, 182, 184, 190
    Detoxification, 35, 78, 80, 81, 105,
        106, 118, 123, 125-127, 133, 146,
        149, 150, 162, 190, 191, 210
    Food and chemical sensitivity/
        intolerance testing, 13, 66, 89, 147,
        157, 192, 230 232- 234
    Hair element analysis, 13, 17, 29, 30,
        48, 52, 69, 81, 96, 190, 209
    Iridology, 23
    Nontoxic dentistry, 22, 23, 64, 159,
        230, 236
    Nontoxic use, 27
    Origin, 16
    Panoramic dental X-rays, 64, 69, 136,
        209, 236
    Saliva, 13, 23, 37, 69, 143, 163, 197, 200
    Thermograms, 13, 23, 39, 209
Bladder infection (See Infections, Urinary
    bladder)
Bladderwrack (*Fucus vesiculosis*)
    Blood type O weight loss and, 67, 230
    Helicobacter pylori infection treatment,
        42, 44, 138, 200, 201
Blood tests (See Biocompatible medicine
    modalities, Blood tests)
Breiner, Mark A., 10, 105
Bronchitis, 54, 212

C
Cadmium, 24, 29, 51, 52, 104, 105, 115,
    197, 198, 211

Calcium, 90, 91, 114, 126, 135, 139, 214
  Absorption, 89, 91
  Arteriosclerosis, caused by, 46, 136
  Blood serum and, 23, 46, 60, 91, 105,
    114, 126, 161
  Bone depletion and, 51, 60, 126, 159,
    161, 192
  Calcium EDTA, 105, 106
  Carbonate, 90, 127
  Channel blockers, 138, 140
  Coral calcium, 90–91
  Crystals, 19, 165, 214
  Free, ionized (See Unbound ["free"]
    calcium)
  Supplementation, 79, 91, 160
Cancer, 19, 22, 69–71, 165, 180, 181,
  183, 212
  Ameliorate, 80, 87, 90, 150, 181
  Causing
    Dementia, 95
  Contributing factors
    Chronic inflammation, 20, 21, 83,
      116, 165
    Chronic stress, 189
    Environmental toxins, 104, 116, 117
    Free radicals, 60, 140, 160
    Obesity, 99
    Oxygen insufficiency, 23, 69, 107, 165
    Toxic metals, 115
    Unbound calcium, 90, 91, 160
  Type
    Breast, 21, 70, 133, 142
    Colon, 70, 86, 89, 112, 137
    Esophageal, 137
    Prostate, 181
    Skin, 185, 186, 211
    Stomach, 42, 116, 138, 199
    Uterine, 179
Candida infections (See Infections, Yeast)
Cat's claw (*Uncaria tomentosa*)
  Treatment for cholesterol, 81
Cayenne (*Capsicum baccatum*)
  Treatment for cholesterol, 81
Chelation (See EDTA)
Chest pain (See also Angina), 123, 134,
  137, 142, 144
Childbirth infections (See Infections,
  Childbirth)
Chinese medicine (See Biocompatible
  medicine modalities, Chinese medicine)

Chloride, 90, 104, 139
Cholecalciferol (See Vitamin D)
Choline (acetylcholine; see also Lecithin),
  111, 112
Chromium, 51, 99, 159, 192
Chromium GTF, 159, 192
Chronic infections (See Infections, Chronic)
Chronic inflammation, 13, 16, 22, 23, 29,
  30, 41, 53, 64, 80, 83–84, 96, 151, 155,
  163, 209, 212
  Arteriosclerosis, 46, 48, 80
  Arthritis, 53
  Dementia, 96, 97
  Dental symptoms, 61, 162
  Heart problems, 136
  Caused by
    Colon toxicity, 38, 101, 116, 210
  Contributing to
    Accelerated aging, 22, 38, 39, 83,
      87, 96, 151
    Acidity, 22, 70, 84, 163, 165, 167, 207
    Jaw infection, 43
    Oxidized cholesterol, 80
    Oxygen insufficiency, 23, 106, 161
    Toxic metal absorption, 29
    Unbound calcium, 60, 161
Chronic stress, 189, 190
Cobalamin (vitamin B_{12}) 175, 176
  Deficiency implicated in
    Anemia, 39, 40, 41
    Tinnitus, 174
  Produced by bacteria, 201
Coenzyme Q10 (See CoQ10)
Colon cancer (See Cancer, Colon)
Colon hydrotherapy (See Biocompatible
  medicine modalities, Colon hydrotherapy)
Colon infections (See Infections, Colon)
Constipation, 29, 58, 68, 88–90, 130, 132,
  192, 195, 206, 210
  Caused by
    "Anger bile," 164
    Back pain, 58, 59
    Dehydration, 88, 94
  Exacerbating
    Colon toxicity, 86, 87
    Diverticulitis, 100, 101
    Gout, 126
    Metal toxicity, 64, 130, 200
Coptis (*Coptis chinensis*) 200
  Treatment for *Helicobacter pylori*, 231

CoQ10 (Coenzyme Q10), 68, 80, 163

Cough, 59, 84
Causing
Hemorrhoids, 89
Symptom of
Toxic metals, 64
Yeast infection, 54
Counseling (See Biocompatible medicine modalities, Counseling)
Cramps
Symptom of
Heat exhaustion, 94
Toxic metals, 63
Type
Menstrual, 132
Muscle, 195

D

D-fucose (bladderwrack sugar), 44, 42, 200
D-mannose (cranberry sugar)
Treatment for urinary bladder infection, 44, 203, 204
D-ribose, 110, 112–115
ATP production and, 112
Cardiac energy and, 113
D'Adamo, Peter J., 65, 67
Dandelion (*Taraxacum*), 81
Liver cleanse, 133
Treatment for
Cholesterol, 81
Headache, 132, 133
Deglycyrrhizinated licorice (DGL)
Treatment for
Adrenal fatigue, 37, 38
Stomach discomfort, 201
Stomach walls, 200
Deqi, 25
Diabetes type II (See also Insulin resistance), 17, 97–99, 133, 144, 147
Comorbidities
ATP production decline, 113
Dehydration, 50, 94
Food intolerance, 24, 66, 98, 161, 212, 213
Gout, 125, 127
Hair loss, 129
Heart attack in women, 133, 134
Complications due to
Blood type O, 67
Childbirth, 74

Fasting, 121
Insulin production, 98
Metabolic imbalance, 98, 99
Pregnancy, 74
Diagnosis, 98, 99
Exacerbated by
Chronic stress, 189
Cow's milk, 40, 41
Emotional trauma, 83
Fungal toxins, 116
Insulin resistance, 83, 98, 149, 161
Native American genetics, 98, 123
Obesity, 65, 98, 99, 144, 157, 161
Oxidative stress, 160–162
Periodontal disease, 61
Sleep deprivation, 188
Toxic metals, 115
Symptoms
Arteriolosclerosis, 47, 161
Dementia, 95
Eye disease, 118, 119
Fatty liver, 112
Foot ulcers, 45
Fungus infections, 116
Leg numbness, 57
Libido loss, 181, 183, 161
Urinary tract infections, 202
Syndrome X, 98, 147
Treatment, 98, 99, 162
Exercise, 149
Diarrhea, 42, 43, 206
Caused by
"Anger bile," 164
Colon infection, 86, 116, 206
Food intolerance, 66, 192
Hemorrhoids, 88
Medication, 126, 200
Niacin deficiency, 111
"Stomach stagnation," 138
Toxic metals, 54, 64, 200
Treatment, 42, 62, 86, 116, 132, 145
Diverticulitis, 100–103
Dizziness, 216
Caused by
Anemia, 40
"Anger bile," 164
Antibiotics, 200
Anxiety or panic attacks, 44
Environmental toxins, 118
Hormone replacement, 142

Toxic metals, 64
Symptom of
Heart attack in women, 134
DL-phenylalanine
Treatment for
Carbohydrate addiction, 192
Obesity, 158

E
Ear infections (See Infections, Ear)
Edema (water retention)
Exacerbated by
Dehydration, 47, 50, 94
Heart attack, 134
Toxic metals, 64
Vascular Insufficiency 47
Treatment for, 47
EDTA (Ethylenediaminetetraacetic acid),
48, 103–106
Suppository, rectal, 70, 106, 216
Treatment for
Arteriosclerosis, 48
Cancer, 70
Toxic metals, 48, 114, 211
Endometriosis, 142
Exacerbated by
Environmental toxins, 24
Hormone imbalance, 141
Symptom of
Yeast infection, 206
Environmental toxin infections (See
Infections, Environmental toxin)
Esophageal cancer (See Cancer,
Esophageal)

F
Fainting, 94, 164
Fenugreek seed (*Foenum-graecum*) 81
Feverfew (*Chrysanthemum parthenium*)
Headaches, treatment for, 132
Folic acid
Deficiency
Caused by oral contraceptives, 142, 144
Symptom of anemia, 40, 41
Glutathione precursor, 175, 176
Prevents spina bifida, 78
Treatment for gout, 126
**Food and chemical sensitivity/Intolerance
testing** (See Biocompatible medicine
modalities)

Free radicals, 51, 163, 165
Caused by
Oxygen, 49, 160, 162, 163
Pesticides, 83
Causing
Accelerated aging, 60
Anaerobic metabolism, 60, 161
Cancer, 6
Diabetes type II, 162
Inflammatory response, 83
Oxidized cholesterol, 80
Yeast infections, 101
Treatment, 87, 96, 140, 150, 155, 162,
163, 165
Fringe Tree, Chinese (*Chionanthus
retusus*), 81

G
G6PD (Glucose-6-phosphate dehydroge-
nase), 40, 41, 165
Causing anemia (See Anemia, G6PD)
EDTA, contraindicated for 106
Gallstones, 80, 112, 123–125
Treatment, 81, 82
Garlic (*Allium sativum*)
Treatment for
Cholesterol, 81
Yeast, 208
**Gastroesophageal reflux disease
(GERD),** 137–140, 199
Ginger (*Zingiber officinale*)
Treatment for
Cholesterol, 81
Morning sickness, 78, 79
Ginkgo biloba (*Ginkgo biloba*)
Treatment for
Arteriosclerosis, 47
Dementia, 96
Tinnitus, 174
Glaucoma, 118, 119
Glucosamine, 52, 59
Glutamic acid
Treatment for
Brain health, 192
Diabetes type II, 97
Fatigue, 192
Glutathione (reduced), 81, 155
Aging, 150, 163
Antioxidant, 87, 96
Liver production and, 87, 96, 97, 155, 162

SAMe metabolite, 70, 82, 175, 176
Suppositories, rectal, 97
Treatment for
    Bell's palsy, 154, 155
    Brain health, 81, 96, 97
    Liver toxicity, 119
    Macrocytic anemia, 40
    Mercury toxicity, 29, 81
    Oxidative stress, 150, 155, 162, 163
Goldenseal (*Hydrastis canadensis*)
Treatment for
    Constipation, 132
    Headaches, 132
    Ulcers, 200
Gout, 125–127, 136
Grapefruit seed extract, 90, 206, 207, 208

H
H. pylori infections (See Infections, *H. pylori*)
Hair element analysis (See Biocompatible medicine modalities, Hair element analysis)
Headache, 3, 44, 82, 131–133, 153, 172, 173, 215, 216
Caused by
    "Anger bile," 164
    Colon toxicity, 86
    Environmental toxins, 64, 118
    Food intolerance, 192
    Oral contraceptives, 142, 144
    Pharmaceutical drugs, 126
    PMS, 141
    Yeast infection, 207
Migraine, 134, 196
Symptom of
    Heart attack in men, 135
    Heart attack in women, 134
Treatment
    Acupuncture, 26, 153
    Sex, 180
Heartburn, 47, 123, 137–140, 206, 207
Helicobacter pylori, 23, 42, 44, 139
Causing
    Back pain, 58
    GERD, 139
    Headaches, 153
    Stomach cancer, 42, 44, 116, 138
    Ulcers, 44, 116, 138, 199–201
Hemorrhoids, 47, 88, 207

High blood pressure (See Hypertension)
High blood sugar (See Hyperglycemia)
Holder, Jay, 10
Horsetail (*Equisetum*)
Treatment for
    Arteriosclerosis, 47, 48
    Hair loss, 130
Hyperglycemia (high blood sugar), 161
Hypertension (high blood pressure), 17, 146–148
Contributing factors
    Colon toxicity, 86
    Libido loss, 181
    Serotonin deficiency, 179
Symptom of
    Tinnitus, 173
Hyperuricemia (See Gout)
Hypoglycemia (low blood sugar), 121, 133, 212
Hypotension (low blood pressure), 146

I
Indian coleus (*Coleus forskohlii*)
Treatment for
    Arteriosclerosis, 47, 48
Indigestion
Caused by
    "Stomach stagnation," 138
    Reflux, 137
    Ulcers, 199
Causing yeast overgrowth, 207
Infections, 21, 23, 29, 36, 37, 43, 46, 48, 55, 84, 94, 116, 151, 161, 162, 164, 172, 177, 206, 207, 208
Affecting
    Childbirth, 72, 74, 75
    Heart, 135
Exacerbated by
    Environmental toxins, 116, 165
    Oxidative Stress 44, 165, 166
Treatment, 145
    Antibiotics, 18, 21, 40, 42
Type
    Amoebic, 63
    Bacterial, 42, 43, 175
    Chronic, 20, 22, 166, 177
    Colon, 38, 100, 101, 145, 147
    Ear, 43, 85, 164
    H. pylori, see *Helicobacter pylori*
    Jaw, 23, 43, 52, 78, 84, 105, 135, 147

Joint, 49, 50
Periodontal, 60, 61, 64, 65, 70, 78,
   116, 146, 135, 136, 151
Sinus, 43, 90, 173
Skin, 62
Stomach, 23, 139
Tuberculosis, 85
Urinary bladder, 42, 44, 58, 202, 203,
   204, 206–208
Viral, 43
Yeast, 26, 54, 90, 125, 202, 207, 208
Inflammation (See Chronic inflammation)
Injection, 99
B-complex, 27
Cell rejuvenating, 120, 151, 152, 169,
   171, 172
EDTA, 211
Glutathione, 97
Institute for Health Realities, 10, 58,
105, 108, 196
Insulin resistance, 98, 114, 161
Caused by
   Age, 188
   Colon toxicity, 80
   Emotional trauma, 83
   Food intolerance, 98, 144, 152, 161
   Sleep deprivation, 188
Control of, 149
Exacerbating
   Diabetes type II, 98, 161, 162
Hypertension and, 147,
Native American genetics and, 98, 212
**International Clinic of Biological
Regeneration** (ICBR), 171
Iodine, 144, 166, 195, 197
Iridology (See Biocompatible medicine
modalities, Iridology)
Iron, 40, 41, 103, 114, 129, 166
Deficiency, 66, 110
Supplementation with, 40, 41, 130

J
Jaw infections (See Infections, Jaws)

L
Lead, 24, 29, 31, 49–60, 62, 104, 105, 114,
115, 127, 209, 211
Lecithin (See also Choline)
Deficiency found in dementia, 96, 112
Instrumental in
   ATP production, 114

Fetal brain development,112
Liver detoxifier, 119, 155
Licorice (See also Deglycyrrhizinated
   licorice [DGL])
Treatment for *H. pylori* infection, 200
Liver "fire," 173
Longhua Hospital, 16, 19, 25, 239
Low back pain (See Back pain)
Low blood pressure (See Hypotension)
Low blood sugar (See Hypoglycemia)
Lutein, 119

M
Magnesium, 91, 114, 160
Alkalizing properties, 166
Deficiency, 108, 135
   Caused by
      Diverticulitis, 102
      Hormone replacement therapy,
         142, 144
      Sugar, 192
Instrumental in ATP production, 68,
   107, 108–109, 114
Prevents dementia, 96
Promotes
   Hydration, 89
   Sodium detoxification, 48
   Weight loss, blood type A, 68
   Weight loss, blood type B, 68
Synergistic with zinc, 109
Treatment for
   Asthma, 55
   Back pain, 59
   Calcium toxicity, 91
   Colon stimulation, 88, 89, 90
   Diabetes type II, 99
   Edema, 48
   Heart attack, 135
   Hypertension, 147
   Oxidative stress, 160
Marsman, Hendrick "Henk," 9
Melatonin, 82, 97, 143, 175,
Controls sleep cycle, 140, 188, 189
Inhibits fluoride damage, 62
Prevents cancer, 70, 140
Mercury, 63–64
Causing
   Decreased thyroid function, 24, 185, 197
   Hair loss, 129
   Headaches, 132

Inflammation, 23, 165
  Joint pain, 51
  Skin problems, 184
Contributing to autism and ADD, 24, 29
Correlation with
  Pathological disorders, 52, 63, 104,
    115, 165
  Psychological disturbances, 69, 104, 115
Detoxified by
  Bile, 79, 155, 211
  EDTA, 48, 105, 211
  Glutathione, 29, 155
Elimination in dentistry, 10, 46, 62, 63
Hair tests measuring, 52, 62, 105, 209
Intoxication among dentists, 35
Sources of, 52, 53, 61, 104, 105, 151
  Amalgams, dental, 23, 48, 51, 52, 61, 62,
    65, 83, 105, 115, 126, 129, 132, 184
  Vaccinations (thimerosal), 29, 30
Toxicity at low concentrations, 51, 105
Methylsulfonylmethane (See MSM)
Migraine (See Headache, Migraine)
Milk thistle (*Silybum marianum*), 81
  Treatment for
    Acetaminophen poisoning, 150
    Liver toxicity, 82, 119, 149
MSM (methylsulfonylmethane), 59

N
Nail fungus, 207
Niacin (vitamin B_3)
  Deficiency caused by sugar, 192
  Deficiency causing pellagra, 111
  Essential cofactor
    Glutathione, 150
Nontoxic dentistry (See Biocompatible
  medicine modalities, Nontoxic dentistry)

O
Olive
  Leaf, 89, 206, 208
  Oil, 81, 124
Oregano (*Origanum vulgare*)
  Causing weight loss, blood type O, 65
Osteoarthritis (See Arthritis, Osteoar-
  thritis)
Osteoporosis, 125, 159–160
  Prevention, 90, 214
  Risk factors for, 125, 126, 192

P
Palpitations, 134, 162
Panoramic dental X-rays (See Biocom-
  patible medicine modalities, Panoramic
  dental X-rays)
Pantothenic acid (vitamin B_5)
  Coenzyme A precursor, 110
  Treatment for
    Aging, 36
    Gout, 127
    Stress reduction, 35
Periodontal infections (See Infections,
  Periodontal)
Phosphate, 62, 90, 91, 107, 165, 166,
  167, 176
Phosphorus, 89, 166
Poly MPV, 70
Potassium, 36, 47, 48, 99, 126, 139, 147,
  148, 163–166, 181, 192, 200
Prostate cancer (See Cancer, Prostate)
Psoriasis, 127, 149, 187, 206
Pyridoxine (vitamin B_6)
  Glutathione production and, 155, 175,
    176
  Treatment for
    Adrenal fatigue, 37
    Aging, 38
    Anemia, 40, 41
    Hair loss, 130
    Nerve problems, 155
    Stress, 37

Q
Queen, H. L. "Sam," 10, 60, 105, 108,
  118, 165, 196, 209

R
Riboflavin (vitamin B_2)
  Glutathione production and, 150
Ringing in the ears (See Tinnitus)

S
S-adenosylmethionine (See SAMe)
SAMe (S-adenosylmethionine), 82,
  175–176
  Glutathione precursor, 70, 97
  Treatment for
    Cancer, 70
    Liver toxicity, 119, 149, 155
    Sleep problems, 188, 189
    Stress, 190

Saliva testing (See Biocompatible medicine modalities, Saliva testing)

Selenium
Treatment for
Aging, 150
Anemia, 40
Arthritis, 52
Asthma, 54
Stress, 37
Weight problems, 99

Shiitake mushrooms
Treatment for cholesterol, 81

Sinus infections (See Infections, Sinus)

Skin cancer (See Cancer, Skin)

Skin infections (See Infections, Skin)

Smith, C. Tom, 10, 171

Sneezeweed (Old man's weed; *Centipeda cunninghamii*), 62

Sodium, 29, 36, 47, 48, 99, 114, 126, 139, 147, 165, 166

St. John's Wort (*Hypericum perforatum*)
Calming effect, 190

Stevia (*Asteraceae stevia*)
Sugar alternative, 192, 193

Stiff neck, 58, 153, 200

Stomach cancer (See Cancer, Stomach)

Stomach infections (See Infections, Stomach)

Stress (See also Chronic stress), 18, 24, 35, 43, 54, 109, 111, 121, 125, 144, 148, 151, 154, 177, 189–191, 214
Ameliorating, 37, 59, 151, 160, 178, 185, 190
Associated factors
Cortisol, 83, 140
Environmental toxins, 79
Hair pulling (trichotillomania), 131
Perception, 151
Sleep deprivation, 188
Uric acid, 127
Viruses, 154
Yeast infections, 205, 208
Exacerbates accelerated aging, 151, 152
Types
Acid, 23, 38, 44, 45, 107, 108, 116, 127, 133, 136, 160, 164, 165, 207
Emotional, 36, 45, 53, 69, 179, 183, 202
Fetal, 74
Heat, 93
Metabolic, 35, 193

Newborn, 77
Oxidative, 18, 44, 136, 151, 160–162, 163, 167
Pathogenic, 85
Relationship, 179, 183

Suppository
EDTA, 105, 216
Glutathione, 97
Vitamin E, 207

Syndrome X (See also Insulin resistance), 98, 147

T
Thalassemia (See Anemia, G6PD)

Thermograms (See also Biocompatible medicine modalities, Thermograms), 13, 23, 39, 209

Thiamine (vitamin B_1), 111

Thimerosal (See Mercury, Sources of)

Tinnitus, 172–174

Tryptophan
Excreted by lactobacilli, 101
Precursor of
5-HTP, 70, 101, 177
Serotonin, 30

Tuberculosis infections (See Infections, Tuberculosis)

Turmeric (*Curcuma longa*),
Cholesterol treatment, 81
Liver cleanse, 82

Tyrosine
Treatment for
Adrenal fatigue, 37, 38
PMS and thyroid, 198

U
Unbound ("free") calcium, 23, 60, 90, 91, 120, 161

Uric acid (See also Gout), 23, 24, 51, 90, 125- 127, 210

Urinary bladder infections (See Infections, Urinary bladder)

Uterine cancer (See Cancer, Uterine)

V
Vanadium, 54

Viana Healing Center, 16, 17, 19, 22, 23, 239

Viana, Manuel, 38

Viral infections (See Infections, Viral)

Vitamin A (retinol)
  Treatment for
    Acne, 186, 187
    Arteriosclerosis, 48
    Sodium removal, 48
    Ulcers, 200
Vitamin B₁ (See Thiamine)
Vitamin B₂ (See Riboflavin)
Vitamin B₃ (See Niacin)
Vitamin B₅ (See Pantothenic acid)
Vitamin B₆ (See Pyridoxine)
Vitamin B₁₂ (See Cobalamin)
Vitamin C (ascorbic acid), 110
  Antioxidant, 83, 96
  Controls inflammatory response, 96, 186
  Deficiency caused by oral contraceptives, 142, 144
  Instrumental in ATP production, 107, 110, 114
  Prevents gallstones, 124
  Treatment for
    Acetaminophen poisoning, 150
    Acne, 187
    Adrenal fatigue, 37
    Hypertension, 147
    Urinary tract infections, 203, 204
Vitamin D₃ (cholecalciferol), 70, 160, 186
Vitamin E (alpha-tocopherol) 80, 83, 187, 200
  Suppository, vaginal, 207
  Treatment for
    Acetaminophen poisoning, 149
    Anemia, macrocytic, 40

W
Water retention (See Edema)

Y
Yeast Infections (See Infections, Yeast)

Z
Zinc 37, 51, 59, 181
  Alkalinity, 166
  Deficiency due to
    Hormone replacement therapy, 142, 144
    Sugar, 192
    Ulcers, 200
  Instrumental in
    ATP production, 107, 109–110, 114
    Prostate health, 181
    Skin health, 187
    Thyroid's zinc-copper ratio, 197, 198
    Weight loss
      Blood type A, 68
      Blood type B, 68
  Prevents
    Asthma, 54
    Dementia, 96
    Gallstones, 124, 155
    Macular degeneration, 119
    Urinary tract infections, 204
    Yeast overgrowth, 208
  Treatment for
    Adrenal fatigue, 37
    Arthritis, 51
    Back pain, 59
    Calcium toxicity, 91
    Hair loss, 130
    Insomnia, 187
    Nerve problems, 155

ABOUT THE AUTHOR

Born in San Jose, Costa Rica, Carlos Manuel Viana Alfaro grew up on Aruba in the Dutch Caribbean. While studying in the Caribbean, Latin America, Europe, and the United States, he aspired to be of public service and early in life wanted to study medicine so he could make it available to all who needed assistance.

Dr. Viana is a medical anthropologist, a specialty dealing in cultural, ethnic, and social barriers to medical assistance. In the 1980s, Dr. Viana worked in New York City developing socially sensitive information campaigns on public health issues. Here he was involved in the study to develop a new legislation for the Mandated Insurance Bill, Fetal Alcohol Syndrome, and for changing the legal drinking age in New York state from eighteen to twenty-one. Here too he was the first instructor to teach First Aid and CPR in a language other than English. He also taught trauma medicine. His contact with "ethnic group healers," including many Asians, exposed him to the teachings of traditional Chinese medicine and its principles of treating the body as a whole.

In the late 1980s, Dr. Viana returned to Aruba and developed a new approach to Baromedicine, or high pressure medicine, based on scuba diving. Then in 1996, he was invited to study at the Shanghai College of Traditional Chinese Medicine and to intern at Longhua Hospital, where he became the 238th "Westerner" to be certified as an Oriental Medical Doctor.

After returning to Aruba once again, Dr. Viana became passionately interested in reducing the inevitable signs of aging—especially cardiovascular disease, loss of cognitive ability, and decreased physical strength—to help people live longer and healthier lives. Toward this end, Dr. Viana continued his studies and is today a Certified Addictionologist (CAd), a Certified Colon Hydro Therapist, a Fellow in Applied Clinical Nutrition, and a member of the International Academy of Oral Medicine and Toxicology (IAOMT), assisting professionals in the developments of biological dentistry. Dr. Viana is also a member of the International and American Association of Clinical Nutritionists (IAACN) and a board-certified Clinical Nutritionist in the United States.

Founder and medical director of the Viana Healing Center, in Aruba, Dr. Viana currently has a live weekly radio program and writes and lectures frequently on health in several languages. He is licensed to practice integrative medicine in Aruba, Dutch West Indies, and in Curaçao, Netherlands Antilles. For more information, please visit www.vianaheal.com.